New Advances in Kidney Transplantation

New Advances in Kidney Transplantation

Editor

Eytan Mor

MDPI • Basel • Beijing • Wuhan • Barcelona • Belgrade • Manchester • Tokyo • Cluj • Tianjin

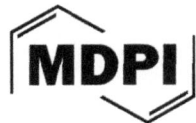

Editor
Eytan Mor
Transplant Center,
Department of Surgery B,
Sheba Medical Center,
Ramat-Gan, Israel

Editorial Office
MDPI
St. Alban-Anlage 66
4052 Basel, Switzerland

This is a reprint of articles from the Special Issue published online in the open access journal *Journal of Clinical Medicine* (ISSN 2077-0383) (available at: https://www.mdpi.com/journal/jcm/special_issues/Advances_Kidney_Transplantation).

For citation purposes, cite each article independently as indicated on the article page online and as indicated below:

LastName, A.A.; LastName, B.B.; LastName, C.C. Article Title. *Journal Name* **Year**, *Volume Number*, Page Range.

ISBN 978-3-0365-5753-3 (Hbk)
ISBN 978-3-0365-5754-0 (PDF)

© 2022 by the authors. Articles in this book are Open Access and distributed under the Creative Commons Attribution (CC BY) license, which allows users to download, copy and build upon published articles, as long as the author and publisher are properly credited, which ensures maximum dissemination and a wider impact of our publications.

The book as a whole is distributed by MDPI under the terms and conditions of the Creative Commons license CC BY-NC-ND.

Contents

About the Editor vii

Eytan Mor
Special Issue: New Advances in Kidney Transplantation
Reprinted from: *J. Clin. Med.* **2022**, *11*, 4190, doi:10.3390/jcm11144190 1

Ximo Garcia-Dominguez, César D. Vera-Donoso, Eric Lopez-Moncholi, Victoria Moreno-Manzano, José S. Vicente and Francisco Marco-Jiménez
Sildenafil Citrate Enhances Renal Organogenesis Following Metanephroi Allotransplantation into Non-Immunosuppressed Hosts
Reprinted from: *J. Clin. Med.* **2022**, *11*, 3068, doi:10.3390/jcm11113068 5

Matteo Righini, Irene Capelli, Marco Busutti, Concettina Raimondi, Giorgia Comai, Gabriele Donati, Maria Laura Cappuccilli, Matteo Ravaioli, Pasquale Chieco and Gaetano La Manna
Impact of the Type of Dialysis on Time to Transplantation: Is It Just a Matter of Immunity?
Reprinted from: *J. Clin. Med.* **2022**, *11*, 1054, doi:10.3390/jcm11041054 19

Ryoichi Imamura, Ryo Tanaka, Ayumu Taniguchi, Shigeaki Nakazawa, Taigo Kato, Kazuaki Yamanaka, Tomoko Namba-Hamano, Yoichi Kakuta, Toyofumi Abe, Koichi Tsutahara, Tetsuya Takao, Hidefumi Kishikawa and Norio Nonomura
Everolimus Reduces Cancer Incidence and Improves Patient and Graft Survival Rates after Kidney Transplantation: A Multi-Center Study
Reprinted from: *J. Clin. Med.* **2022**, *11*, 249, doi:10.3390/jcm11010249 31

Renana Yemini, Ruth Rahamimov, Ronen Ghinea and Eytan Mor
Long-Term Results of Kidney Transplantation in the Elderly: Comparison between Different Donor Settings
Reprinted from: *J. Clin. Med.* **2021**, *10*, 5308, doi:10.3390/jcm10225308 43

Hien Lau, Alberto Jarrin Lopez, Natsuki Eguchi, Akihiro Shimomura, Antoney Ferrey, Ekamol Tantisattamo, Uttam Reddy, Donald Dafoe and Hirohito Ichii
Intraoperative Near-Infrared Spectroscopy Monitoring of Renal Allograft Reperfusion in Kidney Transplant Recipients: A Feasibility and Proof-of-Concept Study
Reprinted from: *J. Clin. Med.* **2021**, *10*, 4292, doi:10.3390/jcm10194292 59

Stephan Kemmner, Christopher Holzmann-Littig, Helene Sandberger, Quirin Bachmann, Flora Haberfellner, Carlos Torrez, Christoph Schmaderer, Uwe Heemann, Lutz Renders, Volker Assfalg, Tarek M. El-Achkar, Pranav S. Garimella, Jürgen Scherberich and Dominik Steubl
Pretransplant Serum Uromodulin and Its Association with Delayed Graft Function Following Kidney Transplantation—A Prospective Cohort Study
Reprinted from: *J. Clin. Med.* **2021**, *10*, 2586, doi:10.3390/jcm10122586 73

Johan Noble, Antoine Metzger, Hamza Naciri Bennani, Melanie Daligault, Dominique Masson, Florian Terrec, Farida Imerzoukene, Beatrice Bardy, Gaelle Fiard, Raphael Marlu, Eloi Chevallier, Benedicte Janbon, Paolo Malvezzi, Lionel Rostaing and Thomas Jouve
Apheresis Efficacy and Tolerance in the Setting of HLA-Incompatible Kidney Transplantation
Reprinted from: *J. Clin. Med.* **2021**, *10*, 1316, doi:10.3390/jcm10061316 85

Małgorzata Kielar, Paulina Dumnicka, Agnieszka Gala-Błądzińska, Alina Będkowska-Prokop, Ewa Ignacak, Barbara Maziarz, Piotr Ceranowicz and Beata Kuśnierz-Cabala
Urinary NGAL Measured after the First Year Post Kidney Transplantation Predicts Changes in Glomerular Filtration over One-Year Follow-Up
Reprinted from: *J. Clin. Med.* **2021**, *10*, 43, doi:10.3390/jcm10010043 . . . . **97**

Natalia Warmuzińska, Kamil Łuczykowski and Barbara Bojko
A Review of Current and Emerging Trends in Donor Graft-Quality Assessment Techniques
Reprinted from: *J. Clin. Med.* **2022**, *11*, 487, doi:10.3390/jcm11030487 . . . . **115**

Maria Irene Bellini, Mikhail Nozdrin, Liset Pengel, Simon Knight and Vassilios Papalois
The Impact of Recipient Demographics on Outcomes from Living Donor Kidneys: Systematic Review and Meta-Analysis [†]
Reprinted from: *J. Clin. Med.* **2021**, *10*, 5556, doi:10.3390/jcm10235556 . . . . **149**

About the Editor

Eytan Mor

Eytan Mor currently holds the position of director of the Transplant Center at Sheba Medical Center. Dr. Mor is a Professor of Surgery at Sackler Medical School, Tel-Aviv University.

Dr. Mor is an active academic surgeon who has published more than 190 peer-reviewed papers and presented more than 100 of his original research works at national and international meetings and congresses. Dr. Mor is a member of several international transplant societies (ESOT, ITS, ASTS, and IPTA) and serves on the editorial board of Pediatric Transplantation Journal and as a reviewer of various leading transplant journals, including American Journal of Transplantation, Transplantation, Liver Transplantation, Journal of Clinical Medicine, and Clinical Gastroenterology and Hepatology. Dr. Mor has served for 25 years as a member on the board of Israel Transplant Center and was a past president of the Israel Transplant Society (2006–2008). He is the Israeli representative at the UEMS (Union European for Medical Sciences) transplant committee.

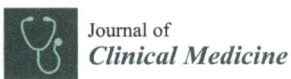

Editorial

Special Issue: New Advances in Kidney Transplantation

Eytan Mor [1,2]

[1] Transplant Center, Department of Surgery B, Sheba Medical Center, Ramat Gan 5266202, Israel; eytan.mor@sheba.health.gov.il
[2] Sackler Medical School, Tel-Aviv University, Tel Aviv 6997801, Israel

This Special Issue in renal transplantation covers a variety of clinical and research areas in kidney transplantation. The recent decade is associated with an ongoing shortage of organs for transplantation with efforts to increase the organ pool with DCDs and extended criteria donors. However, with the increasing success rate of kidney transplants, there is also a growth in the candidate list because of removal of the age barrier and transplantation of high risk patients with other comorbidities. The future seems promising with the development of innovative non-invasive technologies introducing biomarkers for diagnosis of rejection and ischemic reperfusion injury, use of cell therapy for tolerance induction, development of artificial organs, and overcoming immune and non-immune barriers in xenotransplantation. This Special Issue will touch some of these topics that are in the frontiers of the modern era of kidney transplantation.

On the clinical side, there are two papers covering the effect of age and other demographics criteria on long-term outcome after transplant.

The first paper, by Dr Yemini et al., is from my group, and it discusses the "Long-Term Results of Kidney Transplantation in the Elderly: Comparison between Different Donor Settings" [1]. Our paper shows that in a selected population in that age group (>60 y) live-donor transplantation is associated with very good long-term results. As for deceased donor kidney transplantation in the elderly the old-to-old allocation seems to be a rational approach associated with an acceptable outcome.

In a "Systematic Review and Meta-Analysis on The Impact of Recipient Demographics on Outcomes from Living Donor Kidneys" [2], Dr. Bellini et al. shows that gender mismatch between male recipients and female donors has negative impact on graft survival. African ethnicity and obesity do not influence recipient and graft survival but negatively affect DGF and rejection rates.

As for the effect of immunosuppression on malignancy Dr. Imamura et al. preformed a long term multi-center study showing that "Everolimus Reduces Cancer Incidence and Improves Patient and Graft Survival Rates after Kidney Transplantation" [3].

Two other papers focus on pretransplant sensitization. The first paper is by Righini and his colleagues on the "Impact of the Type of Dialysis on Time to Transplantation: Is It Just a Matter of Immunity?" [4]. In that paper, they drew on almost 30 year experience to show that the clinical variables that significantly correlated with longer time to transplantation were the level of presensitization (PRA max and antibodies width) as well as type of dialysis. The lower sensitization rate in the PD population has led to a shorter waiting time until transplant compared to HD group. Another paper, "Apheresis Efficacy and Tolerance in the Setting of HLA-Incompatible Kidney Transplantation" [5] by Dr. Noble and his colleagues, showed that the efficacy of plasmapheresis in lowering preformed anti-HLA antibody levels correlated with the volume of plasma exchanged or filtered and that IA was the most efficient technique for antibody removal compared to plasma exchange (PE) and double filtration plasmapheresis (DFPP). They concluded that apheresis is an effective desensitizing measure that allows kidney transplantation in that high immunological risk group of patients.

Citation: Mor, E. Special Issue: New Advances in Kidney Transplantation. *J. Clin. Med.* **2022**, *11*, 4190. https://doi.org/10.3390/jcm11144190

Received: 4 July 2022
Accepted: 17 July 2022
Published: 19 July 2022

Publisher's Note: MDPI stays neutral with regard to jurisdictional claims in published maps and institutional affiliations.

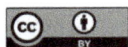

Copyright: © 2022 by the author. Licensee MDPI, Basel, Switzerland. This article is an open access article distributed under the terms and conditions of the Creative Commons Attribution (CC BY) license (https://creativecommons.org/licenses/by/4.0/).

Use of biomarkers in transplantation is another innovative area of interest in recent years. In this Special Issue there are two papers looking at correlation of biomarker and outcome after transplant. The first one is "Pretransplant Serum Uromodulin and Its Association with Delayed Graft Function Following Kidney Transplantation" [6]. In that paper, Dr. Kemmner et al. evaluated the association between serum uromodulin (sUMOD), a potential marker for tubular integrity, with DGF in the clinical setting. They report that higher pretransplant sUMOD was independently associated with lower odds for DGF, potentially serving as a non-invasive marker to stratify patients according to their risk for developing DGF early in the setting of kidney transplantation. The second paper is on the use of "Urinary NGAL Measured after the First Year Post Kidney Transplantation to Predict Changes in Glomerular Filtration over One-Year Follow-Up" [7] by Dr. Keilar and her colleagues. In the clinical setting, we are using biochemical markers in the blood (creatinine levels) and urine (albumin and protein levels) to assess graft function late after transplant. Introduction of new and more sensitive markers are needed in stable patient who may develop quiescent graft injury. In their study, Dr. Keilar and her colleagues assessed the urinary concentrations of neutrophil gelatinase-associated lipocalin (NGAL) as a predictor of changes in kidney transplant function after the first year after transplantation among 109 patients with stable functioning graft. They found that Urinary NGAL measured at baseline was twice higher in patients with at least 10% decrease in eGFR over 1-year follow-up compared to those with stable or improving transplant function. Baseline NGAL significantly predicted the relative and absolute changes in eGFR.

The last few years have seen the emergence of many new technologies designed to examine organ function, including new imaging techniques, transcriptomics, genomics, proteomics, metabolomics, lipidomics, and new solutions in organ perfusion, which has enabled a deeper understanding of the complex mechanisms associated with ischemia-reperfusion injury (IRI), inflammatory process, and graft rejection. This issue includes "A Review of Current and Emerging Trends in Donor Graft-Quality Assessment Technique" [8] written by Ms. Natalia Warmuzińska and her colleagues that summarizes and assesses the strengths and weaknesses of current conventional diagnostic methods and a wide range of new potential strategies with respect to donor graft-quality assessment, the identification of IRI, perfusion control, and the prediction of DGF. One of the new methods to assess graft quality is described in another paper by Dr. lau et al. who used "Intraoperative Near-Infrared Spectroscopy Monitoring of Renal Allograft Reperfusion in Kidney Transplant Recipients" [9]. In their study they used a handheld near-infrared spectroscopy (NIRS) device to quantify regional tissue oxygen saturation levels (rSO_2) in the renal allograft after reperfusion and compared the rSO_2 between recipients of a deceased donor and a living donor. They showed that rSO_2 remained significantly lower in the DDRT group compared to the LDRT group throughout the 50 min after reperfusion and that reperfusion rates were significantly faster in the LDRT group during the first 5 min post-reperfusion. Interestingly, intraoperative rSO_2 strongly correlated with allograft function up to 14 days post-transplantation. They concluded that NIRS may be a useful intra-operative tool to assess the degree of preservation/reperfusion injury and predict early allograft function.

Lastly, future technologies to develop organs to replace the current source of human organs for transplant are in the focus of many research groups around the world. Aiming to achieve future generation of a new kidney Dr. Garcia-Dominguez and his colleagues studied "The effect of Sildenafil Citrate in enhancing renal organogenesis following metanephroi allotransplantation" [10]. Sildenafil citrate (SC) is known as a useful inductor of angiogenesis, offering renoprotective properties due to its anti-inflammatory, antifibrotic, and antiapoptotic effects. In their animal model Dr. Garcia-Dominguez and his colleagues using an animal model performed metanephroi allotransplantation after embedding sildenafil citrate into the retroperitoneal fat. After 21 days the new kidneys' weights become increased significantly. Functionality was proven by renin and erythropoietin gene expression and tubular integrity was evident by highly expressed E-cadherin on Immunofluorescence assay. Histological studies showed mature glomeruli and hydronephrosis showing the new kidney's excretory function.

Conflicts of Interest: The author declares no conflict of interest.

References

1. Yemini, R.; Rahamimov, R.; Ghinea, R.; Mor, E. Long-Term Results of Kidney Transplantation in the Elderly: Comparison between Different Donor Settings. *J. Clin. Med.* **2021**, *10*, 5308. [CrossRef] [PubMed]
2. Bellini, M.I.; Nozdrin, M.; Pengel, L.; Knight, S.; Papalois, V. The Impact of Recipient Demographics on Outcomes from Living Donor Kidneys: Systematic Review and Meta-Analysis. *J. Clin. Med.* **2021**, *10*, 5556. [CrossRef] [PubMed]
3. Imamura, R.; Tanaka, R.; Taniguchi, A.; Nakazawa, S.; Kato, T.; Yamanaka, K.; Namba-Hamano, T.; Kakuta, Y.; Abe, T.; Tsutahara, K.; et al. Everolimus Reduces Cancer Incidence and Improves Patient and Graft Survival Rates after Kidney Transplantation: A Multi-Center Study. *J. Clin. Med.* **2022**, *11*, 249. [CrossRef] [PubMed]
4. Righini, M.; Capelli, I.; Busutti, M.; Raimondi, C.; Comai, G.; Donati, G.; Cappuccilli, M.L.; Ravaioli, M.; Chieco, P.; La Manna, G. Impact of the Type of Dialysis on Time to Transplantation: Is It Just a Matter of Immunity? *J. Clin. Med.* **2022**, *11*, 1054. [CrossRef] [PubMed]
5. Noble, J.; Metzger, A.; Bennani, H.N.; Daligault, M.; Masson, D.; Terrec, F.; Imerzoukene, F.; Bardy, B.; Fiard, G.; Marlu, R.; et al. Apheresis Efficacy and Tolerance in the Setting of HLA-Incompatible Kidney Transplantation. *J. Clin. Med.* **2021**, *10*, 1316. [CrossRef] [PubMed]
6. Kemmner, S.; Holzmann-Littig, C.; Sandberger, H.; Bachmann, Q.; Haberfellner, F.; Torrez, C.; Schmaderer, C.; Heemann, U.; Renders, L.; Assfalg, V.; et al. Pretransplant Serum Uromodulin and Its Association with Delayed Graft Function Following Kidney Transplantation—A Prospective Cohort Study. *J. Clin. Med.* **2021**, *10*, 2586. [CrossRef] [PubMed]
7. Kielar, M.; Dumnicka, P.; Gala-Błądzińska, A.; Będkowska-Prokop, A.; Ignacak, E.; Maziarz, B.; Ceranowicz, P.; Kuśnierz-Cabala, B. Urinary NGAL Measured after the First Year Post Kidney Transplantation Predicts Changes in Glomerular Filtration over One-Year Follow-Up. *J. Clin. Med.* **2021**, *10*, 43. [CrossRef] [PubMed]
8. Warmuzińska, N.; Łuczykowski, K.; Bojko, B. A Review of Current and Emerging Trends in Donor Graft-Quality Assessment Techniques. *J. Clin. Med.* **2022**, *11*, 487. [CrossRef] [PubMed]
9. Lau, H.; Lopez, A.J.; Eguchi, N.; Shimomura, A.; Ferrey, A.; Tantisattamo, E.; Reddy, U.; Dafoe, D.; Ichii, H. Intraoperative Near-Infrared Spectroscopy Monitoring of Renal Allograft Reperfusion in Kidney Transplant Recipients: A Feasibility and Proof-of-Concept Study. *J. Clin. Med.* **2021**, *10*, 4292. [CrossRef] [PubMed]
10. Garcia-Dominguez, X.; Vera-Donoso, C.D.; Lopez-Moncholi, E.; Moreno-Manzano, V.; Vicente, J.S.; Marco-Jiménez, F. Sildenafil Citrate Enhances Renal Organogenesis Following Metanephroi Allotransplantation into Non-Immunosuppressed Hosts. *J. Clin. Med.* **2022**, *11*, 3068. [CrossRef] [PubMed]

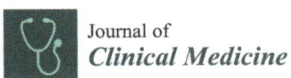

Article

Sildenafil Citrate Enhances Renal Organogenesis Following Metanephroi Allotransplantation into Non-Immunosuppressed Hosts

Ximo Garcia-Dominguez [1], César D. Vera-Donoso [2], Eric Lopez-Moncholi [3], Victoria Moreno-Manzano [3], José S. Vicente [1,†] and Francisco Marco-Jiménez [1,*,†]

1. Laboratory of Biotechnology of Reproduction, Institute for Animal Science and Technology (ICTA), Universitat Politècnica de València, 46022 Valencia, Spain; ximo.garciadominguez@gmail.com (X.G.-D.); jvicent@dca.upv.es (J.S.V.)
2. Servicio de Urología, Hospital Universitari i Politècnic La Fe, 46026 Valencia, Spain; cdveradonoso@gmail.com
3. Neuronal and Tissue Regeneration Laboratory, Centro de Investigación Príncipe Felipe, 46012 Valencia, Spain; elopezm@cipf.es (E.L.-M.); vmorenom@cipf.es (V.M.-M.)
* Correspondence: fmarco@dca.upv.es
† These authors contributed equally to this work.

Abstract: In order to harness the potential of metanephroi allotransplantation to the generation of a functional kidney graft on demand, we must achieve further growth post-transplantation. Sildenafil citrate (SC) is widely known as a useful inductor of angiogenesis, offering renoprotective properties due to its anti-inflammatory, antifibrotic, and antiapoptotic effects. Here, we performed a laparoscopic metanephroi allotransplantation after embedding sildenafil citrate into the retroperitoneal fat of non-immunosuppressed adult rabbit hosts. Histology and histomorphometry were used to examine the morphofunctional changes in new kidneys 21 days post-transplantation. Immunofluorescence of E-cadherin and renin and erythropoietin gene expression were used to assess the tubule integrity and endocrine functionality. After the metanephroi were embedded in a 10 µM SC solution, the new kidneys' weights become increased significantly. The E-cadherin expression together with the renin and erythropoietin gene expression revealed its functionality, while histological mature glomeruli and hydronephrosis proved the new kidneys' excretory function. Thus, we have described a procedure through the use of SC that improves the outcomes after a metanephroi transplantation. This study gives hope to a pathway that could offer a handsome opportunity to overcome the kidney shortage.

Keywords: kidney; metanephros; organogenesis; transplantation; regenerative medicine

1. Introduction

Currently, renal diseases affect epidemic numbers of people worldwide and have continued to escalate in their prevalence globally in recent years [1]. Kidney organs are responsible for vital functions, including the excretion of metabolic wastes and toxins, body fluid regulation, and the endocrine control of the blood pressure and erythrocyte maturation. Hence, when renal degenerative processes end in an organ failure, organ transplantation becomes the ideal method for restoring full physiological organ function [2]. However, the unavailability of suitable organs for transplantation forces end-stage renal patients to decide to take dialysis treatment or die. In Spain, the world's leading country in organ donation for 28 consecutive years [3], only 3423 kidney transplantations were performed in 2019, instead of the 7356 that were necessary according to the waiting list [4]. In 2018, 40% of US patients listed for a kidney transplant were still waiting since 2015, and 34,591 patients were removed from the list due to death or decline in medical condition [5,6]. Therefore, the required organs do not arrive in time for all the patients, and 5–10% of patients die on the waiting list every year [7]. In this precarious situation, emerging technologies in the field of regenerative medicine seek to address the limitations of current treatment strategies, exploring new frontiers. The common idea is to generate kidney grafts on demand to function as native kidneys, based on strategies ranging from stem cell therapy, blastocyst complementation, decellularization-recellularization, or 3D bioprinting [8,9]. However, the kidney is one of the most challenging organs for de novo formation due to its complex architecture and composition, containing numerous highly specialized and differentiated cell types [8,10]. Therefore, to date, cell therapies with individual cells are far from achieving fully functional transplantable renal grafts. As a promising solution for these limitations, the xenotransplantation of embryonic kidneys showed that, if this intact renal primordium was transplanted into adult non-immunosuppressed hosts, then it could mature as if they had not been extracted from the embryo, with a significantly reduced immune response in the hosts [11,12]. These embryonic kidneys (metanephroi) are able to attract the formation of a vascular system from the host, undergoing maturation and exhibiting excretory and endocrine functional properties [11–20]. Glomerular filtration in developing metanephroi was demonstrated firstly in the 1990s [21,22]. Today, metanephroi transplantation remains a promise to treat the renal injury, as metanephroi have been successfully transplanted across concordant and highly disparate xenogeneic barriers [12,20,23,24]. Specifically, Dekel et al. transplanted human and porcine metanephroi into mice, obtaining kidney structures that produce urine [12]. These findings suggest that if embryonic organs are retrieved from pathogen-free animals [9,25], this source could provide an unlimited and elective supply of organs for clinical transplantation.

However, allowing the new kidney to grow larger and sustain life in the long-term is a remaining obstacle to guarantee the feasibility of this strategy for clinical application [18,19,26–29]. Using combinations of growth factors, Hammerman's group have achieved rates of clearance in transplanted metanephroi almost 300 times those measured without any treatment [19]. These values were approximately 6% of the clearance achieved by a normal kidney [27,30], which approximates a renal function level that would be expected to preserve life [30]. Therefore, it is of special importance to investigate whether growth-promoting factors could be used to enhance the growth and function of developing metanephroi. Sildenafil citrate (SC) is a well-known drug used to treat pulmonary hypertension and male erectile dysfunction due to its vasodilatory effect. SC up-regulates cGMP, nitric oxide, and angiogenic systems, causing angiogenesis and renoprotective effects through anti-inflammatory, anti-oxidant, and anti-apoptotic mechanisms [31–35]. SC has demonstrated beneficial properties as a preconditioning or protective drug during kidney transplantation [36,37]. Besides, SC enhances the cartilage graft viability and survival, which is highly dependent on the vascularized host bed, oxygenation of local tissue, and the patient's current systemic status [34]. To some extent, the survival and development of the avascular metanephroi could depend on the same variables, being crucial in its connection to the host vascular system. Therefore, this study was conceived to explore if SC addition during the metanephroi transplantation improves its development.

2. Materials and Methods

All chemicals, unless otherwise stated, were reagent-grade and purchased from Sigma-Aldrich Química SA (Alcobendas, Madrid, Spain).

2.1. Ethical Statements

The study was approved by the Universitat Politècnica de València Ethical Committee (Code: 2015/VSC/PEA/00170). The study followed the Directive 2010/63/EU EEC guidelines. Experimental protocols were conducted under the supervision of the animal welfare committee in charge of this animal facility. An authorisation certificate issued by the Valencian governmental administration to experiment on animals is held by X. GD (code: 2815), F. MJ (code: 2273), and JS. V (code: 0690).

2.2. Experimental Design

New Zealand rabbits were used for the experiment. Metanephroi were recovered from 15-day-old (E15) embryos. Then, the metanephroi were placed in 5 µL drops containing one of the following SC concentrations: 0 µM (0 SC; untreated group), 10 µM (10 SC), and 30 µM (30 SC). After that, metanephroi were laparoscopically transplanted into non-immunosuppressed adult hosts (5 months). Total white blood cells and lymphocytes were estimated to identify any immunological response. After 21 days, the transplantation efficiency (recovery rate: kidneys recovered/metanephroi transplanted), nascent kidney growth (weight), its excretory function (histology, histomorphometry, and hydronephrosis), the tubule integrity (E-Cadherin), and its endocrine function (mRNA) were assessed. Kidneys originated from neonatal rabbits (1 week-old, coeval with metanephroi age) were used as control. The experimental design is summarized in Figure 1.

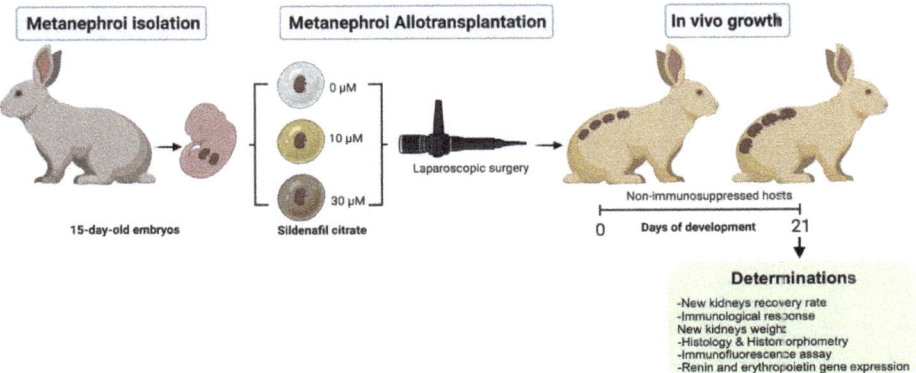

Figure 1. Experimental design. Metanephroi were recovered, embedded in 5 µL drops of sildenafil citrate (0, 10, 30 µM), and laparoscopically transplanted into non-immunosuppressed hosts. The immunological response, recovery rate (kidneys recovered/metanephroi transplanted), and the new kidneys weight and function (excretory and endocrine) were assessed (figure created with BioRender.com).

2.3. Metanephroi Recovery and Transplantation

Metanephroi were carefully dissected from E15 rabbit embryos under a dissecting microscope. One embryo was fixed directly for histological examination. Just before its allotransplantation, metanephroi were deposited in 5-µL droplets of phosphate-buffered saline (PBS) solution containing SC concentrations of 0 µM (untreated group), 10 µM, or 30 µM. All manipulations were performed at room temperature (25 ± 1 °C). The allotransplantation was performed using a minimally invasive laparoscopic technique, as previously described [38], within 45 min after the metanephroi were retrieved. Briefly, animals were placed on an operating table in a vertical position (head down at a 45-degree angle). Only one endoscope trocar was inserted into the abdominal cavity. Then, an epidural needle was inserted into the inguinal region. After a renal vessel was identified in the retroperitoneal fat, a hole (as a pouch) was performed adjacent to the vessel. Then, each metanephros was aspirated with 5 µL of each SC solution (0 SC, 10 SC, or 30 SC) in an epidural catheter (Vygon corporate, Paterna, Valencia, Spain), introduced into the inguinal region through an epidural needle, and deposited (transplanted) into the pouch previously created. Between 5 to 9 metanephroi were transplanted in each host (one metanephros per hole). A total of seven adult rabbits were used as hosts in three sessions, without immunosuppressive therapy (2, 2 and 3 hosts for 0, 10 and 30 SC, respectively). Anaesthesia, analgesia, and the postoperative care were performed as we previously described for laparoscopic procedures [39].

2.4. Determination of Peripheral White Blood Cells

Before the transplantation (day 0), a blood sample of each host ($n = 7$) was collected from the central ear artery and dispensed into an EDTA-coated tube (Deltalab S.L., Barcelona, Spain). Then, basal levels of total white blood cells and lymphocytes were estimated at most 10 min after blood collection, using an automated veterinary haematology analyser (MS 4e automated cell counter, MeletSchloesing Laboratories, Osny, France) and according to the manufacturer's instructions. After metanephroi transplantation, two blood extractions were analysed weekly along the experiment to detect significant variations of the total white blood cell and lymphocyte populations.

2.5. Metanephroi Development and Histomorphometry of the Renal Corpuscle

All animals were euthanized 3 weeks after transplantation, retrieving all the new kidneys developed to annotate the recovery rate (recovered kidneys/transplanted metanephroi). Then, renal structures were weighted, fixed in formaldehyde solution, and embedded in paraffin wax for histological analysis. Samples for histology were cut into 5-µm sections and stained with haematoxylin and eosin. The stained sections were observed with light microscopy for histological and histomorphometric examination. To measure histomorphometric parameters, a minimum of 25 renal corpuscles and glomeruli were evaluated (area and perimeter) for each experimental group. Photomicrographs were taken at a total magnification of ×400. Measurements were determined using ImageJ software (public domain http://rsb.info.nih.gov/ij/, accessed 1 April 2022). In addition, the glomerular tuft cellularity was estimated by counting the total number of nuclei of each glomerulus. Kidneys originating from a 5-week-old rabbit (coeval with the metanephroi age) were used as controls.

2.6. Tubule Integrity by Targeting E-Cadherin

Immunofluorescence for paraffin-embedded kidney 5-µm sections required prior dewaxing, rehydration, and antigen retrieval (immersion in tris-EDTA buffer (10 mM Tris, pH 9.0) for 25 min at 97 °C) steps. Then, samples were incubated with blocking solution (5% horse serum, 10% fetal bovine serum in phosphate buffer solution with 0.1% Triton X-100) for 1 h at room temperature and incubated with the primary antibody mouse anti-E-Caherin (Cat. C20820; BD bioscience, Franklin Lakes, NJ, USA) overnight in a humidified chamber at 4 °C. After washing, the sample was incubated with the secondary antibody (Alexa-Fluor 555; 1:400; Invitrogen, Waltham, MA, USA) at room temperature for 2 h. All cells were counterstained by incubation with 4,6-diamidino-2-phenylindole dihydrochloride (DAPI; Invitrogen). After a final wash, the sections were evaluated by using the Apotome Inverted Fluorescence Microscope (Zeiss, Jena, Germany). Consistent exposures were applied for all images.

2.7. Renin and Erythropoietin mRNA Gene Expression

After euthanasia, developed metanephroi samples were obtained by retrieving biopsies randomly from different sites. Immediately, samples were washed with PBS to remove blood remnants and stored in RNA-later (Ambion Inc., Huntingdon, UK) at −20 °C until the analysis. Five samples were analysed in each experimental group (control, 0 SC, 10 SC, and 30 SC). Host kidneys (under the same physiological environment as nascent kidneys) were used as the control. RNA was extracted with a Dynabeads kit (Invitrogen Life Technology) according to the manufacturer's instructions and treated with DNase I to eliminate genomic DNA contamination. Then, reverse transcription was carried out using a Reverse Transcriptase Quantitect kit (Qiagen, Hilden, Germany). Real-time quantitative PCR (RT-qPCR) reactions were conducted in an Applied Biosystems 7500 (Applied Biosystems, Foster City, CA, USA). Every RT-qPCR was performed from 5 µL of diluted 1:40 cDNA template, 250 nM of forward and reverse primers (Table 1), and 10 µL of PowerSYBR Green PCR Master Mix (Fermentas GMBH, Madrid, Spain) in a final volume of 20 µL. The PCR protocol included an initial step of 50 °C (2 min), followed by 95 °C (10 min), and 42 cycles of 95 °C (15 s) and 60 °C (60 s). After RT-qPCR, a melting curve analysis was performed by slowly increasing the temperature from 65 °C to 95 °C, with the continuous recording of changes in fluorescent emission intensity. The amplification products were confirmed by SYBR Green-stained 2% agarose gel electrophoresis in 1X Bionic buffer. Serial dilutions of the cDNA pool made from several samples were conducted to assess RT-qPCR efficiency. A ΔΔCt method adjusted for RT-qPCR efficiency was used [40], employing the geometric average of glyceraldehyde-3-phosphate dehydrogenase (GAPDH) as the housekeeping normalization factor [41]. Relative expression of the cDNA pool from various samples was used as the calibrator to normalise all samples within one RT-qPCR run or between several runs.

Table 1. Primer sequences.

Genes	Sequence (5'-3')	Product Size (bp)
REN	Forward: 5'-GGGACTCCTGCTGGTACTCT-3' Reverse: 5'-CTGAGGGCATTTTCTTGAGG-3'	100
EPO	Forward: 5'-ACGTGGACAAGGCTGTCAGT-3' Reverse: 5'-TGGAGTAGATGCGGAAAAGC-3'	162
GAPDH	Forward: 5'-GCCGCTTCTTCTCGTGCAG-3' Reverse: 5'-ATGGATCATTGATGGCGACAACAT-3'	144

REN: renin; EPO: erythropoietin; GAPDH: glyceraldehyde-3-phosphate dehydrogenase.

2.8. Statistical Analyses

Differences in the recovery rates between groups were assessed using a probit link model with binomial error distribution, including the experimental group as a fixed effect. Variations in the peripheral blood cells were evaluated using a general linear model (GLM), including the day post-transplant as a fixed factor. The experimental group was non-significant and was removed from the model. The new kidney weight, hitomorphometric measures (area and perimeter), and the glomerular tuft cellularity were compared using a GLM, including the experimental group as a fixed effect and a replicate as a random factor. The replicate was non-significant and was removed from the model. Data of relative mRNA abundance were normalized by a Napierian logarithm transformation and evaluated using a GLM as previously described. Data were expressed as least square means ± standard error of means. Differences of $p \leq 0.05$ were considered significant. All statistical analyses were performed with SPSS 21.0 software package (SPSS Inc., Chicago, IL, USA).

3. Results

3.1. Allotransplanted Metanephroi Form Adult Organs

Three New Zealand white rabbits were used as embryo donors, obtaining a total of 28 E15 embryos. Metanephroi were carefully micro-dissected and transplanted into seven adult non-immunosuppressed hosts (5-month-old animals). A total of 49 whole metanephroi were allotransplanted: 15 in 0 SC (untreated group), 17 in 10 SC, and 17 in 30 SC. The peripheral circulating white blood cell count (total, lymphocytes, monocytes, and eosinophils) remained unchanged after allotransplantation (Figure 2).

Twenty-one days after transplantation, we observed that the transplanted metanephroi grew and promoted angiogenesis (Figure 3). Metanephroi treated with SC exhibited a macroscopic view of deeper vascular integration than the untreated ones (Figure 3). A similar recovery rate was observed for all the groups: 10/15 (67%), 9/17 (53%), and 8/17 (47%) for 0 SC, 10 SC, and 30 SC groups, respectively.

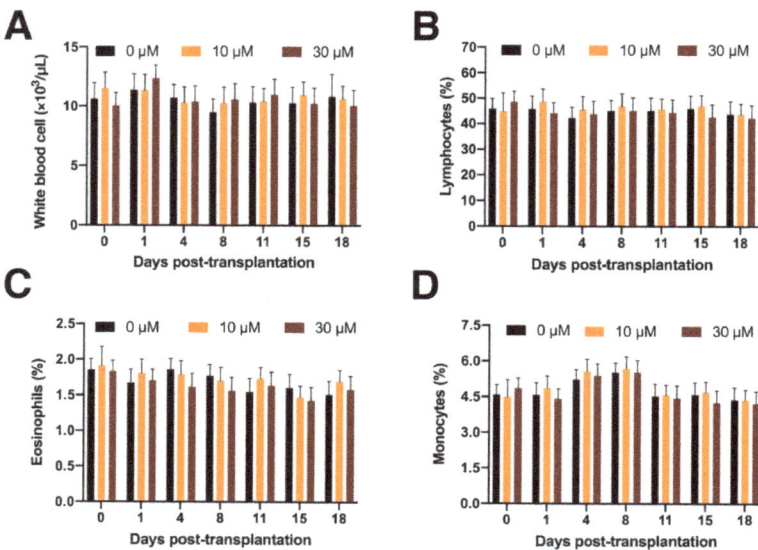

Figure 2. White blood cell counts after metanephroi allotransplantation: (**A**) total white blood cells; (**B**) lymphocytes; (**C**) eosinophils; (**D**) monocytes.

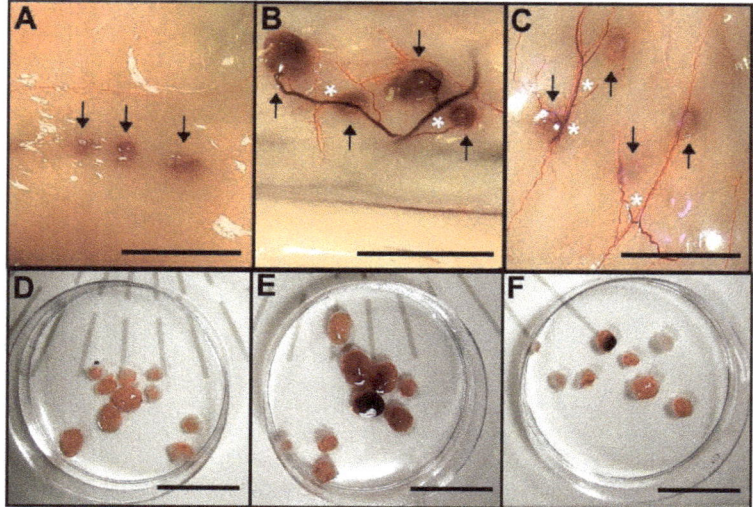

Figure 3. Development of new kidney recovery 21 days after metanephroi allotransplantation with or without sildenafil citrate (SC). (**A**) Nascent kidney from metanephroi without SC treatment. Arrows indicate the growing metanephroi. (**B**) Developing kidney from metanephroi treated with the 10 μM SC solution. Asterisk indicates neoangiogenesis. Arrows indicate the growing metanephroi. (**C**) Developing kidney from metanephroi treated with the 30 μM SC solution. Asterisk indicates neoangiogenesis. Arrows indicate the growing metanephroi. (**D–F**) New kidneys recovered from transplanted metanephroi (**D**) without SC treatment, (**E**) with the 10 μM SC solution, and (**F**) with the 30 μM SC solution. Scale bars: 2 cm.

3.2. Comparative Renal Weight and Histomorphometry Study

Significant increase in developing kidney weight was observed for the 10 SC group (0.13 ± 0.021 g), compared with the 30 SC (0.07 ± 0.025 g) and the 0 SC (0.08 ± 0.020 g) groups. All nascent kidney weights were lower than the control samples (0.74 ± 0.028 g), independently of the experimental group ($p < 0.05$, Figure 4).

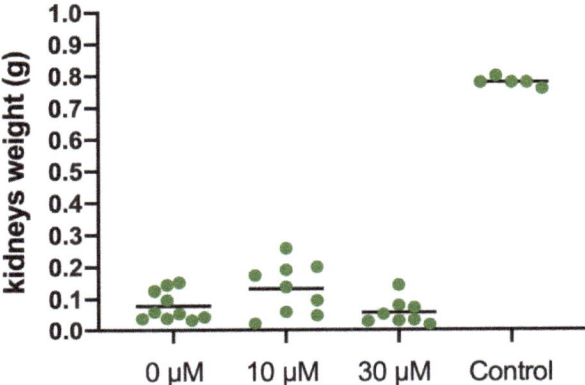

Figure 4. Kidney weight recovery 21 days after metanephroi allotransplantation embedding in sildenafil citrate (0, 10 and 30 µM). The control kidney originated from a neonatal rabbit (1 week-old).

All nascent kidneys became hydronephrotic, demonstrating its excretory function. Concordantly, in all the groups, metanephroi underwent differentiation and developed new kidney graft explants with histologically mature glomeruli (Figure 5), whose histomorphometric analysis is shown in Table 2.

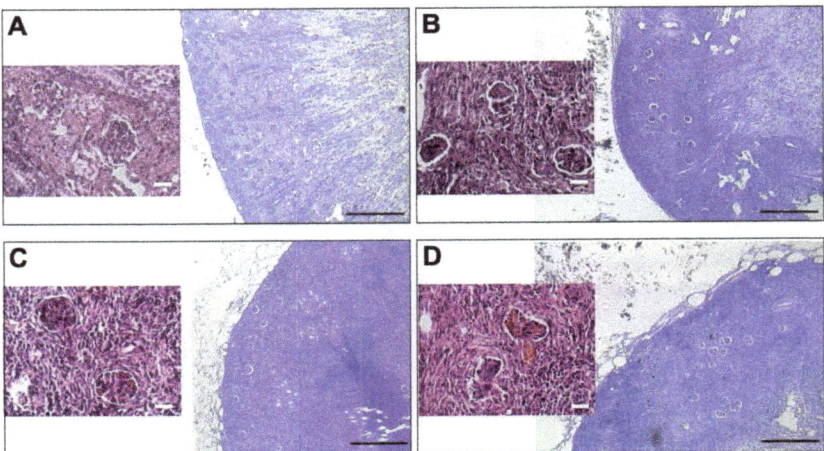

Figure 5. Histology of developing kidneys with or without sildenafil citrate. (**A**) Micrograph showing the glomerulus details (original magnification, ×400) and the outer renal cortex (original magnification, ×40) of the control kidney originating from a neonatal rabbit (1 week-old). (**B–D**) Micrograph showing the glomerulus details (original magnification, ×400) and the outer renal cortex (original magnification, x40) of a new kidney after metanephroi transplantation: (**B**) without sildenafil citrate (SC) treatment, (**C**) with a 10 µM SC solution, and (**D**) with a 30 µM SC solution.

Table 2. Histomorphometric quantification of the renal corpuscle of kidneys developed after metanephroi allotransplantation.

Sildenafil Citrate	n	Renal Corpuscle		Glomerulus		
		Area (μm^2)	Perimeter (μm)	Area (μm^2)	Perimeter (μm)	Cell Number
0 μM SC	10	3034.6 ± 176.44 [b]	201.1 ± 6.06 [b]	2132.5 ± 142.56 [b]	170.9 ± 5.70 [b]	41.0 ± 2.22 [b]
10 μM SC	9	3639.7 ± 179.94 [a]	218.5 ± 6.18 [a]	2749.5 ± 145.39 [a]	192.0 ± 5.81 [a]	49.9 ± 2.26 [a]
30 μM SC	8	3582.44 ± 187.59 [a]	218.3 ± 6.45 [a]	2655.7 ± 151.85 [a]	190.2 ± 6.06 [a]	48.3 ± 2.36 [a]
Control	6	2633.4 ± 92.31 [c]	184.2 ± 3.17 [c]	2104.7 ± 74.58 [b]	165.3 ± 2.98 [b]	52.7 ± 1.16 [a]

n: Number of new kidneys or control kidneys. Data are expressed as least-square means ± standard error of the mean. [a,b,c] Data in the same column with uncommon letters are different ($p < 0.05$).

The histomorphometric data showed that all the metanephroi-developed kidneys exhibited higher renal corpuscle values (area and perimeter) than the control samples, demonstrating the hydronephrotic state of the former and its filtering activity. Moreover, both renal corpuscle and glomerulus measurements were increased in the 10 SC and 30 SC groups compared to the untreated one, suggesting that SC increased both the capillary dilatation and glomerular filtration. Tuft cell density in the 10 SC and 30 SC groups' developed metanephroi were also higher than in the untreated one, and similar to the control samples, they showed a trophic effect of the SC on the glomeruli development.

3.3. Tubule Integrity in the New Kidneys

Immunofluorescence assay results showed that E-cadherin was highly expressed in new kidneys (Figure 6B–D). E-cadherin expression reflected the reduced tubule size in the 30 SC group (Figure 6D).

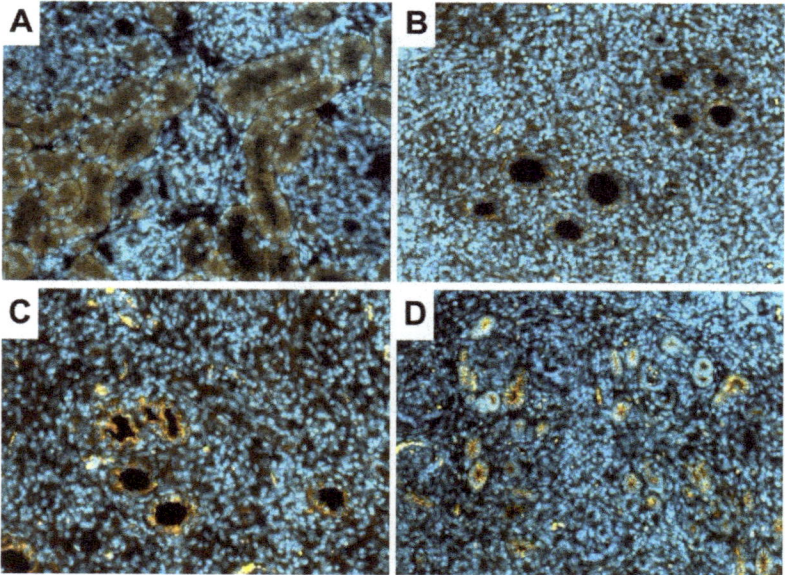

Figure 6. Immunofluorescence and confocal microscopy assay for the detection of tubular integrity marker E-Cadherin. (A) Micrograph showing tubular integrity of the control kidney originating from a neonatal rabbit (1 week-old). (B–D) Micrograph tubular integrity of the new kidney after metanephroi transplantation: (B) without sildenafil citrate (SC) treatment, (C) with a 10-μM SC solution, and (D) with a 30-μM SC solution. Original view: × 20.

3.4. Glomerular Renin and Erythropoietin Production in the New Kidneys

Renin and erythropoietin mRNA levels were similar between metanephroi-developed kidneys and the control samples (host's kidney), regardless of the experimental group (Figure 7).

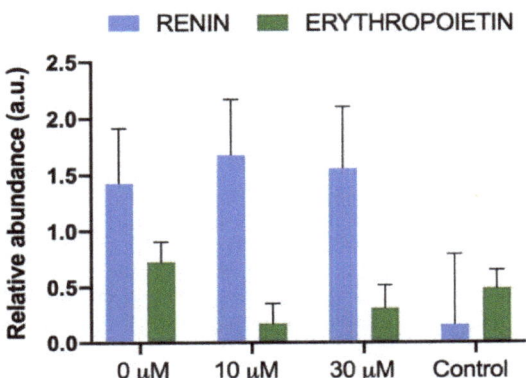

Figure 7. Renal gene expression levels of the renin and erythropoietin in the new kidney recovery 21 days after metanephroi allotransplantation embedding in sildenafil citrate (0, 10, and 30 µM), and the kidneys originated from a neonatal rabbit (1 week-old, control group).

4. Discussion

Herein, we have established a protocol to obtain an enlarged kidney after the use of SC during metanephroi transplantation. Moreover, our findings revealed that SC also positively affects glomerular development and function without affecting the tubule integrity and the endocrine properties. Besides, our data provide that there are no substantial changes in the magnitude of lymphocyte population, regardless of the SC concentration used. Altogether, our results represent firm evidence of the SC trophic effects for metanephroi development. Looking for the strategies that allow obtaining life-sustaining renal structures, SC's use becomes a potential factor towards the clinical translation of metanephroi transplantation therapy.

Severely damaged kidneys possess a limited regenerative potential, and therapeutic interventions are not sufficient to restore renal function in patients with ESRD, turning transplantation into the ideal method to restore full physiological functions [8,42]. Given the graft shortage, either from living or deceased donors, well recognized by WHO [43], some regenerative and bioengineering strategies are trying to generate kidney grafts on demand [8,9,44]. Metanephroi transplantation remains one of the most promising approaches, but obtaining larger and life-sustaining renal structures after its transplantation remains an obstacle for its therapeutic potential [19,26–29]. In this sense, we evaluated the SC effect during a metanephroi transplantation on their in vivo development. Previously, Rostaing et al. demonstrated that SC exerts a dilatation of glomerular afferent arterioles, promoting an increase in the filtration process [45]. Likewise, our histomorphometric data showed that SC increases the area and perimeter of the glomerulus and the renal corpuscle. If SC promotes glomerular filtration in nascent kidneys, they must accumulate more filtrate in the bowman's space due to the lack of a urine-excretion channel (hydronephrosis). Taking into account that SC acts as a potent inductor of VEGF (vascular endothelial growth factor) release [46–48], our results support those of Hammerman's group, who indicated that urine volumes were increased significantly in VEGF-treated metanephroi [27]. However, although VEGF treatment did not affect the weights of transplanted metanephroi [27], SC treatment allows us to obtain larger renal structures. As a possible explanation, it has been proven that low SC doses resulted in more angiogenic responses than those produced by a saturating VEGF concentration [46]. Besides, SC has been previously proposed as a helpful agent in instances where neo-vascularization is desired [46], enhancing graft viability [34]. On the other hand, the renoprotective effects attributable to SC could retard hydronephrosis-related damages [31–35], allowing metanephroi growth for longer. However, this overgrowth appeared in the 10 SC group but not in the 30 SC one. As hydronephrosis turns metanephroi not viable [18], maybe high SC doses could accelerate glomerular filtration, exacerbating a hydronephrotic state that arrests the metanephroi growth earlier. Similar results were observed by Yardimci et al. [49], which allow us to speculate that metanephroi development could be better in the 30 SC group before urine production was started. Therefore, the use of 10 SC allows us to recover larger renal structures with a higher degree of glomerular development and function. Moreover, developed metanephroi showed glomerular filtration activity and endocrine functions, which are consistent with the previous literature [12,14,15,17–19,27]. We have identified the expression of E-cadherin in the renal tubules of the new kidneys. E-cadherin is a key adherent protein in the formation of adhesion junctions, which are critical to tubule integrity in normal kidneys [50]. In addition, the renin and erythropoietin gene expression levels were similar between new and host kidneys. Interestingly, this study was consistent with previous reports showing that harvesting metanephroi at the optimal age avoids the immunological response from hosts [38,51]. Compared to coeval native organs, developed metanephroi reach a diminished renal mass that could incur potential life-sustaining limitations. However, it has been demonstrated that the survival time of anephric recipients transplanted with metanephroi is proportional to the renal mass developed [52]. This concept is similar to that used in kidney transplantation from paediatric donors, in which both kidneys are transplanted in bloc into adult recipients to guarantee acceptable glomerular filtration rates [53,54]. This strategy should be combined with those designed to avoid hydronephrosis [18], or others developed in our group, such as the minimally invasive laparoscopic transplantation procedure [38,55], effective banking protocols [56–58], and, now, the use of SC. All these strategies, in conjunction, could constitute a path increasingly consolidated by which metanephroi xenotransplantation could provide transplantable renal grafts to treat patients with ESRD.

5. Conclusions

In conclusion, we have reported a procedure based on SC's addition during the metanephroi transplantation that promotes the nascent kidneys' growth and glomerular filtration. This treatment enhances the glomerular developmental degree without compromising either the endocrine activity or the new renal structures' immunological silence. This study gives hope to a pathway that could offer a handsome opportunity to overcome the kidney shortage.

Author Contributions: Conceptualization, C.D.V.-D. and F.M.-J.; methodology, X.G.-D., J.S.V., F.M.-J., E.L.-M. and V.M.-M.; software, X.G.-D.; validation, X.G.-D. and F.M.-J.; formal analysis, X.G.-D., J.S.V., and F.M.-J.; investigation, X.G.-D., J.S.V. and F.M.-J.; resources, C.D.V.-D., J.S.V. and F.M.-J.; data curation, X.G.-D.; writing—original draft preparation, X.G.-D.; writing—review and editing, X.G.-D., C.D.V.-D., J.S.V. and F.M.-J.; supervision, C.D.V.-D. and F.M.-J.; project administration, C.D.V.-D. and F.M.-J.; funding acquisition, C.D.V.-D. and F.M.-J. All authors have read and agreed to the published version of the manuscript.

Funding: This research was funded by Alcer-turia foundation, Astellas pharma inc., and Precipita crowdfunding. X.G.-D. was supported by a research grant from the Ministry of Economy, Industry and Competitiveness of Spain (BES-2015-072429).

Institutional Review Board Statement: The study was conducted according to the guidelines of the Directive 2010/63/EU EEC, and approved by the Universitat Politècnica de València Ethical Committee (Code: 2015/VSC/PEA/00170).

Informed Consent Statement: Not applicable.

Data Availability Statement: The datasets analysed during the current study are available from the corresponding author on reasonable request.

Conflicts of Interest: The authors declare no conflict of interest. The funders had no role in the design of the study; in the collection, analyses, or interpretation of data; in the writing of the manuscript; or in the decision to publish the results.

References

1. Chambers, J.M.; McKee, R.A.; Drummond, B.E.; Wingert, R.A. Evolving technology: Creating kidney organoids from stem cells. *AIMS Bioeng.* **2016**, *3*, 305–318. [CrossRef] [PubMed]
2. Salvatori, M.; Peloso, A.; Katari, R.; Orlando, G. Regeneration and Bioengineering of the Kidney: Current Status and Future Challenges. *Curr. Urol. Rep.* **2014**, *15*, 1–10. [CrossRef] [PubMed]
3. Organización Nacional de Trasplantes (ONT). Nota de Prensa. Available online: http://www.ont.es/prensa/NotasDePrensa/07.09.2020NPONTRegistroMundial.pdf (accessed on 14 October 2020).
4. Organización Nacional de Trasplantes (ONT). Memoria Actividad Donación Y Trasplante Renal. España. 2019. Available online: http://www.ont.es/infesp/Memorias/Actividad_de_Donación_y_Trasplante_Renal_2019.pdf (accessed on 13 October 2020).
5. Organ Procurement and Transplantation Network (OPTN) Web Site. Available online: https://optn.transplant.hrsa.gov/ (accessed on 10 October 2020).
6. Hart, A.; Smith, J.M.; Skeans, M.A.; Gustafson, S.K.; Wilk, A.R.; Castro, S.; Foutz, J.; Wainright, J.L.; Snyder, J.J.; Kasiske, B.L.; et al. OPTN/SRTR 2018 Annual Data Report: Kidney. *Am. J. Transplant.* **2020**, *20*, 20–130. [CrossRef] [PubMed]
7. Heilman, R.L.; Smith, M.L.; Smith, B.H.; Kumar, A.; Srinivasan, A.; Huskey, J.L.; Khamash, H.A.; Jadlowiec, C.C.; Mathur, A.K.; Moss, A.A.; et al. Long-term Outcomes Following Kidney Transplantation From Donors With Acute Kidney Injury. *Transplantation* **2019**, *103*, e263–e272. [CrossRef]
8. García-Domínguez, X.; Vicente, J.S.; Vera-Donoso, C.D.; Marco-Jimenez, F. Current Bioengineering and Regenerative Strategies for the Generation of Kidney Grafts on Demand. *Curr. Urol. Rep.* **2017**, *18*, 1–8. [CrossRef]
9. Peired, A.J.; Mazzinghi, B.; De Chiara, L.; Guzzi, F.; Lasagni, L.; Romagnani, P.; Lazzeri, E. Bioengineering strategies for nephrologists: Kidney was not built in a day. *Expert Opin. Biol. Ther.* **2020**, *20*, 467–480. [CrossRef]
10. Montserrat, N.; Garreta, E.; Belmonte, J.C.I. Regenerative strategies for kidney engineering. *FEBS J.* **2016**, *283*, 3303–3324. [CrossRef]
11. Hammerman, M.R. Transplantation of renal primordia: Renal organogenesis. *Pediatr. Nephrol.* **2007**, *22*, 1991–1998. [CrossRef]
12. Dekel, B.; Burakova, T.; Arditti, F.D.; Reich-Zeliger, S.; Milstein, O.; Aviel-Ronen, S.; Rechavi, G.; Friedman, N.; Kaminski, N.; Passwell, J.H.; et al. Human and porcine early kidney precursors as a new source for transplantation. *Nat. Med.* **2003**, *9*, 53–60. [CrossRef]
13. Takeda, S.-I.; Rogers, S.A.; Hammerman, M.R. Differential origin for endothelial and mesangial cells after transplantation of pig fetal renal primordia into rats. *Transpl. Immunol.* **2006**, *15*, 211–215. [CrossRef]
14. Matsumoto, K.; Yokoo, T.; Yokote, S.; Utsunomiya, Y.; Ohashi, T.; Hosoya, T. Functional development of a transplanted embryonic kidney: Effect of transplantation site. *J. Nephrol.* **2012**, *25*, 50–55. [CrossRef] [PubMed]
15. Yokote, S.; Yokoo, T.; Matsumoto, K.; Utsunomiya, Y.; Kawamura, T.; Hosoya, T. The effect of metanephros transplantation on blood pressure in anephric rats with induced acute hypotension. *Nephrol. Dial. Transplant.* **2012**, *27*, 3449–3455. [CrossRef] [PubMed]
16. Yokote, S.; Yokoo, T.; Matsumoto, K.; Ohkido, I.; Utsunomiya, Y.; Kawamura, T.; Hosoya, T. Metanephros Transplantation Inhibits the Progression of Vascular Calcification in Rats with Adenine-Induced Renal Failure. *Nephron Exp. Nephrol.* **2012**, *120*, 32–40. [CrossRef] [PubMed]
17. Matsumoto, K.; Yokoo, T.; Matsunari, H.; Iwai, S.; Yokote, S.; Teratani, T.; Gheisari, Y.; Tsuji, O.; Okano, H.; Utsunomiya, Y.; et al. Xenotransplanted Embryonic Kidney Provides a Niche for Endogenous Mesenchymal Stem Cell Differentiation into Erythropoietin-Producing Tissue. *Stem Cells* **2012**, *30*, 1228–1235. [CrossRef]
18. Yokote, S.; Matsunari, H.; Iwai, S.; Yamanaka, S.; Uchikura, A.; Fujimoto, E.; Matsumoto, K.; Nagashima, H.; Kobayashi, E.; Yokoo, T. Urine excretion strategy for stem cell-generated embryonic kidneys. *Proc. Natl. Acad. Sci. USA* **2015**, *112*, 12980–12985. [CrossRef]
19. Rogers, S.A.; Lowell, J.A.; Hammerman, N.A.; Hammerman, M.R. Transplantation of developing metanephroi into adult rats. *Kidney Int.* **1998**, *54*, 27–37. [CrossRef]
20. Rogers, S.A.; Talcott, M.; Hammerman, M.R. Transplantation of Pig Metanephroi. *ASAIO J.* **2003**, *49*, 48–52. [CrossRef]
21. Woolf, A.S.; Palmer, S.J.; Snow, M.L.; Fine, L.G. Creation of a functioning chimeric mammalian kidney. *Kidney Int.* **1990**, *38*, 991–997. [CrossRef]
22. Abrahamson, D.R.; St. John, P.L.; Pillion, D.J.; Tucker, D.C. Glomerular development in intraocular and intrarenal grafts of fetal kidneys. *Lab. Investig.* **1991**, *64*, 629–639.
23. Rogers, S.A.; Hammerman, M.R. Transplantation of rat metanephroi into mice. *Am. J. Physiol. Regul. Integr. Comp. Physiol.* **2001**, *280*, R1865–R1869. [CrossRef]

24. Hammerman, M.R. Xenotransplantation of developing kidneys. *Am. J. Physiol. Ren. Physiol.* **2002**, *283*, 601–606. [CrossRef] [PubMed]
25. Noordergraaf, J.; Schucker, A.; Martin, M.; Schuurman, H.-J.; Ordway, B.; Cooley, K.; Sheffler, M.; Theis, K.; Armstrong, C.; Klein, L.; et al. Pathogen elimination and prevention within a regulated, Designated Pathogen Free, closed pig herd for long-term breeding and production of xenotransplantation materials. *Xenotransplantation* **2018**, *25*, e12428. [CrossRef] [PubMed]
26. Rogers, S.A.; Liapis, H.; Hammerman, M.R. Transplantation of metanephroi across the major histocompatibility complex in rats. *Am. J. Physiol. Regul. Integr. Comp. Physiol.* **2001**, *280*, 132–136. [CrossRef]
27. Hammerman, M.R. Transplantation of renal precursor cells: A new therapeutic approach. *Pediatr. Nephrol.* **2000**, *14*, 513–517. [CrossRef]
28. Rogers, S.A.; Powell-Braxton, L.; Hammerman, M.R. Insulin-like growth factor I regulates renal development in rodents. *Dev. Genet.* **1999**, *24*, 293–298. [CrossRef]
29. Rogers, S.A.; Hammerman, M.R. Prolongation of Life in Anephric Rats following de novo Renal Organogenesis. *Organogenesis* **2004**, *1*, 22–25. [CrossRef]
30. Hammerman, M.R. Organogenesis of kidneys following transplantation of renal progenitor cells. *Transpl. Immunol.* **2004**, *12*, 229–239. [CrossRef]
31. Zahran, M.H.; Barakat, N.; Khater, S.; Awadalla, A.; Mosbah, A.; Nabeeh, A.; Hussein, A.M.; Shokeir, A.A. Renoprotective effect of local sildenafil administration in renal ischaemia–reperfusion injury: A randomised controlled canine study. *Arab J. Urol.* **2019**, *17*, 150–159. [CrossRef]
32. Georgiadis, G.; Zisis, I.-E.; Docea, A.O.; Tsarouhas, K.; Fragkiadoulaki, I.; Mavridis, C.; Karavitakis, M.; Stratakis, S.; Stylianou, K.; Tsitsimpikou, C.; et al. Current Concepts on the Reno-Protective Effects of Phosphodiesterase 5 Inhibitors in Acute Kidney Injury: Systematic Search and Review. *J. Clin. Med.* **2020**, *9*, 1284. [CrossRef]
33. Koneru, S.; Penumathsa, S.V.; Thirunavukkarasu, M.; Vidavalur, R.; Zhan, L.; Singal, P.K.; Engelman, R.M.; Das, D.K.; Maulik, N. Sildenafil-mediated neovascularization and protection against myocardial ischaemia reperfusion injury in rats: Role of VEGF/angiopoietin-1. *J. Cell. Mol. Med.* **2008**, *12*, 2651–2664. [CrossRef]
34. Kemaloğlu, C.A.; Tekin, Y. The effect of sildenafil on fascia-wrapped diced cartilage grafts. *Laryngoscope* **2015**, *125*, E168–E172. [CrossRef] [PubMed]
35. Bae, E.H.; Kim, I.J.; Joo, S.Y.; Kim, E.Y.; Kim, C.S.; Choi, J.S.; Ma, S.K.; Kim, S.H.; Lee, J.U.; Kima, S.W. Renoprotective Effects of Sildenafil in DOCA-Salt Hypertensive Rats. *Kidney Blood Press. Res.* **2012**, *36*, 248–257. [CrossRef] [PubMed]
36. Lledó-García, E.; Subirá-Ríos, D.; Rodríguez–Martínez, D.; Dulín, E.; Alvarez-Fernández, E.; Hernández-Fernández, C.; Del Cañizo-López, J.F. Sildenafil as a Protecting Drug for Warm Ischemic Kidney Transplants: Experimental Results. *J. Urol.* **2009**, *182*, 1222–1225. [CrossRef] [PubMed]
37. Lledo-Garcia, E.; Rodriguez-Martinez, D.; Cabello-Benavente, R.; Moncada-Iribarren, I.; Tejedor-Jorge, A.; Dulin, E.; Hernandez-Fernandez, C.; Del Canizo-Lopez, J.F. Sildenafil Improves Immediate Posttransplant Parameters in Warm-Ischemic Kidney Transplants: Experimental Study. *Transplant. Proc.* **2007**, *39*, 1354–1356. [CrossRef] [PubMed]
38. Vera-Donoso, C.D.; García-Dominguez, X.; Jiménez-Trigos, E.; García-Valero, L.; Vicente, J.S.; Marco-Jiménez, F. Laparoscopic transplantation of metanephros: A first step to kidney xenotransplantation. *Actas Urológicas Españolas (Engl. Ed.)* **2015**, *39*, 527–534. [CrossRef]
39. Garcia-Dominguez, X.; Marco-Jimenez, F.; Viudes-De-Castro, M.P.; Vicente, J.S. Minimally Invasive Embryo Transfer and Embryo Vitrification at the Optimal Embryo Stage in Rabbit Model. *J. Vis. Exp.* **2019**, *147*, e58055. [CrossRef]
40. Weltzien, F.-A.; Pasqualini, C.; Vernier, P.; Dufour, S. A quantitative real-time RT-PCR assay for European eel tyrosine hydroxylase. *Gen. Comp. Endocrinol.* **2005**, *141*, 134–142. [CrossRef]
41. Llobat, L.; Marco-Jiménez, F.; Peñaranda, D.S.; Saenz-de-Juano, M.D.; Vicente, J.S. Effect of Embryonic Genotype on Reference Gene Selection for RT-qPCR Normalization. *Reprod. Domest. Anim.* **2012**, *47*, 629–634. [CrossRef]
42. Imberti, B.; Corna, D.; Rizzo, P.; Xinaris, C.; Abbate, M.; Longaretti, L.; Cassis, P.; Benedetti, V.; Benigni, A.; Zoja, C.; et al. Renal Primordia Activate Kidney Regenerative Events in a Rat Model of Progressive Renal Disease. *PLoS ONE* **2015**, *10*, e0120235. [CrossRef]
43. Organ Donation and Transplantation Activities 2018 Report. Global Observatory on Donation and Transplantation (GODT). Available online: http://www.transplant-observatory.org/wp-content/uploads/2020/10/glorep2018-2.pdf (accessed on 10 October 2020).
44. Yamanaka, S.; Yokoo, T. Current Bioengineering Methods for Whole Kidney Regeneration. *Stem Cells Int.* **2015**, *2015*, 1–10. [CrossRef]
45. Rostaing, L.; Tran-Van, T.; Ader, J.-L. Increased Glomerular Filtration Rate in Kidney-Transplant Recipients Who Take Sildenafil. *N. Engl. J. Med.* **2000**, *342*, 1679–1680. [CrossRef] [PubMed]
46. Pyriochou, A.; Zhou, Z.; Koika, V.; Petrou, C.; Cordopatis, P.; Sessa, W.C.; Papapetropoulos, A. The phosphodiesterase 5 inhibitor sildenafil stimulates angiogenesis through a protein kinase G/MAPK pathway. *J. Cell. Physiol.* **2007**, *211*, 197–204. [CrossRef] [PubMed]
47. Vidavalur, R.; Penumathsa, S.V.; Zhan, L.; Thirunavukkarasu, M.; Maulik, N. Sildenafil induces angiogenic response in human coronary arteriolar endothelial cells through the expression of thioredoxin, hemeoxygenase and vascular endothelial growth factor. *Vasc. Pharmacol.* **2006**, *45*, 91–95. [CrossRef] [PubMed]

48. Liu, G.; Sun, X.; Dai, Y.; Zheng, F.; Wang, D.; Huang, Y.; Bian, J.; Deng, C. Chronic Administration of Sildenafil Modified the Impaired VEGF System and Improved the Erectile Function in Rats with Diabetic Erectile Dysfunction. *J. Sex. Med.* **2010**, *7*, 3868–3878. [CrossRef]
49. Yardimci, S.; Bostanci, E.B.; Ozer, I.; Dalgic, T.; Surmelioglu, A.; Aydog, G.; Akoglu, M. Sildenafil Accelerates Liver Regeneration after Partial Hepatectomy in Rats. *Transplant. Proc.* **2012**, *44*, 1747–1750. [CrossRef]
50. Gao, L.; Liu, M.-M.; Zang, H.-M.; Ma, Q.-Y.; Yang, Q.; Jiang, L.; Ren, G.-L.; Li, H.-D.; Wu, W.-F.; Wang, J.-N.; et al. Restoration of E-cadherin by PPBICA protects against cisplatin-induced acute kidney injury by attenuating inflammation and programmed cell death. *Lab. Investig.* **2018**, *98*, 911–923. [CrossRef]
51. Hammerman, M.R. Windows of opportunity for organogenesis. *Transpl. Immunol.* **2005**, *15*, 1–8. [CrossRef]
52. Marshall, D.; Dilworth, M.R.; Clancy, M.; Bravery, C.A.; Ashton, N. Increasing renal mass improves survival in anephric rats following metanephros transplantation. *Exp. Physiol.* **2007**, *92*, 263–271. [CrossRef]
53. Andersen, O.S.; Jonasson, O.; Merkel, F.K. En Bloc Transplantation of Pediatric Kidneys Into Adult Patients. *Arch. Surg.* **1974**, *108*, 35–37. [CrossRef]
54. Damji, S.; Callaghan, C.J.; Loukopoulos, I.; Kessaris, N.; Stojanovic, J.; Marks, S.D.; Mamode, N. Utilisation of small paediatric donor kidneys for transplantation. *Pediatr. Nephrol.* **2019**, *34*, 1717–1726. [CrossRef]
55. García-Domínguez, X.; Vera-Donoso, C.D.; García-Valero, L.; Vicente, J.S.; Marco-Jimenez, F. Embryonic Organ Transplantation: The New Era of Xenotransplantation. In *Frontiers in Transplantology*; Abdeldayem, H., El-Kased, A.F., El-Shaarawy, A., Eds.; InTech: London, UK, 2016; pp. 25–46.
56. Marco-Jiménez, F.; García-Domínguez, X.; Jiménez-Trigos, E.; Vera-Donoso, C.D.; Vicente, J.S. Vitrification of kidney precursors as a new source for organ transplantation. *Cryobiology* **2015**, *70*, 278–282. [CrossRef] [PubMed]
57. Garcia-Dominguez, X.; Vicente, J.S.; Vera-Donoso, C.D.; Marco-Jimenez, F. Successful development of vitrified embryonic kidney after laparoscopy transplantation into non-immunosuppressed hosts. *Trends Transplant.* **2017**, *10*, 1–5. [CrossRef]
58. Garcia-Dominguez, X.; Vera-Donoso, C.D.; Jimenez-Trigos, E.; Vicente, J.S.; Marco-Jimenez, F. First steps towards organ banks: Vitrification of renal primordial. *Cryo Lett.* **2016**, *37*, 47–52.

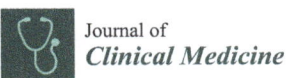

Article

Impact of the Type of Dialysis on Time to Transplantation: Is It Just a Matter of Immunity?

Matteo Righini [1,2], Irene Capelli [1], Marco Busutti [1], Concettina Raimondi [1], Giorgia Comai [1], Gabriele Donati [1], Maria Laura Cappuccilli [3], Matteo Ravaioli [4], Pasquale Chieco [3] and Gaetano La Manna [1,*]

[1] Nephrology, Dialysis and Transplantation Unit, IRCCS—Azienda Ospedaliero Universitaria di Bologna, Alma Mater Studiorum, University of Bologna, 40100 Bologna, Italy; matteo.righini5@unibo.it (M.R.); irene.capelli@gmail.com (I.C.); marco.busutti@live.it (M.B.); concettina.raimondi@aosp.bo.it (C.R.); giorgia.comai@aosp.bo.it (G.C.); gabriele.donati@aosp.bo.it (G.D.)

[2] Nephrology and Dialysis Unit, Santa Maria delle Croci Hospital, 48100 Ravenna, Italy

[3] Department of Experimental, Diagnostic and Specialty Medicine (DIMES), University of Bologna, 40126 Bologna, Italy; maria.cappuccilli@unibo.it (M.L.C.); pasquale.chieco@unibo.it (P.C.)

[4] Department of General Surgery and Transplantation, Policlinico di Sant' Orsola, 40138 Bologna, Italy; matteo.ravaioli@aosp.bo.it

* Correspondence: gaetano.lamanna@unibo.it; Tel.: +39-0512143255; Fax: +39-051340871

Abstract: Background: Renal transplantation represents the therapeutic gold standard in patients with end stage renal disease (ESRD). Still the role of pre-transplant dialysis in affecting time to transplantation has yet to be determined. We wanted to verify whether the type of renal replacement therapy (hemodialysis vs. peritoneal dialysis) affects time to transplantation and to identify clinical features related to the longer time to transplantation. Methods: We performed a retrospective single-center observational study on patients who had received a transplant in the Bologna Transplant Unit from 1991 to 2019, described through the analysis of digital transplant list documents for sex, age, body mass index (BMI), blood group, comorbidities, underlying disease, serology, type of dialysis, time to transplantation, Panel Reactive Antibodies (PRA) max, number of preformed anti Human Leukocyte Antigens (HLA) antibodies. A p-value < 0.05 was considered statistically significant. Results: In the 1619 patients analyzed, we observed a significant difference in time to transplant, PRA max and Preformed Antibodies Number between patients who received Hemodialysis (HD) and Peritoneal dialysis (PD). Then we performed a multiple regression analysis with all the considered factors in order to identify features that support these differences. The clinical variables that independently and directly correlate with longer time to transplantation are PRA max ($p < 0.0001$), Antibodies number ($p < 0.0001$) and HD ($p < 0.0001$); though AB blood group ($p < 0.0001$), age ($p < 0.003$) and PD ($p < 0.0001$) inversely correlate with time to transplantation. Conclusions: In our work, PD population received renal transplants in a shorter period of time compared to HD and turned out to be less immunized. Considering immunization, the type of dialysis impacts both on PRA max and on anti HLA antibodies.

Keywords: peritoneal dialysis; hemodialysis; kidney transplantation; autoimmunity

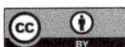

1. Introduction

Hemodialysis (HD) and Peritoneal Dialysis (PD) are the two most common forms of renal replacement therapy, life-saving treatment for patients with End Stage Renal Disease (ESRD). Despite there being contraindications for each treatment, nowadays the choice of the kind of treatment depends on several features, mainly the specific experience of the Clinical Unit and the patient's choice [1]. Although PD is a well-established treatment modality it is underused in Western countries, with a prevalence in Italy of 15% [2,3]. Recently, several studies showed a relative survival advantage for patients receiving PD lasting one to two years after dialysis initiation [4–8]. Renal transplantation represents the therapeutic "gold standard" in patients with ESRD ensuring better outcomes compared with dialysis both in patient survival and quality of life [2,9–11]. The role of pre-transplant dialysis choice in affecting transplant outcomes has been the subject of long-standing interest [12–15]. For those who could not stand the prospect of living donor transplantation, being on the waiting list for kidney transplantation from a deceased donor is a vital choice. According to CNT (National Transplant Centre) data, in our country a patient who signs up for renal transplant waiting list normally waits 3.3 years before getting a transplant [16]. There are several known demographic and clinical factors that affect time to transplantation (age, blood group, and level of antibody sensitization) [14] but many other factors are implied.

We wanted to verify whether the type of renal replacement therapy (HD vs. PD) affects time to transplantation and we wanted to identify clinical features related to longer time to transplantation.

2. Materials and Methods

We performed a retrospective study on patients who have received a transplant in the Bologna Transplant Unit from 1991 to 2019, described through the analysis of digital transplant list documents for sex, age, BMI, blood group, hypertension, diabetes, cardiovascular disease, neoplastic disease, underlying disease, serology (HBV, HCV, HIV, CMV, Toxo, EBV, LUE), type of dialysis, time to transplantation, Panel Reactive Antibodies (PRA max), and number of preformed anti Human Leukocyte Antigens (HLA) antibodies. Immunologic data were collected regarding typing of HLA, PRA max that represent the maximal value of PRA in the considered waiting time to transplant. PRA was expressed as the percentage of lymphocyte panel members against which the patient's serum reacts and thus against which the patient has HLA class I or II antibodies. Since 2012 all the PRA was tested with the complement-dependent cytotoxicity test (PRA-CDC) for monitoring the degree of immunization in kidney transplant candidates on active waiting lists, after that year patients were tested with the use of Labscreen PRA class I and II on a Luminex platform. The number of preformed antibodies expressed the quantity of specific preformed HLA class I or II that the recipient patient presented. Levels of normalized, mean fluorescence intensity >1000 were considered to be positive.

We excluded patients who had received a previous transplant, who were recorded in the national hyperimmune program supposing that those patients were too immunized and they have been on the waiting list a very long time, patients transplanted or signed up in pre-emptive modality, and patients who received a combined transplant (Figure 1).

We used survival curves to analyze time to transplantation with transplantation as an end point.

Data were taken from the digital medical records and was imported to create a database specifically for the study. The study was approved by the Local Ethical Committee.

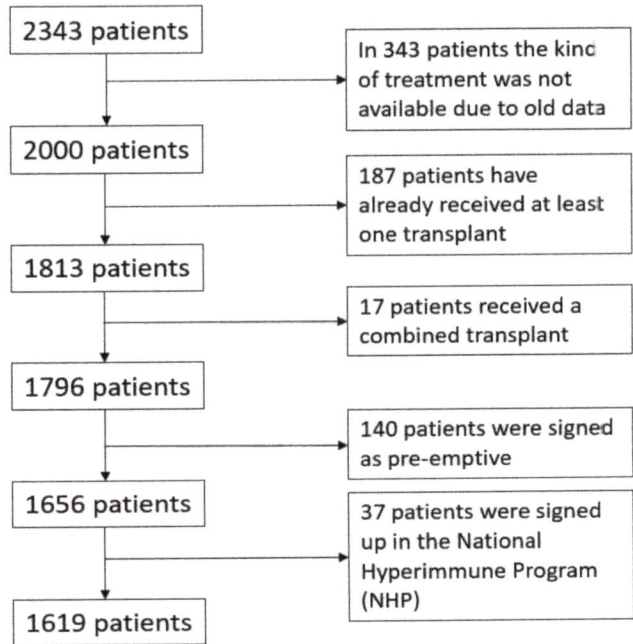

Figure 1. Patients who received a kidney transplant in Bologna Transplant Unit between 1991 and 2019 and exclusion criteria.

3. Statistical Analysis

The aim of statistical analysis in this observational study was to find factors associated with time to transplantation. The proper test of statistical significance depends on the nature of the examined variables. Student's t-test or ANOVA followed by Tukey post-hoc test, corrected for heteroscedasticity, when necessary, were used for real outcome variables. For non-parametric outcomes we used Mann-Whitney test or Kruskal-Wallis ANOVA followed by Dunn's test for pair-wise comparisons. Categorical data were analyzed using contingency tables and χ^2. Linear associations using one or more covariate were explored with linear regression. Survival curves were computed by Kaplan-Meier estimate [17] and compared by a log-rank test. Continuous variables are presented as mean ± Standard Deviation or as median and Interquartile interval (IQR) when appropriated. All statistical tests were two-tailed, and we used JMP 13 (SAS Institute Inc., Cary NC, USA) for data management and analysis. p-values were not corrected for multiplicity and the findings should be interpreted as exploratory. A p-value < 0.05 was considered statistically significant.

4. Results

We considered in our analysis 2343 patients who received a transplant in Bologna from 1991 to 2019. According to exclusion criteria (Figure 1), we analyzed 1619 patients. As is shown in Table 1, our population presented 1053 (65%) men, mean age at transplantation was 61.9 ± 12.4 years, mean years of dialysis before transplantation were 4.4 ± 6.5 years (1618.34 ± 2376.75 days), 554 (34.2%) patients had hypertension, 214 (13.2%) had diabetes, 79 (4.9%) had cardiovascular disease, 18 (1.1%) had a history of neoplastic disease. Mean BMI was 24.1 ± 3.5. There were 1347 patients who received HD and 271 (16.7%) received PD, latency from the beginning of dialysis to the enrolment on the transplant waiting list resulted in 354.5 days (IQR 108.6 days); 901 (55.6%) patients presented with HbsAb; 1037 (64%) patients had positive CMV IgG; 653 (40.3%) patients had Blood Group A;

180 (11.1%) had B; 705 (43.5%) had 0; and only 78 (4.8%) had AB. In our cohort 169 (10.4%) patients had IgA nephropathy; 161 (9.9%) had hypertensive nephropathy; 328 (20.3%) presented with Polycystic Kidney Disease; 153 (9.4%) had Diabetic Nephropathy; 374 (23.1%) patients presented with other nephropathies while 433 (26.7%) patients had an unknown diagnosis. In total, 554 patients presented with hypertension. Mean time to transplantation was 2.4 ± 2.6 years (889.3 ± 945.7 days), PRA max resulted in 21.04 ± 31.5 and number of preformed antibodies resulted in 4.6 ± 12.9.

Table 1. Features of the study population and according to the type of dialysis.

	Population	Hemodialysis	Peritoneal Dialysis	p Value
No. of patients	1619	1347 (83.2%)	271 (16.8%)	
Sex				
• Male	1053 (65%)	898 (66.7%)	155 (57.2%)	0.002 *
• Female	565 (35%)	449 (33.3%)	116 (42.8%)	
Age (years)	61.9 ± 12.4	61.9 ± 12.3	62.2 ± 12.5	ns
Blood group				
• A	651 (40.2%)	533 (39.6%)	118 (43.5%)	
• B	179 (11.1%)	150 (11.1%)	29 (10.7%)	0.007 *
• AB	76 (4.7%)	54 (4%)	22 (8.1%)	
• O	705 (43.5%)	605 (44.9%)	100 (36.9%)	
BMI	24.1 ± 3.5	23.9 ± 3.5	24.7 ± 3.4	0.001 *
Diabetes	214 (13.2%)	182 (13.5%)	32 (11.8%)	ns
Hypertension	554 (34.2%)	452 (33.6%)	102 (37.6%)	ns
Cardiovascular disease	79 (4.9%)	56 (4.2%)	23 (8.5%)	ns
Neoplastic disease	18 (1.1%)	15 (1.1%)	3 (1.1%)	ns
Nephropathy				
• Unknown	433 (26.7%)	366 (27.2%)	67 (24.7%)	
• IgA nephropathy	169 (10.4%)	138 (10.2%)	31 (11.4%)	
• Hypertensive	161 (9.9%)	127 (9.4%)	34 (12.5%)	ns
• ADPKD	328 (20.3%)	284 (21.1%)	44 (16.2%)	
• Diabetic	153 (9.4%)	126 (9.3%)	27 (10%)	
• Other	374 (23.1%)	306 (22.7%)	68 (25.1%)	
Prior time of dialysis until listing for transplantation Med [IQR]	354.5 [108.6] days	383 [118.3] days	225 [271.8] days	ns
HCV IgG	61 (3.8%)	58 (4.3%)	3 (1.1%)	ns
HBsAb	901 (55.6%)	753 (55.9%)	148 (54.6%)	ns
HbcAb	220 (13.6%)	186 (13.8%)	34 (12.5%)	ns
CMV IgG	1037 (64.1%)	839 (62.3%)	198 (73.1%)	ns
PRA max (%)				
• 0	477 (29.5%)	350 (26%)	127 (46.9%)	
• 1–19	472 (29.1%)	395 (29.3%)	77 (28.4%)	
• 20–79	258 (15.9%)	230 (17.1%)	28 (10.3%)	
• >80	157 (9.7%)	145 (10.8%)	12 (4.4%)	

Features of the study population described as Sex, Age at the time of transplantation, BMI, underlying nephropathy, prior time of dialysis until listing for transplantation, serology for HCV, HBV and CMV. Cardiovascular disease was considered as patients who had heart failure or previous myocardial infarction. All the variables were compared through Student's t-test or ANOVA followed by Tukey post-hoc test, corrected for heteroscedasticity. BMI: Body Mass Index. ADPKD: Autosomic Dominant Polycystic Kidney Disease. * A p value was considered significant when p < 0.05.

As previously described, we aimed to analyze whether the type of dialysis could influence time to transplant. Indeed, we observed a significant difference in time to transplant (933 ± 25.6 days in HD and 667.3 ± 57.1 days in PD, $p < 0.001$), PRA max (23.1 ± 0.9 in HD and 11.4 ± 1.9 in PD, $p < 0.001$) and Preformed Antibodies Number (5.1 ± 0.3 in HD and 2 ± 0.7 in PD, $p < 0.001$) between patients who received HD and PD. Then we performed a multiple regression analysis with all the considered factors in order to identify features that support these differences. In Table 2 the clinical variables that independently and directly correlates with longer time to transplantation are listed: PRA max ($p < 0.0001$), Antibodies number ($p < 0.0001$) and HD ($p < 0.0001$). Other features inversely correlate with time to transplantation: AB blood group ($p < 0.0001$), age ($p < 0.003$) and PD ($p < 0.0001$).

Table 2. Multiple regression for Time to transplant.

Source	LogWorth		p Value
PRAmax	17.382		0.00000
Blood group	13.148		0.00000
Type of dialysis	4.808		0.00002
Antibodies Number	4.080		0.00008
Age	1.332		0.04654
CMV IgG	0.611		0.24496
Diagnosis	0.200		0.63037
BMI	0.187		0.65032
Sex	0.037		0.91757
HBsAb	0.023		0.94883

We can observe that the variables that directly correlate with time to transplantation are PRA max, Antibodies Number and HD; factors that inversely correlate are AB blood group, age and PD. These results are confirmed even in the Multivariate analysis. PRA = Panel Reactive Antibodies. HD = Hemodialysis. PD = Peritoneal Dialysis.

Assuming that immunization is a key factor in determining time to transplant, though we analyzed our PRA max data according to the model that Bostock et al. used [18] (Figure 2). Then we performed a multiple regression on PRA max: the only parameters that correlate with PRA max values are the type of dialysis ($p = 0.0015$), AB blood group ($p = 0.0017$) and BMI ($p = 0.0079$) (Table 3). Another way to describe immunization is through antibodies' expression: as shown in Table 4, in performing a multiple regression analysis on antibodies number we evidenced that the only features that correlate with a higher number of pre-formed antibodies were age ($p = 0.0001$) and type of dialysis ($p = 0.0004$).

Table 3. Multiple regression for PRA max.

Source	LogWorth		p Value
Type of dialysis	2.831		0.00148
Blood group	2.759		0.00174
BMI	1.733		0.01848
Age	0.989		0.10251
HBsAb	0.959		0.11001
CMV IgG	0.249		0.56355

Factors that correlate with elevated PRA max are Type of dialysis, AB blood group and, slightly, BMI. These factors are confirmed even in the multivariate analysis.

Considering time to transplantation to be our first goal we represent our results in Figure 3. Then we created subgroups according to Age, BMI, Blood Group, and Diagnosis, exploring whether these differences persisted in all the subgroups. Data are presented in Table 3.

Table 4. Multiple regression for Antibodies Number.

Source	LogWorth		p Value
Age	2.771		0.00169
Type of dialysis	1.985		0.01034
BMI	0.812		0.15432
HBsAb	0.784		0.16447
Blood Group	0.407		0.39161
CMV IgG	0.197		0.63481

Factors that correlate with Antibodies Number are Type of dialysis and Age. These factors are confirmed even in the multivariate analysis.

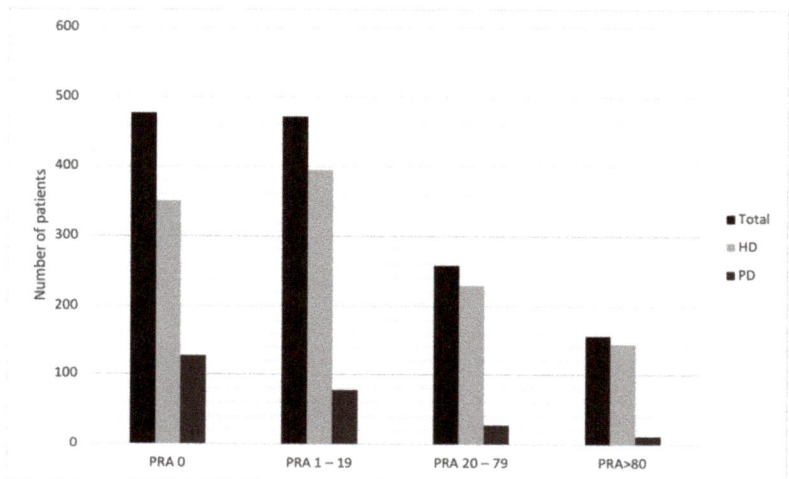

Figure 2. Patients divided according to PRA max. The classes were selected according to the study conducted by Bostock IC et al. [18]. HD: hemodialysis. PD: peritoneal dialysis.

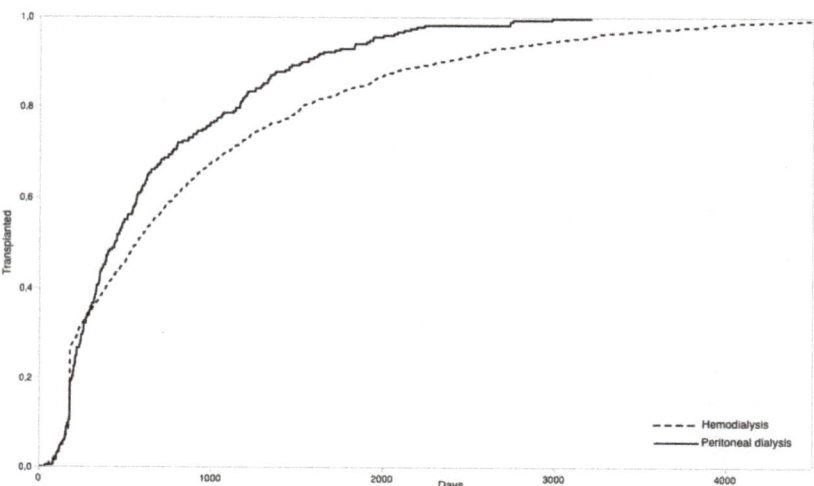

Figure 3. Patients who received kidney transplant divided by type of dialysis. Those who received PD (271 patients) reached the goal (kidney transplant) far earlier than those who received HD (1347 patients) (Log-Rank ChiSquare 21.99, $p < 0.0001$, Wilcoxon ChiSquare 5.77, $p = 0.0163$).

4.1. Age

Considering age, we analyzed the population divided into 5 groups: Group 1 Age $\leq$ 45; Group 2 45 < Age $\leq$ 55; Group 3 55 < Age $\leq$ 65; Group 4 65 < Age $\leq$ 75; Group 5 Age > 75. In the HD population we found significant differences between group 3 (1117 $\pm$ 49.4 days) and 5 (680.4 $\pm$ 72.9 days, $p < 0.0001$), and between group 3 and 4 (854.5 $\pm$ 50.4 days, $p = 0.002$).

In the PD population we pointed out significant differences only between group 2 (815.1 $\pm$ 84.4 days) and 4 (521.1 $\pm$ 60.9 days, $p = 0.04$).

Considering age to be a factor that independently correlates with Antibodies number, we performed the same analysis, showing that in the HD population there existed a significant difference between group 2 (7.2 $\pm$ 0.9) and group 5 (1.9 $\pm$ 1, $p < 0.001$); group 1 (6.8 $\pm$ 1.2) and group 5 ($p < 0.01$); group 3 (5.9 $\pm$ 0.7) and group 5 ($p < 0.01$); and group 2 and group 4 (3.8 $\pm$ 0.7, $p < 0.02$). Conversely, in the PD population we evidenced no differences.

4.2. BMI

Considering BMI, we analyzed the two populations divided into 4 groups: Group 1 BMI $\leq$ 20, Group 2 20 < BMI $\leq$ 25, Group 3 25 < BMI $\leq$ 30, Group 4 BMI > 30. We did not found any significant difference among groups both in HD as in PD.

Since BMI resulted in an independent factor that influenced PRA max, we performed the same analysis showing that in the HD group there existed significant differences between group 1 (26.1 $\pm$ 33.5) and group 2 (20.2 $\pm$ 30.6, $p < 0.048$), and between group 1 and group 3 (19.2 $\pm$ 28.7, $p < 0.02$). In the PD population we highlighted no differences among groups.

4.3. Blood Group

Considering blood group, we analyzed the population according to the 4 groups: A, AB, B, O. In the HD population we evidenced significant differences between 0 (1124.5 $\pm$ 39.7 days) and AB (426 $\pm$ 131.7 days, $p < 0.0001$), B (957.3 $\pm$ 79.5 days) and AB ($p = 0.003$), 0 and A (765.2 $\pm$ 42.3 days, $p < 0.0001$). The difference between A and AB is nearly significant ($p = 0.06$). In the PD group differences occurred between O (840.3 $\pm$ 59 days) and AB (433.9 $\pm$ 122.9 days, $p = 0.01$) and between O and A (590.1 $\pm$ 54 days, $p = 0.01$).

Since blood group represented a category that influence the PRA max, we performed the same group analysis but we did not evidence differences both in HD as in PD.

Between HD and PD there existed in our whole population a significant difference in PRA max for the A group (mean HD PRAmax 20.7 $\pm$ 1.4, mean PD PRAmax 8.9 $\pm$ 2.9, $p = 0.0004$), AB group (mean HD PRAmax 22.2 $\pm$ 4.2, mean PD PRAmax 3 $\pm$ 6, $p = 0.01$) and O group (mean HD PRAmax 25.9 $\pm$ 1.4, mean PD PRAmax 15.1 $\pm$ 3.4, $p = 0.003$).

4.4. Diagnosis

Considering diagnosis, we analyzed the population divided into 6 groups: IgA nephropathy, Hypertensive, ADPKD, Diabetic, Other nephropathies, Unknown origin.

Both in the HD as in the PD population we evidenced no differences among groups.

Considering that ESA could have substantially reduced the use of blood transfusions, we divided our population in two groups, before 2000 (old group) and after 2000 (new group), considering that ESA were introduced in 1990 and in the following years achieved global distribution. We compared the Antibodies numbers of two groups showing that there was no significant difference (HD group $p = 0.068$, PD group $p = 0.290$) but the statistical difference remained if we compared the HD old group vs. PD old group ($p = 0.029$) and the HD new group vs. PD new group ($p = 0.018$).

5. Discussion

Prolonged dialysis exposure casts a long shadow and negatively impacts patient and graft survival even after transplantation [19–21]. Despite similar results in terms of outcome,

PD is far less used as renal replacement therapy compared to HD [2,3]. Decisions regarding dialysis choice should be individualized, considering several important outcomes including patient survival and quality of life. A study conducted by Heaf et al. analyzed the relative survival of PD compared to HD, showing that PD has a relatively better prognosis for younger and non-diabetic patients, and for no subgroup was worse than HD; one possible cause is the better preservation of residual renal function in PD [22,23]. A shorter time to transplant could be one of the drives that lead the patient's choice. Several studies analyzed kidney transplant outcomes according to dialysis modality; most studies revealed that PD was associated with shorter time on dialysis, better graft and patient survival [24–31].

Recent works reported that the transplant list waiting time is reduced in PD compared to those on HD [13,15] and the results in our cohort confirm this data. What causes these differences is yet to be proven: some explanations can be hypothesized.

As reported by several studies, sensitization is a known barrier to transplantation and sensitized patients have substantially longer waiting times; the breadth of sensitization against HLAs is routinely monitored in wait-listed patients with ESRD using panel reactive antibody (PRA) assays [32–35]. Previous transplant, in addition to pregnancies and blood transfusions, is a known cause of immune sensitization against "non-self" human leukocyte antigens (HLAs). Moreover, PRA is an independent predictor of mortality in wait-listed kidney transplant candidates [36]. There is good epidemiologic evidence showing a direct relationship between pretransplant PRA levels and adverse graft outcomes [37–39]. Our study confirms that an elevated PRA is associated with longer time to transplant, but also shows that even patients on PD have a lower mean PRA compared to those on HD ($p < 0.0001$).

Considering anti-HLA antibodies, our study shows that they are related to an increased time to transplantation, as supported by a large cohort study, where the authors suggest that anti-HLA antibodies are associated with an increased sensitization and mortality in waitlisted kidney transplant candidates [36]. In our cohort, PD patients presented less anti-HLA antibodies than HD patients ($p < 0.001$). A reason may lie in the fact that HD patients had a greater tendency to anemia and more likely may require blood transfusions, which can determine an increase in panel reactive antibody percentage [15,40]. Other explanations may be further investigated. Our results suggest that BMI is a factor that influences kidney transplant recipient immunization. Lots of studies have investigated obesity in kidney transplant recipients, recognizing its importance as a risk factor for chronic allograft dysfunction, exposing to a major risk of delayed graft function and considering some cases an exclusion criteria for transplantation [41–43]. Several mechanisms exert negative metabolic effects of raised BMI and adiposity, and recent studies demonstrated that higher BMI was associated with higher inflammation, that correlates with mortality [44–46].

Indeed, in our cohort, PD patients presented a significantly reduced waiting time for kidney transplant even eliminating the impact of immunization: so we have to wonder that other non-immunological factors may have an impact on this result.

Patients who undergo PD tend to be more empowered, to have a strong social support network and to pursue their care plan by themselves [47]. Moreover, our PD group had a lower pretransplant dialysis vintage compared with the HD group (PD 225–271.8 vs. HD 383–118.3, $p = 0.06$), leading to a different exposure to dialysis-related immune dysfunction. Nonetheless, the latency from the beginning of dialysis to the enrolment on the transplant waiting list resulted in differences between the PD group and the HD group, though nearly significant ($p = 0.06$). This could once more be explained by the strong social support network of patients who chose PD.

Age is a considering factor in transplant recipients and up to twenty years ago, lots of patients would have been excluded due to being elderly. The "old to old" allocation system in the Eurotransplant [48,49] community has shown to be effective in increasing the number of transplants; thus, in our population 45 to 65 years old patients were the most represented age groups, therefore they present a longer mean time to transplantation. These results are in line with literature [50].

Regarding the relationship between blood groups and time to transplant, Chang et al. [51] reported that blood group AB have the highest likelihood of deceased donor transplantation, followed by patients with blood groups A, O and B; within blood groups, the likelihood of transplantation was inversely related to the level of sensitization (PRA max). Our study confirms previous work showing longer waiting times for blood group O patients [14,52] and that AB recipients were more likely to receive deceased donor kidneys [53]. Thus, AB patients represent a small population, though not sufficient to draw conclusions on time to transplant.

Our study presents some limitations: in addition to the retrospective nature of the analysis due to the long-considered time and to patients' dialysis center variability, the precise number of blood transfusions was not available. Since the study covers 30 years of experience, variability in dialysis practice (HD vs. PD) between different referral centers made the population less homogeneous.

6. Conclusions

In our work, the PD population received renal transplant in a shorter period of time compared to the HD, turned out to be less immunized, considering immunization to be the number of antibodies and PRA. Time to transplant is mostly a matter of immunity but other factors can influence it, such as age, blood group and type of dialysis. Considering immunization, the type of dialysis impacted both on PRA max (together with BMI and blood group) as on anti HLA antibodies (together with age). Our study supports the choice of PD for patients who can afford it, particularly for those who would like to receive a kidney transplant.

Author Contributions: M.R. (Matteo Righini), I.C. and C.R. designed the work, M.R. (Matteo Righini); I.C. and M.B. researched literature and conceived the study. G.D., G.C. and M.R. (Matteo Ravaioli) were involved in patients' recruitment and data interpretation; M.L.C. revised the English language and performed statistical analysis; P.C. performed the statistical analysis; M.R. (Matteo Righini), I.C., M.B. and P.C. wrote the first draft of the manuscript; G.L.M. revised the work critically and revised data interpretation. All authors have read and agreed to the published version of the manuscript.

Funding: This research received no specific grant from any funding agency in the public, commercial, or not-for-profit sectors.

Institutional Review Board Statement: The study was conducted in accordance with the principles of the Declaration of Helsinki and was approved by the local Ethical Committee.

Informed Consent Statement: All the patients signed an informed consent when they entered on the transplant list. The informed consent, according to the national and regional transplantation protocol, let the data be used for research.

Data Availability Statement: Data can be found on the Donor Manager transplant program.

Conflicts of Interest: The authors declare no conflict of interest.

References

1. Desai, A.A.; Bolus, R.; Nissenson, A.; Bolus, S.; Solomon, M.D.; Khawar, O.; Gitlin, M.; Talley, J.; Spiegel, B.M. Identifying best practices in dialysis care: Results of cognitive interviews and a national survey of dialysis providers. *Clin. J. Am. Soc. Nephrol. CJASN* **2008**, *3*, 1066–1076. [CrossRef]
2. Khawar, O.; Kalantar-Zadeh, K.; Lo, W.K.; Johnson, D.; Mehrotra, R. Is the declining use of long-term peritoneal dialysis justified by outcome data? *Clin. J. Am. Soc. Nephrol. CJASN* **2007**, *2*, 1317–1328. [CrossRef] [PubMed]
3. Zaza, G.; Rugiu, C.; Trubian, A.; Granata, S.; Poli, A.; Lupo, A. How has peritoneal dialysis changed over the last 2015, 30 years: Experience of the Verona dialysis center. *BMC Nephrol.* **2015**, *16*, 53. [CrossRef] [PubMed]
4. Weinhandl, E.D.; Foley, R.N.; Gilbertson, D.T.; Arneson, T.J.; Snyder, J.J.; Collins, A.J. Propensity-matched mortality comparison of incident hemodialysis and peritoneal dialysis patients. *J. Am. Soc. Nephrol.* **2010**, *21*, 499–506. [CrossRef] [PubMed]
5. Quinn, R.R.; Hux, J.E.; Oliver, M.J.; Austin, P.C.; Tonelli, M.; Laupacis, A. Selection bias explains apparent differential mortality between dialysis modalities. *J. Am. Soc. Nephrol.* **2011**, *22*, 1534–1542. [CrossRef]
6. Yeates, K.; Zhu, N.; Vonesh, E.; Trpeski, L.; Blake, P.; Fenton, S. Hemodialysis and peritoneal dialysis are associated with similar outcomes for end-stage renal disease treatment in Canada. *Nephrol. Dial. Transplant.* **2012**, *27*, 3568–3575. [CrossRef] [PubMed]

7. Vonesh, E.F.; Snyder, J.J.; Foley, R.N.; Collins, A.J. The differential impact of risk factors on mortality in hemodialysis and peritoneal dialysis. *Kidney Int.* **2004**, *66*, 2389–2401. [CrossRef]
8. Termorshuizen, F.; Korevaar, J.C.; Dekker, F.W.; Van Manen, J.G.; Boeschoten, E.W.; Krediet, R.T. Hemodialysis and peritoneal dialysis: Comparison of adjusted mortality rates according to the duration of dialysis: Analysis of The Netherlands Cooperative Study on the Adequacy of Dialysis 2. *J. Am. Soc. Nephrol.* **2003**, *14*, 2851–2860. [CrossRef] [PubMed]
9. Wolfe, R.A.; Ashby, V.B.; Milford, E.L.; Ojo, A.O.; Ettenger, R.E.; Agodoa, L.Y.; Held, P.J.; Port, F.K. Comparison of mortality in all patients on dialysis, patients on dialysis awaiting transplantation, and recipients of a first cadaveric transplant. *N. Engl. J. Med.* **1999**, *341*, 1725–1730. [CrossRef] [PubMed]
10. Port, F.K.; Wolfe, R.A.; Mauger, E.A.; Berling, D.P.; Jiang, K. Comparison of survival probabilities for dialysis patients vs. cadaveric renal transplant recipients. *JAMA* **1993**, *270*, 1339. [CrossRef]
11. Gaston, R.S.; Danovitch, G.M.; Adams, P.L.; Wynn, J.J.; Merion, R.M.; Deierhoi, M.H.; Metzger, R.A.; Cecka, J.M.; Harmon, W.E.; Leichtman, A.B.; et al. The report of a national conference on the wait list for kidney transplantation. *Am. J. Transplant.* **2003**, *3*, 775. [CrossRef]
12. Held, P.J.; Turenne, M.N.; Liska, D.W.; Zobel, D.L.; Webb, R.L.; Alexander, S.R.; Jones, C. Treatment modality patterns and transplantation among the United States pediatric end-stage renal disease population: A longitudinal study. *Clin. Transplant.* **1991**, 71–85. [PubMed]
13. Snyder, J.J.; Kasiske, B.L.; Gilbertson, D.T.; Collins, A.J. A comparison of transplant outcomes in peritoneal and hemodialysis patients. *Kidney Int.* **2002**, *62*, 1423–1430. [CrossRef] [PubMed]
14. Sanfilippo, F.P.; Vaughn, W.K.; Peters, T.G.; Shield, C.F.; Adams, P.L.; Lorber, M.I.; Williams, G.M. Factors affecting the waiting time of cadaveric kidney transplant candidates in the USA. *JAMA* **1992**, *267*, 247. [CrossRef] [PubMed]
15. Rigoni, M.; Torri, E.; Nollo, G.; Zarantonello, D.; Laudon, A.; Sottini, L.; Guarrera, G.M.; Brunori, G. Survival and time-to-transplantation of peritoneal dialysis versus hemodialysis for ESRD patients: Competing-risks regression model in a single Italian center experience. *J. Nephrol.* **2017**, *30*, 441–447. [CrossRef]
16. Report CNT. 2019. Available online: http://www.trapianti.salute.gov.it/ (accessed on 11 November 2021).
17. Kaplan, E.L.; Meier, P. Nonparametric estimation for incomplete observations. *J. Am. Statist. Assoc.* **1958**, *53*, 457–481. [CrossRef]
18. Bostock, I.C.; Alberu, J.; Arvizu, A.; Hernández-Mendez, E.A.; De-Santiago, A.; Gonzalez-Tableros, N.; López, M.; Castelán, N.; Contreras, A.G.; Morales-Buenrostro, L.E.; et al. Probability of deceased donor kidney transplantation based on % PRA. *Transpl. Immunol.* **2013**, *28*, 154–158. [CrossRef]
19. Abecassis, M.; Bartlett, S.T.; Collins, A.J.; Davis, C.L.; Delmonico, F.L.; Friedewald, J.J.; Hays, R.; Howard, A.; Jones, E.; Leichtman, A.B.; et al. Kidney transplantation as primary therapy for end-stage renal disease: A National Kidney Foundation/Kidney Disease Outcomes Quality Initiative (NKF/KDOQITM) conference. *Clin. J. Am. Soc. Nephrol.* **2008**, *3*, 471–480. [CrossRef]
20. Knoll, G.; Cockfield, S.; Blydt-Hansen, T.; Baran, D.; Kiberd, B.; Landsberg, D.; Rush, D.; Cole, E. Canadian Society of transplantation consensus guidelines on eligibility for kidney transplantation. *CMAJ* **2005**, *173*, S1–S25. [CrossRef]
21. Huang, Y.; Samaniego, M. Preemptive kidney transplantation: Has it come of age? *Nephrol. Ther.* **2012**, *8*, 428–432. [CrossRef]
22. Moist, L.M.; Port, F.K.; Orzol, S.M.; Young, E.W.; Ostbye, T.; Wolfe, R.A.; Hulbert-Shearon, T.; Jones, C.A.; Bloembergen, W.E. Predictors of loss of residual renal function among new dialysis patients. *J. Am. Soc. Nephrol.* **2000**, *11*, 556–564. [CrossRef] [PubMed]
23. Heaf, J.G.; Wehberg, S. Relative survival of peritoneal Dialysis and Hemodialysis Patients: Effect of Cohort and Mode of Dialysis Initiation. *PLoS ONE* **2014**, *9*, e90119. [CrossRef] [PubMed]
24. Martins, L.S.; Malheiro, J.; Pedroso, S.; Almeida, M.; Dias, L.; Henriques, A.C.; Silva, D.; Davide, J.; Cabrita, A.; Noronha, I.L.; et al. Pancreas-kidney transplantation: Impact of dialysis modality on the outcome. *Transpl. Int.* **2015**, *28*, 972–979. [CrossRef] [PubMed]
25. López-Oliva, M.O.; Rivas, B.; Pérez-Fernández, E.; Ossorio, M.; Ros, S.; Chica, C.; Aguilar, A.; Bajo, M.A.; Escuin, F.; Hidalgo, L.; et al. Pretransplant peritoneal dialysis relative to hemodialysis improves long-term survival of kidney transplant patients: A single-center observational study. *Int. Urol. Nephrol.* **2014**, *46*, 825–832. [CrossRef]
26. Tang, M.; Li, T.; Liu, H. A comparison of transplant outcomes in peritoneal and hemodialysis patients: A meta-analysis. *Blood Purif.* **2016**, *42*, 170–176. [CrossRef]
27. Dipalma, T.; Fernández-Ruiz, M.; Praga, M.; Polanco, N.; González, E.; Gutiérrez-Solis, E.; Gutiérrez, E.; Andrés, A. Pre-transplant dialysis modality does not influence short- or long-term outcome in kidney transplant recipients: Analysis of paired kidneys from the same deceased donor. *Clin. Transplant.* **2016**, *30*, 1097–1107. [CrossRef]
28. Kramer, A.; Jager, K.J.; Fogarty, D.G.; Ravani, P.; Finne, P.; Pérez-Panadés, J.; Prütz, K.G.; Arias, M.; Heaf, J.G.; Wanner, C.; et al. Association between pre-transplant dialysis modality and patient and graft survival after kidney transplantation. *Nephrol. Dial. Transplant.* **2012**, *27*, 4473–4480. [CrossRef]
29. Molnar, M.Z.; Mehrotra, R.; Duong, U.; Bunnapradist, S.; Lukowsky, L.R.; Krishnan, M.; Kovesdy, C.P.; Kalantar-Zadeh, K. Dialysis modality and outcomes in kidney transplant recipients. *Clin. J. Am. Soc. Nephrol.* **2012**, *7*, 332–341. [CrossRef] [PubMed]
30. Goldfarb-Rumyantzev, A.S.; Hurdle, J.F.; Scandling, J.D.; Baird, B.C.; Cheung, A.K. The role of pretransplantation renal replacement therapy modality in kidney allograft and recipient survival. *Am. J. Kidney Dis.* **2005**, *46*, 537–549. [CrossRef] [PubMed]

31. Schwenger, V.; Döhler, B.; Morath, C.; Zeier, M.; Opelz, G. The role of pretransplant dialysis modality on renal allograft outcome. *Nephrol. Dial. Transplant.* **2011**, *26*, 3761–3766. [CrossRef]
32. Katznelson, S.; Bhaduri, S.; Cecka, J.M. Clinical aspects of sensitization. *Clin. Transpl.* **1997**, 285–296. [PubMed]
33. Barama, A.; Oza, U.; Panek, R.; Belitsky, P.; MacDonald, A.S.; Lawen, J.; McAlister, V.; Kiberd, B. Effect of recipient sensitization (peak PRA) on graft outcome in haploidentical living related kidney transplants. *Clin. Transplant.* **2000**, *14*, 212–217. [CrossRef]
34. Gebel, H.M.; Bray, R.A.; Nickerson, P. Pre-transplant assessment of donor-reactive, HLA-specific antibodies in renal transplantation: Contraindication vs. risk. *Am. J. Transpl.* **2003**, *3*, 1488–1500. [CrossRef]
35. Tambur, A.R.; Leventhal, J.R.; Walsh, R.C.; Zitzner, J.R.; Friedewald, J.J. HLA- DQ barrier: Effects on cPRA calculations. *Transplantation* **2013**, *96*, 1065–1072. [CrossRef] [PubMed]
36. Sapir-Pichhadze, R.; Tinckam, K.J.; Laupacis, A.; Logan, A.G.; Beyene, J.; Kim, S.J. Immune sensitization and mortality in Wait-Listed Kidney Transplant Candidates. *J. Am. Soc. Nephrol.* **2016**, *27*, 570–578. [CrossRef]
37. Registry, A. ANZDATA Report 2011 Chapter 8 Transplantation. 2012. Available online: https://www.anzdata.org.au/report/anzdata-35th-annual-report-2012/ (accessed on 11 November 2021).
38. Faravardeh, A.; Eickhoff, M.; Jackson, S.; Spong, R.; Kukla, A.; Issa, N.; Matas, A.J.; Ibrahim, H.N. Predictors of graft failure and death in elderly kidney transplant recipients. *Transplantation* **2013**, *96*, 1089. [CrossRef] [PubMed]
39. Lim, W.H.; Chapman, J.R.; Wong, G. Peak panel reactive antibody, cancer, graft, and patient outcomes in kidney transplant recipients. *Transplantation* **2015**, *99*, 1043–1050. [CrossRef]
40. Wetmore, J.B.; Peng, Y.; Monda, K.L.; Kats, A.M.; Kim, D.H.; Bradbury, B.D.; Collins, A.J.; Gilbertson, D.T. Trends in anemia management practices in patients receiving hemodialysis and peritoneal dialysis: A retro- spective cohort analysis. *Am. J. Nephrol.* **2015**, *41*, 354–361. [CrossRef]
41. Hoogeveen, E.K.; Aalten, J.; Rothman, K.J.; Roodnat, J.I.; Mallat, M.J.; Borm, G.; Weimar, W.; Hoitsma, A.J.; de Fijter, J.W. Effect of Obesity on the Outcome of Kidney Transplantation: A 20-Year Follow-Up. *Transplantation* **2011**, *91*, 869–874. [CrossRef]
42. Streja, E.; Molnar, M.Z.; Kovesdy, C.P.; Bunnapradist, S.; Jing, J.; Nissenson, A.R.; Mucsi, I.; Danovitch, G.M.; Kalantar-Zadeh, K. Associations of Pretransplant Weight and Muscle Mass with Mortality in Renal Transplant Recipients. *Clin. J. Am. Soc. Nephrol.* **2011**, *6*, 1463–1473. [CrossRef]
43. Chan, W.L.W.; Bosch, J.A.; Jones, D.; McTernan, P.; Philips, A.; Borrows, R. Obesity in kidney transplantation. *J. Ren. Nutr.* **2014**, *24*, 1–12. [CrossRef] [PubMed]
44. Abedini, S.; Holme, I.; März, W.; Weihrauch, G.; Fellström, B.; Jardine, A.; Cole, E.; Maes, B.; Neumayer, H.H.; Grønhagen-Riska, C.; et al. Inflammation in Renal Transplantation. *Clin. J. Am. Soc. Nephrol.* **2009**, *4*, 1246–1254. [CrossRef] [PubMed]
45. Kaisar, M.O.; Armstrong, K.; Hawley, C.; Campbell, S.; Mudge, D.; Johnson, D.W.; Prins, J.B.; Isbel, N.M. Adiponectin is associated with cardiovascular disease in male renal transplant recipients: Baseline results from the LANDMARK 2 study. *BMC Nephrol.* **2009**, *10*, 29. [CrossRef] [PubMed]
46. Winkelmayer, W.C.; Schaeffner, E.S.; Chandraker, A.; Kramar, R.; Rumpold, H.; Sunder-Plassmann, G.; Födinger, M. A J-shaped association between high- sensitivity C-reactive protein and mortality in kidney transplant recipients. *Transplant. Int.* **2007**, *20*, 505–511. [CrossRef]
47. Chanouzas, D.; Ng, K.P.; Fallouh, B.; Baharani, J. What influ- ences patient choice of treatment modality at the pre-dialysis stage? *Nephrol. Dial. Transpl.* **2012**, *27*, 1542–1547. [CrossRef]
48. Frei, U.; Noeldeke, J.; Machold-Fabrizii, V.A.; Arbogast, H.; Margreiter, R.; Fricke, L.; Voiculescu, A.; Kliem, V.; Ebel, H.; Albert, U.; et al. Prospective age- matching in elderly kidney transplant recipients—A 5-year analysis of Eurotransplant Senior Program. *Am. J. Transplant.* **2008**, *8*, 50–57. [CrossRef] [PubMed]
49. Neri, F.; Furian, L.; Cavallin, F.; Ravaioli, M.; Silvestre, C.; Donato, P.; La Manna, G.; Pinna, A.D.; Rigotti, P. How does age affect the outcome of kidney transplantation in elderly recipients? *Clin. Transplant.* **2017**, *31*, e13036. [CrossRef]
50. United States Renal Data System. *2020 USRDS Annual Data Report: Epidemiology of Kidney Disease in the United States*; National Institutes of Health, National Institute of Diabetes and Digestive and Kidney Diseases: Bethesda, MD, USA, 2020.
51. Chang, P.; Gill, J.; Dong, J.; Rose, C.; Yan, H.; Landsberg, D.; Cole, E.H.; Gill, J.S. Living donor age and kidney allograft half-life: Implications for living donor paired exchange programs. *Clin. J. Am. Soc. Nephrol.* **2012**, *7*, 835–841. [CrossRef] [PubMed]
52. Phelan, P.J.; O'Kelly, P.; O'Neill, D.; Little, D.; Hickey, D.; Keogan, M.; Walshe, J.; Magee, C.; Conlon, P.J. Analysis of waiting times on Irish renal Transplant list. *Clin. Transpl.* **2010**, *24*, 381–385. [CrossRef]
53. Ng, M.S.Y.; Ullah, S.; Wilson, G.; McDonald, S.; Sypek, M.; Mallett, A.J. ABO blood group relationships to kidney transplant recipient and graft outcomes. *PLoS ONE* **2020**, *15*, e0236396. [CrossRef] [PubMed]

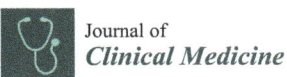

Article

Everolimus Reduces Cancer Incidence and Improves Patient and Graft Survival Rates after Kidney Transplantation: A Multi-Center Study

Ryoichi Imamura [1,*], Ryo Tanaka [1], Ayumu Taniguchi [1], Shigeaki Nakazawa [1], Taigo Kato [1], Kazuaki Yamanaka [1], Tomoko Namba-Hamano [2], Yoichi Kakuta [3], Toyofumi Abe [1], Koichi Tsutahara [3], Tetsuya Takao [3], Hidefumi Kishikawa [4] and Norio Nonomura [1]

1. Department of Urology, Graduate School of Medicine, Osaka University, Osaka 565-0871, Japan; ryotnk0302@gmail.com (R.T.); taniguchi@uro.med.osaka-u.ac.jp (A.T.); nakazawa@uro.med.osaka-u.ac.jp (S.N.); kato@uro.med.osaka-u.ac.jp (T.K.); yamanaka@uro.med.osaka-u.ac.jp (K.Y.); abe@uro.med.osaka-u.ac.jp (T.A.); nono@uro.med.osaka-u.ac.jp (N.N.)
2. Department of Nephrology, Graduate School of Medicine, Osaka University, Osaka 565-0871, Japan; namba@kid.med.osaka-u.ac.jp
3. Osaka General Medical Center, Department of Urology, Osaka 558-8558, Japan; ykakuta17@gmail.com (Y.K.); k.tsuta@gmail.com (K.T.); tetsuyatakao@gmail.com (T.T.)
4. Department of Urology, Hyogo Prefectural Nishinomiya Hospital, Nishinomiya 662-0918, Japan; hidefumi69@hotmail.com
* Correspondence: imamura@uro.med.osaka-u.ac.jp; Tel.: +81-6-6879-3531

Abstract: Kidney transplantation can prevent renal failure and associated complications in patients with end-stage renal disease. Despite the good quality of life, de novo cancers after kidney transplantation are a major complication impacting survival and there is an urgent need to establish immunosuppressive protocols to prevent de novo cancers. We conducted a multi-center retrospective study of 2002 patients who underwent kidney transplantation between 1965 and 2020 to examine patient and graft survival rates and cumulative cancer incidence in the following groups categorized based on specific induction immunosuppressive therapies: group 1, antiproliferative agents and steroids; group 2, calcineurin inhibitors (CNIs), antiproliferative agents and steroids; group 3, CNIs, mycophenolate mofetil, and steroids; and group 4, mammalian target of rapamycin inhibitors including everolimus, CNIs, mycophenolate mofetil, and steroids. The patient and graft survival rates were significantly higher in groups 3 and 4. The cumulative cancer incidence rate significantly increased with the use of more potent immunosuppressants, and the time to develop cancer was shorter. Only one patient in group 4 developed de novo cancer. Potent immunosuppressants might improve graft survival rate while inducing de novo cancer after kidney transplantation. Our data also suggest that everolimus might suppress cancer development after kidney transplantation.

Keywords: cumulative incidence; everolimus; de novo cancer; kidney transplantation; mammalian target of rapamycin; survival

1. Introduction

In patients with end-stage renal disease, kidney transplantation is a promising treatment to prevent renal failure and associated complications [1]. The introduction of new immunosuppressants has led to improved short-term patient and graft survival rates, with most recipients achieving a better quality of life after kidney transplantation [2]. However, long-term patient and graft survival rates remain insufficient [3]. Improvement of patient and graft survival rates requires the resolution of not only immunological but also non-immunological complications. Specifically, de novo cancer formation after kidney transplantation is a major complication associated with patients as well as graft survival.

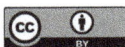

The incidence of de novo cancers is 3–10-fold higher in patients with organ transplants than in the general population [4]. One approach to reducing cancer risk is early detection by cancer screening [5] which, in addition to treatment, is important to protect both the patient and the kidney graft. We previously demonstrated that the overall survival rate was significantly lower in kidney transplant recipients not undergoing routine cancer screening compared to those undergoing cancer screening, highlighting the additional need for immunosuppressive protocols for cancer prevention [5]. In addition, there is an urgent need to establish immunosuppressive protocols to inhibit carcinogenesis.

The phosphatidylinositol 3-kinase (PI3K)/Akt/mammalian target of rapamycin (mTOR) signaling pathway is a major critical node for a wide range of normal cellular functions. Moreover, activation of the PI3K/Akt/mTOR pathway contributes to carcinogenesis [6] and plays a major role in regulating the growth of angiogenic tumors [7,8]. Conversely, phosphatase and tensin homolog negatively regulates the PI3K/Akt/mTOR pathway [9] and acts as a tumor suppressor. The mTOR inhibitors (mTORis), such as rapamycin, have been gaining increasing attention because of their anticancer effects, with recent studies showing their therapeutic role in angiogenic tumors such as renal cell carcinoma [8,10] and endocrine cancers [11]. Several clinical trials have demonstrated the anticancer effects of rapamycin and its analogs, including temsirolimus and everolimus [12].

The mTORis are also used as immunosuppressive agents to prevent allograft rejection in transplant patients [13,14]. Immunosuppressive induction therapy consisting of calcineurin inhibitors (CNIs), mycophenolate mofetil (MMF), and corticosteroids, is associated with improved patient and graft survival rates compared with previous treatment approaches. However, the subsequent increase in cancer prevalence has led to the consideration of adding mTORis to conventional triplet immunosuppression therapy to prevent cancer development while maintaining good immunosuppression [15].

In the present study, we aimed to investigate cancer trends and cancer-specific and all-cause mortality rates in kidney transplant recipients receiving different induction immunosuppression protocols. In addition, we examined the efficacy of the mTORi, everolimus, in cancer prevention.

2. Materials and Methods
2.1. Patient Characteristics

In this multi-center retrospective study, we reviewed the medical records of 2002 patients who underwent kidney transplantation in Osaka University Hospital ($n = 933$), Hyogo Prefectural Nishinomiya Hospital ($n = 654$), and Osaka General Medical Center ($n = 415$) between 1 June 1965 and 30 June 2020. All data were collected and analyzed on 30 September 2020 using the REDCap® electronic registration software (Vanderbilt University, Nashville, TN, USA). We performed cancer screening including computed tomography and abdominal ultrasonography for all recipients once a year and registered the results to the software.

The patients were categorized into the following groups based on the type of induction immunosuppressive therapy: group 1, patients who received antiproliferative agents (azathioprine or mizoribine) and prednisolone; group 2, patients who received CNIs (cyclosporine A or tacrolimus), antiproliferative agents (azathioprine or mizoribine), and prednisolone; group 3, patients who received CNIs, mycophenolate mofetil (MMF), and prednisolone; and group 4, patients who received CNIs, MMF, mTORi, and prednisolone. This group targeted patients who started taking mTORis immediately after the kidney transplantation and continued for more than a year. But in some patients, mTORis were added at least three months after the kidney transplantation. Moreover, 21 patients who received CNIs, mTORis, and prednisolone for induction immunosuppressive therapy were included in group 4. The target trough levels of CNIs at one year after kidney transplantation were 80–100 ng/mL (cyclosporine A, group 2 and 3) and 4–6 ng/mL (tacrolimus, group 2–4).

The collected data included relevant information such as transplant and cancer history; dialysis duration before kidney transplantation; renal allograft conditions including rejection; and history of transplantation, transfusion, and comorbidities for the analyses of demographic characteristics. In addition, data were collected to determine the rates of patient survival, graft survival, cumulative cancer incidence, and cancer types.

Antilymphocyte globulin and the anti-CD25 antibody basiliximab were added to induction immunosuppressive therapy in patients undergoing kidney transplantation from 1993 to 2003 and from 2004 to 2019, respectively. Splenectomy or rituximab infusion was performed in patients undergoing ABO-incompatible kidney transplantation. Additionally, kidney biopsies were routinely performed at 3 and 12 months after kidney transplantation in patients with elevated serum creatinine levels. In patients with biopsy-proven rejection, methylprednisolone was administered for three days. The same approach was used in patients who could not be evaluated by kidney biopsy but were clinically diagnosed with rejection (e.g., >20% elevation of serum creatinine level). In patients with steroid-resistant rejection, gusperimus hydrochloride or anti-CD3 monoclonal antibody was used after methylprednisolone treatment until 2010. Starting in 2011, thymoglobulin was used as an alternative therapy for T cell-mediated rejection. For antibody-mediated rejection, plasma exchange, rituximab infusion, and intravenous immunoglobulin therapy were used.

The primary study outcome was all-cause mortality, and the secondary study outcomes were cancer-specific mortality, death-censored allograft survival rate, and cumulative cancer incidence rate. The study protocol was approved by the Institutional Review Board of Osaka University Hospital (approval no, 19475), Hyogo Prefectural Nishinomiya Hospital (approval no, H28-19), and Osaka General Medical Center (approval no, 28-2034). All procedures were performed in accordance with the 1975 Helsinki Declaration.

2.2. Statistical Analysis

The SPSS statistical software version 27 (IBM, Armonk, NY, USA) was used for all analyses. Categorical variables were presented as percentages or frequencies, and continuous variables were presented as means with standard deviation. Differences in group characteristics, graft survival, and overall survival among groups were compared. Univariate analyses were performed using the Mann–Whitney, Kruskal–Wallis, chi-square, and Fisher's exact tests to compare continuous and categorical variables, as appropriate. The Kaplan–Meier method with the log-rank test was used to compare patient and graft survival rates. The statistical significance level was defined as a two-tailed p-value of <0.05.

3. Results

3.1. Cohort Characteristics

Of a total of 2002 recipients, 15 patients who received induction immunosuppressive monotherapy with steroids were excluded from the study. Therefore, 1987 patients were included in the final analysis (Figure 1). The summary of patient characteristics is presented in Table 1. The median follow-up durations were 21.6 ± 15.0, 18.8 ± 10.0, 10.7 ± 5.8, and 4.9 ± 2.2 years in groups 1, 2, 3, and 4, respectively. Although 24 recipients started mTORis as prescribed, they could not take it for more than a year and were included in group 3. The reasons for discontinuing oral administration were stomatitis (58.3%), followed by proteinuria, leg edema, and diarrhea. The number of elderly patients was particularly high in groups 3 and 4 ($p < 0.001$, between each group). Moreover, the number of transplantations from ABO-incompatible ($p < 0.001$, between each group) or unrelated donors (primarily spouses, $p < 0.001$, between each group) and the number of preemptive kidney transplantations ($p < 0.001$, between group 1, 2, and 3, and 1, 2, and 4, respectively) were statistically significantly higher in recent years.

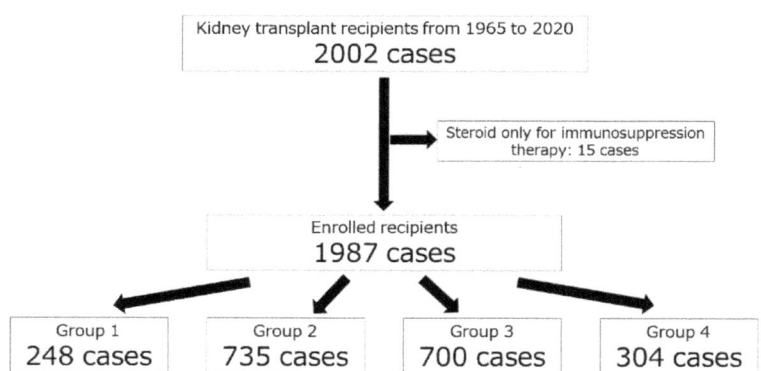

Figure 1. A diagram describing the study population.

Table 1. Demographic characteristics of transplant recipients.

		Group 1	Group 2	Group 3	Group 4	p-Value
The Number of Patients		248	735	700	304	
Follow-up duration (yr)		21.6 (15.0)	18.8 (10.0)	10.7 (5.8)	4.9 (2.2)	<0.001
Recipient age (yr)	<30	141 (63.2)	248 (36.1)	108 (16.3)	25 (9.5)	<0.001
	30–45	100 (34.2)	367 (47.6)	265 (33.8)	89 (30.4)	
	46–60	7 (2.6)	113 (15.5)	234 (35.7)	128 (36.7)	
	>61	0 (0.0)	7 (0.8)	93 (14.2)	62 (23.4)	
Recipient sex	Female	89 (35.9)	294 (40.0)	268 (38.3)	113 (37.2)	0.648
	Male	159 (64.1)	441 (60.0)	432 (61.7)	191 (62.8)	
Donor type	living	214 (86.3)	539 (73.3)	615 (87.9)	273 (89.8)	<0.001
	deceased	34 (13.7)	196 (26.7)	85 (12.1)	31 (10.2)	
Blood relation	Yes	214 (86.3)	530 (72.1)	432 (61.7)	146 (48.0)	<0.001
ABO blood-type	compatible	248 (100.0)	715 (97.3)	548 (78.3)	201 (66.1)	<0.001
	incompatible	0 (0.0)	20 (2.7)	152 (21.7)	103 (33.9)	
Number of HLA mismatches	A, B, DR	0.64 (1.01)	1.39 (1.06)	1.80 (1.26)	1.79 (1.29)	<0.001
Body mass index (kg/m^2)		21.5 (1.47)	21.3 (1.55)	21.3 (2.57)	21.4 (3.33)	0.417
Dialysis duration (yr)	0	7 (3.1)	17 (2.6)	109 (18.6)	89 (26.6)	<0.001
	<1, ≤1	91 (36.8)	202 (27.0)	153 (21.7)	59 (20.3)	
	1–3, ≤3	92 (25.0)	215 (17.1)	147 (12.3)	61 (16.5)	
	3–5, ≤5	38 (27.6)	111 (28.0)	69 (16.3)	23 (17.7)	
	5–10, ≤10	19 (7.0)	130 (17.3)	86 (12.3)	31 (7.0)	
	10–20, ≤20	1 (0.4)	51 (6.8)	94 (13.1)	29 (8.2)	
	>20	0 (0.0)	9 (1.1)	42 (5.7)	12 (3.8)	
Calcineurin inhibitors	Cyclosporine	0 (0.0)	552 (75.1)	212 (30.3)	17 (5.6)	<0.001
	Tacrolimus	0 (0.0)	183 (24.9)	488 (69.7)	287 (94.4)	
	none	248 (100.0)	0 (0.0)	0 (0.0)	0 (0.0)	
Antiproliferative agents	Azathioprine	248 (100.0)	361 (49.1)	0 (0.0)	1 (0.3)	<0.001
	Mizoribine	0 (0.0)	321 (43.7)	0 (0.0)	3 (1.0)	
	Mycophenolate mofetil	0 (0.0)	0 (0.0)	700 (100.0)	300 (98.7)	
	none	0 (0.0)	53 (7.2)	0 (0.0)	0 (0.0)	
mTOR inhibitor (everolimus)	induction therapy	0 (0.0)	0 (0.0)	0 (0.0)	155 (51.0)	<0.001
	add-on within 3 months	0 (0.0)	0 (0.0)	0 (0.0)	149 (49.0)	
History of rejection	Yes	145 (58.5)	519 (70.6)	165 (23.6)	31 (10.2)	<0.001
History of transplantation	Yes	6 (2.4)	17 (2.3)	42 (6.0)	21 (7.6)	<0.001
History of transfusion	Yes	87 (35.1)	116 (15.8)	148 (21.1)	70 (23.0)	<0.001

Categorical variables are presented as frequencies and/or percentages, and continuous variables are presented as means with standard deviation.

In the overall cohort, 242 patients were diagnosed with de novo cancers, including 30 patients who developed two primary cancers and three patients who developed three primary cancers after transplantation (Table 2). The mean intervals between kidney transplantation and cancer diagnosis were 21.9 ± 9.7, 14.5 ± 7.2, and 6.9 ± 4.6 years in groups 1, 2, and 3, respectively. In group 4, there was only one patient who suffered de novo cancer, and the interval was 1.2 years. The mean period from transplantation to cancer diagnosis was significantly different among the four groups ($p < 0.001$). Moreover, the age of cancer diagnosis was significantly different among the four groups ($p < 0.001$). The patient with cancer in group 4 was diagnosed at 47 years of age, previously received kidney transplantation in 2013, and received multidrug immunosuppressive therapy with tacrolimus, MMF, and prednisolone for six years after the first transplantation. Finally, there was no significant difference in sex among the four groups.

Table 2. Demographic characteristics of transplant recipients with de novo cancers after kidney transplantation.

		Group 1	Group 2	Group 3	Group 4	p-Value
The Number of Patients		42 (16.9)	119 (16.2)	80 (11.7)	1 (0.3)	
Number of yrs from KTP to diagnosis of cancer (yr)		21.9 (9.7)	14.5 (7.2)	6.9 (4.6)	1.2 (-)	<0.001
Recipient age (yr)	<30	20 (47.6)	23 (19.3)	10 (12.5)	0 (0.0)	<0.001
	30–45	19 (45.2)	72 (60.5)	25 (31.2)	0 (0.0)	
	46–60	3 (7.2)	23 (19.3)	32 (40.0)	1 (100.0)	
	>61	0 (0.0)	1 (0.9)	13 (16.3)	0 (0.0)	
Recipient sex	Female	15 (35.7)	52 (43.7)	38 (47.5)	0 (0.0)	0.501
	Male	27 (64.3)	67 (56.3)	42 (52.5)	1 (100.0)	
Donor type	living	36 (85.7)	81 (68.1)	72 (90.0)	1 (100.0)	0.02
	deceased	6 (14.3)	38 (31.9)	8 (10.0)	0 (0.0)	
Blood relation	Yes	36 (85.7)	81 (67.8)	48 (60.0)	1 (100.0)	0.028
ABO blood-type	compatible	42 (100.0)	117 (98.3)	59 (73.8)	1 (100.0)	<0.001
	incompatible	0 (0.0)	2 (1.7)	21 (26.2)	0 (0.0)	
Number of HLA mismatches	A, B, DR	1.17 (1.32)	2.02 (1.02)	2.99 (1.51)	3.00 (-)	<0.001
Body mass index (kg/m^2)		21.8 (1.28)	21.3 (1.58)	21.3 (2.36)	27.64 (-)	0.11
Dialysis duration (yr)	0	2 (4.8)	3 (2.5)	6 (7.5)	1 (100.0)	0.02
	≤1	9 (21.4)	22 (18.5)	13 (16.3)	0 (0.0)	
	1<, ≤2	10 (23.8)	18 (15.1)	9 (11.3)	0 (0.0)	
	2<, ≤5	13 (31.0)	32 (26.9)	20 (25.0)	0 (0.0)	
	5<, ≤10	6 (14.3)	23 (19.3)	13 (16.3)	0 (0.0)	
	10<, ≤20	0 (0.0)	12 (10.1)	13 (16.3)	0 (0.0)	
	>20	0 (0.0)	3 (2.5)	6 (7.5)	0 (0.0)	
Calcineulin inhibitors	Cyclosporine	0 (0.0)	88 (73.9)	34 (41.4)	0 (0.0)	<0.001
	Tacrolimus	0 (0.0)	31 (26.1)	46 (58.5)	1 (100.0)	
	none	42 (100.0)	0 (0.0)	0 (0.0)	0 (0.0)	
Antiproliferative agents	Azathioprine	42 (100.0)	69 (58.0)	0 (0.0)	0 (0.0)	<0.001
	Mizoribine	0 (0.0)	44 (42.0)	0 (0.0)	0 (0.0)	
	Mcophenolatemofetil	0 (0.0)	0 (0.0)	80 (100.0)	1 (100.0)	
	none	0 (0.0)	6 (5.1)	0 (0.0)	0 (0.0)	
mTOR inhibitor	everolimus	0 (0.0)	0 (0.0)	0 (0.0)	1 (100.0)	
History of rejection	Yes	24 (57.1)	85 (71.4)	24 (30.5)	0 (0.0)	<0.001
History of transplantation	Yes	1 (2.4)	4 (3.4)	6 (8.5)	1 (100.0)	<0.001
History of transfusion	Yes	23 (54.8)	26 (21.8)	15 (23.2)	1 (100.0)	<0.001

Categorical variables are presented as frequencies and/or percentages, and continuous variables are presented as means with standard deviation.

The comparison of cancer types among the four group is presented in Table 3. Briefly, skin cancer (non-melanoma) was the most common malignant neoplasm in group 1 ($n = 10$, 23.8%) whereas post-transplant lymphoproliferative disorders ($n = 21$, 17.6% in group 2; $n = 13$, 16.3% in group 3), renal cell carcinoma ($n = 12$, 10.1% in group 2; $n = 13$, 16.3% in group 3), and breast cancer ($n = 13$, 10.9% in group 2; $n = 11$, 13.8% in group 3) were the most common malignant neoplasms in groups 2 and 3. Hepatocellular carcinoma ($n = 5$, 11.9% in group 1; $n = 7$, 5.9% in group 2) and gastric cancer ($n = 5$, 11.9% in group 1; $n = 8$, 6.7% in group 2), two frequent malignant neoplasms in groups 1 and 2, were less common in group 3 (hepatocellular carcinoma, $n = 1$, 1.3%; gastric cancer, $n = 5$, 6.3%). The number of patients with prostate cancer increased gradually, with 1 (2.4%), 4 (3.4%), and 5 (6.3%) patients in groups 1, 2, and 3, respectively. Lung cancer, one of the most common cancers in the general population, was diagnosed in only a few patients in each of the groups 1 ($n = 2$, 4.8%) and 2 ($n = 1$, 0.8%).

Table 3. Distribution of cancer types.

	Group 1	Group 2	Group 3	Group 4
The number of recipients	248	735	700	304
Total cancer-positive recipients	42 (16.9)	119 (16.2)	80 (11.7)	1 (0.3)
Double cancer-positive recipients	6	12	9	0
Triple cancer-positive recipients	4	1	0	0
Type of cancer				
PTLD	3	21	13	1
renal cell carcinoma	2	12	13	0
breast cancer	4	13	13	0
skin cancer (melanoma)	0	0	1	0
skin cancer (non-melanoma)	10	12	9	0
prostate cancer	1	5	5	0
colorectal cancer	5	7	6	0
uterus cancer	2	10	5	0
gastric cancer	5	8	5	0
urothelial cancer	2	6	4	0
thyroid cancer	1	6	3	0
tongue cancer	3	7	2	0
pancreas cancer	0	2	2	0
hepatocellular carcinoma	5	7	1	0
lung cancer	2	1	0	0
ovarian cancer	1	1	0	0
vaginal cancer	0	1	0	0
anal cancer	0	1	0	0
others	10	13	7	0
Total	56	133	89	1

PTLD, post-transplant lymphoproliferative disorders.

3.2. Cumulative de Novo Cancer Incidence Rates after Kidney Transplantation According to the Type of Induction Immunosuppressive Therapy

The 5-year cumulative de novo all cancer incidence rates after kidney transplantation were 0.0%, 1.0%, 5.3%, and 0.4% in groups 1, 2, 3, and 4, respectively (Figure 2a). Moreover, the 10- and 15-year cumulative de novo cancer incidence rates were 3.3% and 6.8% in group 1, 5.6% and 11.8% in group 2, and 11.5% and 19.3% in group 3, respectively. There were significant differences among the groups ($p = 0.007$, Gray's test). This result suggested that the addition of mTORi to conventional immunosuppressive therapy may reduce the cancer incidence rate. Since the prognosis of skin cancer except melanoma is unlikely to generate a clinically relevant change in survival, the cumulative cancer incidence excluding non-melanoma skin cancers was also calculated. The 5-year survival rates were 0.0%, 1.1%, 4.7%, and 0.4% in groups 1, 2, 3, and 4, respectively (Figure 2b). The 10- and 15-year cumulative de novo cancer incidence rates were 3.3% and 6.9% in group 1, 5.5% and 11.3% in group 2, and 10.0% and 17.9% in group 3, respectively. Even if excluded the non-melanoma skin cancers, there were significant differences among the groups ($p = 0.006$, Gray's test).

3.3. Overall and Cancer-Specific Survival Rates According to the Type of Induction Immunosuppressive Therapy

As shown in Figure 3a, the 5-year overall survival rates after kidney transplantation were 87.2%, 93.6%, 95.6%, and 96.8% in groups 1, 2, 3, and 4, respectively, with significant differences among the groups ($p < 0.001$, log-rank test) except for that between groups 3 and 4 ($p = 0.252$). Moreover, the 5-year cancer-specific survival rates after kidney transplantation were 100%, 99.4%, 99.1%, and 100% in groups 1, 2, 3, and 4, respectively (Figure 3b). The differences among the groups were not statistically significant ($p = 0.832$, log-rank test).

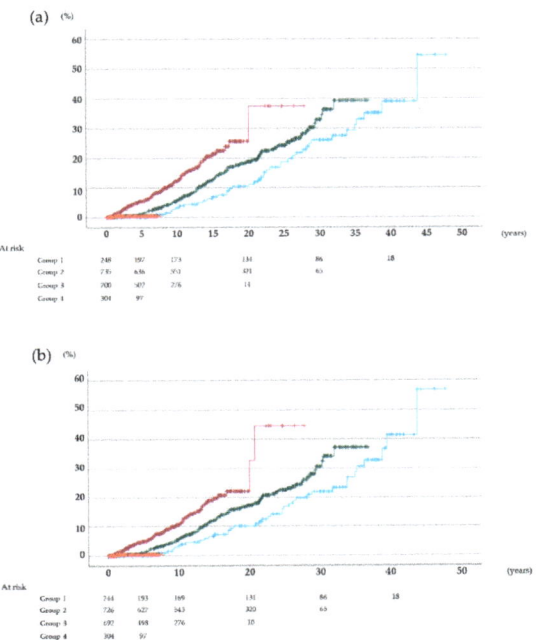

Figure 2. Cumulative cancer incidence rates after kidney transplantation. (**a**) all cancers, (**b**) all cancers except non-melanoma skin cancer: Blue, group 1; green, group 2; dark red, group 3; vermilion, group 4.

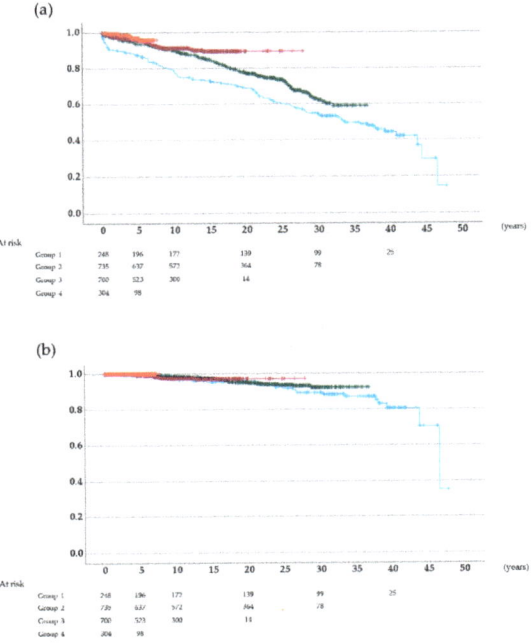

Figure 3. (**a**) Overall and (**b**) cancer-specific survival rates after kidney transplantation: Blue, group 1; green, group 2; dark red, group 3; vermilion, group 4.

3.4. Graft Survival Rate According to the Type of Induction Immunosuppressive Therapy

The 5- and 10-year death-censored graft survival rates after kidney transplantation were 69.4% and 60.3% in group 1, 84.2% and 73.0% in group 2, and 92.8% and 85.9% in group 3, respectively (Figure 4). The 5-year graft survival rate was 97.5% in group 4, and there were no patients who had been followed up for more than 10 years in this group. The graft survival rates were significantly different among the groups ($p < 0.001$, log-rank test).

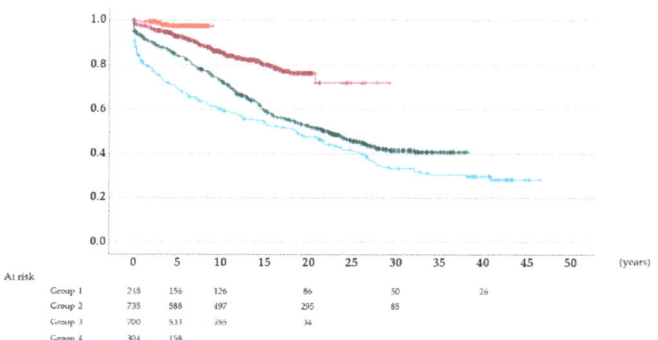

Figure 4. Death-censored graft survival rates after kidney transplantation: Blue, group 1; green, group 2; dark red, group 3; vermilion, group 4.

4. Discussion

In the present multi-center, retrospective study of 1987 patients who underwent kidney transplantation during a long time period between 1965 and 2020, we found that the cumulative cancer incidence rate after kidney transplantation increased with the introduction of new and more effective immunosuppressive drugs. These results lend further support to our previous report revealing that the aggressiveness of immunosuppressive treatment regimens or the use of potent immunosuppressives might increase the risk of de novo cancer after kidney transplantation despite the improvement of graft survival rates [16].

De novo cancer after kidney transplantation is one of the most threatening complications that reduces graft survival [16] and is a leading cause of kidney transplantation-associated mortality [17,18]. It is therefore critical to establish safe and effective immunosuppressive therapies that prevent allograft rejection as well as cancer development in patients undergoing kidney transplantation. Importantly, kidney transplant recipients who develop cancer before graft loss, i.e., those with a functioning graft at the time of cancer diagnosis, are at more than 9-fold risk of death compared to those without cancer and over 50% of recipients with cancer lose their grafts within five years following cancer diagnosis [18]. Therefore, prevention and early treatment of cancer are essential. However, discontinuation of potential cancer-promoting immunosuppressive drugs increases the risk of allograft rejection, posing a significant clinical dilemma. To address this concern, we, the authors, have started using the mTORi everolimus for induction and maintenance therapies, in addition to conventional therapies. mTORis are commonly prescribed for maintenance immunosuppression after kidney transplantation [19], and the combined use of CNIs and mTORi was reported to prevent nonmelanoma skin cancers [20–23]. Basu et al. [24] indicated that mTORis could prevent the rapid progression of post-transplantation renal cancer through the downregulation of the angiogenic cytokine vascular endothelial growth factor and the chemokine receptor CXCR3 and its ligands. mTORis act by forming a complex with the FK506-binding protein 12, and the complex inhibits mTOR, a serine-threonine kinase in the PI3K pathway, to eventually inhibit the antigenic and interleukin-stimulated activation and proliferation of T cells [25]. Several other mechanisms of cancer prevention by mTORis were also reported. For example, mTORis induce cell cycle arrest at the G1 checkpoint [26]. Additionally, everolimus, the mTORi included in the present study, has also been approved for use in several malignancies including advanced metastatic renal cell cancer [10,27]; gastric, intestinal, and pancreatic neuroendocrine tumors [11]; and subependymal giant cell astrocytoma [28].

A study previously reported that patients on mTORi-based therapy had a 59% reduced relative risk of developing new cancers (relative risk, 0.412; 95% confidence interval, 0.256–0.663) than those on CNI-based therapy [23], suggesting the possibility of replacing CNIs with mTORis in kidney transplant recipients. However, this approach may not be appropriate. Complete avoidance or withdrawal of CNIs could be associated with a greater risk of acute or chronic rejection and graft failure [29,30]. Conversion from mTORis to CNIs has been reported to be associated with increased risk of donor-specific antibody production and reduced allograft survival rate because of chronic antibody-mediated rejection [31]. Therefore, we recognize that conversion from CNIs to mTORis may not be effective in improving graft survival rate. Moreover, MMF is effective in suppressing deoxyribonucleic acid production and the onset of antibody-mediated rejection, which is difficult not only in early diagnosis but also in treatment [32,33]. In the present study, we found that quadruple induction immunosuppressive therapy, including the three drugs used in group 3 plus everolimus, was associated with not only a reduction in cancer incidence but also with an improvement in recipient and graft survival rates. The quadruple therapy appears to provide strong, albeit brief, immunosuppression; however, since the introduction of MMF and prednisolone, the CNI dose has been reduced (5–8 ng/mL within 3 months, 4–5 ng/mL at 4–12 months after kidney transplantation). Therefore, complications, such as infectious diseases, caused by potent immunosuppressive status did not increase (data not shown).

Of course, incidence and survival rates of specific cancers are not determined by whether mTORi is used for induction immunosuppressive therapy. The background characteristics contributing to specific cancer incidences should be carefully considered. For example, our results indicated that the incidence of hepatocellular carcinoma (HCC) was lower in group 3 than in groups 1 and 2. Hepatitis B and C virus infections are the main causes of HCC. Our data also showed that 11 of 13 cases were infected with at least hepatitis B or C. (type B only; $n = 2$, type C only; $n = 6$, both; $n = 3$, respectively). Blood transfusion associated with end-stage renal disease is also a cause of hepatitis. It is strongly likely that the decrease in the rate of hepatitis due to the development of erythropoiesis-stimulating agents and direct-acting antivirals has led to a decrease in the rate of HCC after kidney transplantation. On the other hand, the rates of renal cell carcinoma and prostate cancer increased in group 3 compared to groups 1 and 2. The duration of hemodialysis before kidney transplantation was also significantly longer in group 3. The preoperative dialysis period before kidney transplantation was previously reported to be correlated with the rate of renal cell carcinoma [34], as reflected in our findings. Conversely, the increase in the number of elderly recipients in recent years was likely linked to the increase in the incidence of prostate cancer observed in the present study. The average recipient age at the time of kidney transplantation was significantly higher in group 4 than that in other groups. Therefore, it is possible that mTORis might suppress the development of prostate cancer.

We have performed cancer screening on most patients so far, including the current cohort [5]. It is not possible to detect cancer by screening in all patients. However, we believe that cancer screening is a major underlying cause of the lack of a difference in cancer-specific survival rates among the study groups. In addition to cancer screening, we believe that suppressing the onset of de novo cancers using mTORis in combination with aggressive immunosuppressive therapy after kidney transplantation is critical. Several studies have also reported the beneficial effect of mTORis in cardiovascular diseases [35,36] and infections [37–39]. Cancers, cardiovascular diseases, and infections are leading causes of death after kidney transplantation [40]. Therefore, mTORis might contribute to the further improvement of survival rates by suppressing the onset of these diseases.

mTORi was previously used as a treatment for renal cell carcinoma (10 mg/day). However, various adverse events (e.g., stomatitis; 40–60%) occurred at high rates, and it was often difficult to continue [27,41,42]. Fortunately, when used as an immunosuppressant, the dose (1.5 mg/day) is about one-eighth, and the incidence of adverse events is relatively low [43]. In our study, mTORi was able to continue for a long time without interruption in most cases. However, mTORi adverse events can significantly impair the recipient's quality of life and should be carefully considered for risks and benefits and discontinued if necessary.

The present study has several notable strengths. This study was based on a large population of kidney transplant recipients from several high-volume centers. The study analyses were based on a comprehensive dataset with a long duration and very few missing values. The completeness of the dataset suggests that selection and ascertainment biases in exposure and study factors were minimal. However, the present study has several limitations that should also be acknowledged. First, this was a retrospective study, and the observation period of group 4 was notably shorter than that of the other groups. Therefore, although mTORi has been shown to reduce cancer morbidity with short-term observations, we believe that the efficacy of mTORi needs to be reassessed at long-term observations. Second, despite the adjustment for all confounding factors, there may be unmeasured residual effects such as details on the dose and duration of immunosuppressants used for the treatment of primary disease and incomplete details on smoking habits and alcohol consumption, which might have altered the strength and magnitude of association of cancer risk after transplantation. Third, some patients in groups 1, 2, and 3 received mTORis after the cancer diagnosis, although the treatment was initiated several years after the kidney transplantation. Finally, cancer treatment approaches and reductions in immunosuppressant doses in patients who developed cancer were determined by the attending physician in each case. However, despite these limitations, the current study findings are important as they are based on the largest Japanese cancer registry data of patients with kidney transplants. Especially, it is noteworthy that in group 4, the prevalence of de novo cancers at the early phase after kidney transplantation was clearly lower than in the other groups, despite the significantly older recipients.

5. Conclusions

Despite the improvement of patient and graft survival rates with the increasing potency of immunosuppressants, the cumulative cancer incidence rate after kidney transplantation increased, with a tendency for a shorter time from kidney transplantation to cancer development. The addition of mTORis to conventional induction immunosuppressive therapy was not only associated with improved patient and graft survival rates but also with reduced cancer incidence, at least in the short term after kidney transplantation. The current study findings have potential clinical significance, including the optimization of effective immunosuppressive therapies to prevent the development of post-transplantation cancer, which requires further long-term studies.

Author Contributions: Conceptualization, R.I. and N.N.; methodology, R.I.; software, R.I., R.T., A.T. and S.N.; validation, T.K., K.Y., T.N.-H., Y.K., T.A. and K.T.; formal analysis, R.I.; investigation, R.I.; Resources, R.I.; data curation, R.T., A.T., S.N. and T.A.; writing—original draft preparation, R.I.; writing—review and editing, R.I.; visualization, R.I.; supervision, T.T., H.K. and N.N.; project administration, T.T., H.K. and N.N.; funding acquisition, N.N. All authors have read and agreed to the published version of the manuscript.

Funding: This research received no external funding.

Institutional Review Board Statement: The study was conducted according to the guidelines of the Declaration of Helsinki and approved by the Institutional Review Board of Osaka University Hospital (approval No. 19475), Hyogo Prefectural Nishinomiya Hospital (approval No. H28-19), and Osaka General Medical Center (approval No. 28-2034).

Informed Consent Statement: Informed consent was obtained from all subjects involved in the study.

Data Availability Statement: The data presented in this study are available upon request from the corresponding author. The data are not publicly available due to privacy restrictions.

Acknowledgments: We would like to thank Yukito Kokado (Takahashi Clinic), Saki Utsumi and Shiro Takahara (Kansai Medical Hospital), and Miyaji Kyakuno (Takatsuki Hospital) for collection of data from medical records.

Conflicts of Interest: The authors declare no conflict of interest.

References

1. Abecassis, M.; Bartlett, S.T.; Collins, A.J.; Davis, C.L.; Delmonico, F.L.; Friedewald, J.; Hays, R.; Howard, A.; Jones, E.; Leichtman, A.B.; et al. Kidney Transplantation as Primary Therapy for End-Stage Renal Disease: A National Kidney Foundation/Kidney Disease Outcomes Quality Initiative (NKF/KDOQI™) Conference. *Clin. J. Am. Soc. Nephrol.* **2008**, *3*, 471–480. [CrossRef]
2. Luan, F.L.; Ding, R.; Sharma, V.K.; Chon, W.J.; Lagman, M.; Suthanthiran, M. Rapamycin is an effective inhibitor of human renal cancer metastasis. *Kidney Int.* **2003**, *63*, 917–926. [CrossRef]
3. Viklicky, O.; Novotny, M.; Hruba, P. Future developments in kidney transplantation. *Curr. Opin. Organ Transplant.* **2020**, *25*, 92–98. [CrossRef]
4. Campistol, J. Minimizing the Risk of Posttransplant Malignancy. *Transplant. Proc.* **2008**, *40*, S40–S43. [CrossRef]
5. Kato, T.; Kakuta, Y.; Abe, T.; Yamanaka, K.; Imamura, R.; Okumi, M.; Ichimaru, N.; Takahara, S.; Nonomura, N. The benefits of cancer screening in kidney transplant recipients: A single-center experience. *Cancer Med.* **2016**, *5*, 153–158. [CrossRef]
6. Bellacosa, A.; Kumar, C.C.; Di Cristofano, A.; Testa, J.R. Activation of AKT Kinases in Cancer: Implications for Therapeutic Targeting. *Adv. Cancer Res.* **2005**, *94*, 29–86. [CrossRef] [PubMed]
7. Bjornsti, M.-A.; Houghton, P.J. The tor pathway: A target for cancer therapy. *Nat. Rev. Cancer* **2004**, *4*, 335–348. [CrossRef] [PubMed]
8. Hudes, G.; Carducci, M.; Tomczak, P.; Dutcher, J.; Figlin, R.; Kapoor, A.; Staroslawska, E.; Sosman, J.; McDermott, D.; Bodrogi, I.; et al. Temsirolimus, Interferon Alfa, or Both for Advanced Renal-Cell Carcinoma. *N. Engl. J. Med.* **2007**, *356*, 2271–2281. [CrossRef] [PubMed]
9. Sansal, I.; Sellers, W.R. The Biology and Clinical Relevance of the PTEN Tumor Suppressor Pathway. *J. Clin. Oncol.* **2004**, *22*, 2954–2963. [CrossRef]
10. Motzer, R.J.; Escudier, B.; Oudard, S.; Hutson, T.E.; Porta, C.; Bracarda, S.; Grünwald, V.; Thompson, J.A.; Figlin, R.A.; Hollaender, N.; et al. Efficacy of everolimus in advanced renal cell carcinoma: A double-blind, randomised, placebo-controlled phase III trial. *Lancet* **2008**, *372*, 449–456. [CrossRef]
11. Yao, J.C.; Shah, M.H.; Ito, T.; Bohas, C.L.; Wolin, E.M.; Van Cutsem, E.; Hobday, T.J.; Okusaka, T.; Capdevila, J.; de Vries, E.; et al. Everolimus for Advanced Pancreatic Neuroendocrine Tumors. *N. Engl. J. Med.* **2011**, *364*, 514–523. [CrossRef]
12. Meric-Bernstam, F.; Gonzalez-Angulo, A.M. Targeting the mTOR Signaling Network for Cancer Therapy. *J. Clin. Oncol.* **2009**, *27*, 2278–2287. [CrossRef]
13. Dantal, J.; Soulillou, J.-P. Immunosuppressive Drugs and the Risk of Cancer after Organ Transplantation. *N. Engl. J. Med.* **2005**, *352*, 1371–1373. [CrossRef]
14. Monaco, A.P. The Role of mTOR Inhibitors in the Management of Posttransplant Malignancy. *Transplantation* **2009**, *87*, 157–163. [CrossRef] [PubMed]
15. Rousseau, B.; Guillemin, A.; Duvoux, C.; Neuzillet, C.; Tlemsani, C.; Compagnon, P.; Azoulay, D.; Salloum, C.; Laurent, A.; de la Taille, A.; et al. Optimal oncologic management and mTOR inhibitor introduction are safe and improve survival in kidney and liver allograft recipients with de novo carcinoma. *Int. J. Cancer* **2019**, *144*, 886–896. [CrossRef]
16. Imamura, R.; Nakazawa, S.; Yamanaka, K.; Kakuta, Y.; Tsutahara, K.; Taniguchi, A.; Kawamura, M.; Kato, T.; Abe, T.; Uemura, M.; et al. Cumulative cancer incidence and mortality after kidney transplantation in Japan: A long-term multicenter cohort study. *Cancer Med.* **2021**, *10*, 2205–2215. [CrossRef] [PubMed]
17. Farrugia, D.; Mahboob, S.; Cheshire, J.; Begaj, I.; Khosla, S.; Ray, D.; Sharif, A. Malignancy-related mortality following kidney transplantation is common. *Kidney Int.* **2014**, *85*, 1395–1403. [CrossRef]
18. Lim, W.H.; Badve, S.V.; Wong, G. Long-term allograft and patient outcomes of kidney transplant recipients with and without incident cancer-a population cohort study. *Oncotarget* **2017**, *8*, 77771–77782. [CrossRef]
19. Badve, S.V.; Pascoe, E.; Burke, M.; Clayton, P.A.; Campbell, S.B.; Hawley, C.; Lim, W.H.; McDonald, S.P.; Wong, G.; Johnson, D.W. Mammalian Target of Rapamycin Inhibitors and Clinical Outcomes in Adult Kidney Transplant Recipients. *Clin. J. Am. Soc. Nephrol.* **2016**, *11*, 1845–1855. [CrossRef]
20. Campbell, S.B.; Walker, R.; Tai, S.S.; Jiang, Q.; Russ, G.R. Randomized Controlled Trial of Sirolimus for Renal Transplant Recipients at High Risk for Nonmelanoma Skin Cancer. *Arab. Archaeol. Epigr.* **2012**, *12*, 1146–1156. [CrossRef]
21. Lim, W.H.; Eris, J.; Kanellis, J.; Pussell, B.; Wiid, Z.; Witcombe, D.; Russ, G.R. A Systematic Review of Conversion from Calcineurin Inhibitor to Mammalian Target of Rapamycin Inhibitors for Maintenance Immunosuppression in Kidney Transplant Recipients. *Arab. Archaeol. Epigr.* **2014**, *14*, 2106–2119. [CrossRef] [PubMed]
22. Ying, T.; Wong, G.; Lim, W.; Kanellis, J.; Pilmore, H.; Campbell, S.; Masterson, R.; Walker, R.; O'Connell, P.; Russ, G.; et al. De novo or early conversion to everolimus and long-term cancer outcomes in kidney transplant recipients: A trial-based linkage study. *Arab. Archaeol. Epigr.* **2018**, *18*, 2977–2986. [CrossRef] [PubMed]

23. Kauffman, H.M.; Cherikh, W.S.; Cheng, Y.; Hanto, D.W.; Kahan, B.D. Maintenance Immunosuppression with Target-of-Rapamycin Inhibitors is Associated with a Reduced Incidence of De Novo Malignancies. *Transplantation* **2005**, *80*, 883–889. [CrossRef]
24. Basu, A.; Liu, T.; Banerjee, P.; Flynn, E.; Zurakowski, D.; Datta, D.; Viklicky, O.; Gasser, M.; Waaga-Gasser, A.M.; Yang, J.; et al. Effectiveness of a combination therapy using calcineurin inhibitor and mTOR inhibitor in preventing allograft rejection and post-transplantation renal cancer progression. *Cancer Lett.* **2012**, *321*, 179–186. [CrossRef]
25. Andrassy, J.; Graeb, C.; Rentsch, M.; Jauch, K.-W.; Guba, M. mTOR Inhibition and its Effect on Cancer in Transplantation. *Transplantation* **2005**, *80*, S171–S174. [CrossRef]
26. Hashemolhosseini, S.; Nagamine, Y.; Morley, S.J.; Desrivières, S.; Mercep, L.; Ferrari, S. Rapamycin inhibition of the G1 to S transition is mediated by effects on cyclin D1 mRNA and protein stability. *J. Biol. Chem.* **1998**, *273*, 14424–14429. [CrossRef] [PubMed]
27. Motzer, R.J.; Escudier, B.; Oudard, S.; Hutson, T.E.; Porta, C.; Bracarda, S.; Grünwald, V.; Thompson, J.A.; Figlin, R.A.; Hollaender, N.; et al. Phase 3 trial of everolimus for metastatic renal cell carcinoma: Final results and analysis of prognostic factors. *Cancer* **2010**, *116*, 4256–4265. [CrossRef]
28. Franz, D.N.; Belousova, E.; Sparagana, S.; Bebin, E.M.; Frost, M.; Kuperman, R.; Witt, O.; Kohrman, M.H.; Flamini, J.R.; Wu, J.Y.; et al. Efficacy and safety of everolimus for subependymal giant cell astrocytomas associated with tuberous sclerosis complex (EXIST-1): A multicentre, randomised, placebo-controlled phase 3 trial. *Lancet* **2013**, *381*, 125–132. [CrossRef]
29. Ekberg, H.; Tedesco-Silva, H.; Demirbas, A.; Vítko, Š.; Nashan, B.; Guerkan, A.; Margreiter, R.; Hugo, C.; Grinyó, J.M.; Frei, U.; et al. Reduced Exposure to Calcineurin Inhibitors in Renal Transplantation. *N. Engl. J. Med.* **2007**, *357*, 2562–2575. [CrossRef] [PubMed]
30. Ponticelli, C.; Scolari, M. Calcineurin Inhibitors in Renal Transplantation Still Needed but in Reduced Doses: A Review. *Transplant. Proc.* **2010**, *42*, 2205–2208. [CrossRef]
31. Croze, L.E.; Tetaz, R.; Roustit, M.; Malvezzi, P.; Janbon, B.; Jouve, T.; Pinel, N.; Masson, D.; Quesada, J.L.; Bayle, F.; et al. Conversion to mammalian target of rapamycin inhibitors increases risk of de novo donor-specific antibodies. *Transpl. Int.* **2014**, *27*, 775–783. [CrossRef]
32. Lederer, S.R.; Friedrich, N.; Banas, B.; Welser, G.; Albert, E.D.; Sitter, T. Effects of mycophenolate mofetil on donor-specific antibody formation in renal transplantation. *Clin. Transplant.* **2005**, *19*, 168–174. [CrossRef]
33. Terasaki, P.I.; Ozawa, M. Predicting Kidney Graft Failure by HLA Antibodies: A Prospective Trial. *Arab. Archaeol. Epigr.* **2004**, *4*, 438–443. [CrossRef] [PubMed]
34. Wong, G.; Turner, R.M.; Chapman, J.R.; Howell, M.; Lim, W.H.; Webster, A.C.; Craig, J.C. Time on Dialysis and Cancer Risk After Kidney Transplantation. *Transplantation* **2013**, *95*, 114–121. [CrossRef] [PubMed]
35. Andrés, V.; Castro, C.; Campistol, J.M. Potential role of proliferation signal inhibitors on atherosclerosis in renal transplant patients. *Nephrol. Dial. Transplant.* **2006**, *21*, iii14–iii17. [CrossRef]
36. Zeier, M.; van der Giet, M. Calcineurin inhibitor sparing regimens using m-target of rapamycin inhibitors: An opportunity to improve cardiovascular risk following kidney transplantation? *Transpl. Int.* **2010**, *24*, 30–42. [CrossRef]
37. Nashan, B.; Curtis, J.; Ponticelli, C.; Mourad, G.; Jaffe, J.; Haas, T. Everolimus and Reduced-Exposure Cyclosporine in de novo Renal-Transplant Recipients: A Three-Year Phase II, Randomized, Multicenter, Open-Label Study. *Transplantation* **2004**, *78*, 1332–1340. [CrossRef]
38. Silva, H.T., Jr.; Cibrik, D.; Johnston, T.; Lackova, E.; Mange, K.; Panis, C.; Walker, R.; Wang, Z.; Zibari, G.B.; Kim, Y.S. Everolimus Plus Reduced-Exposure CsA versus Mycophenolic Acid Plus Standard-Exposure CsA in Renal-Transplant Recipients. *Arab. Archaeol. Epigr.* **2010**, *10*, 1401–1413. [CrossRef] [PubMed]
39. Vítko, Š.; Margreiter, R.; Weimar, W.; Dantal, J.; Kuypers, D.; Winkler, M.; Øyen, O.; Viljoen, H.G.; Filiptsev, P.; Sadek, S.; et al. Three-Year Efficacy and Safety Results from a Study of Everolimus Versus Mycophenolate Mofetil in de novo Renal Transplant Patients. *Arab. Archaeol. Epigr.* **2005**, *5*, 2521–2530. [CrossRef] [PubMed]
40. Kahwaji, J.; Bunnapradist, S.; Hsu, J.-W.; Idroos, M.L.; Dudek, R. Cause of Death With Graft Function Among Renal Transplant Recipients in an Integrated Healthcare System. *Transplantation* **2011**, *91*, 225–230. [CrossRef]
41. Sánchez-Fructuoso, A.; Ruiz, J.; Pérez-Flores, I.; Alamillo, C.G.; Romero, N.C.; Arias, M. Comparative Analysis of Adverse Events Requiring Suspension of mTOR Inhibitors: Everolimus versus Sirolimus. *Transplant. Proc.* **2010**, *42*, 3050–3052. [CrossRef] [PubMed]
42. Eertwegh, A.J.V.D.; Karakiewicz, P.; Bavbek, S.; Rha, S.Y.; Bracarda, S.; Bahl, A.; Ou, Y.-C.; Kim, D.; Panneerselvam, A.; Anak, O.; et al. Safety of Everolimus by Treatment Duration in Patients With Advanced Renal Cell Cancer in an Expanded Access Program. *Urology* **2013**, *81*, 143–149. [CrossRef] [PubMed]
43. Ventura-Aguiar, P.; Campistol, J.M.; Diekmann, F. Safety of mTOR inhibitors in adult solid organ transplantation. *Expert Opin. Drug Saf.* **2016**, *15*, 303–319. [CrossRef] [PubMed]

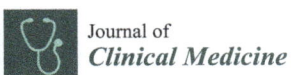

Article

Long-Term Results of Kidney Transplantation in the Elderly: Comparison between Different Donor Settings

Renana Yemini [1,2], Ruth Rahamimov [3,4], Ronen Ghinea [4,5] and Eytan Mor [3,4,*,†]

1. Department of Surgery, Samson Assuta Ashdod University Hospital, Ashdod 7747629, Israel; renanayemini@gmail.com
2. Faculty of Health Sciences, Ben Gurion University of the Negev, Be'er Sheva 8410501, Israel
3. Institute of Nephrology, Beilinson Medical Center, Petach-Tikva 49100, Israel; rutir@clalit.org.il
4. Sackler Medical School, Tel-Aviv University, Tel-Aviv 6997801, Israel; rghinea@hotmail.com
5. Transplant Unit, Department of Surgery B, Sheba Medical Center, Ramat Gan 52621, Israel
* Correspondence: eytan.mor@sheba.health.gov.il
† Previous address: Department of Transplant Surgery, Beilinson Medical Center, Petach-Tikva 49100, Israel, affiliated to the Sackler Faculty of Medicine, Tel-Aviv University, Tel-Aviv 6997801, Israel.

Abstract: With scarce organ supply, a selection of suitable elderly candidates for transplant is needed, as well as auditing the long-term outcomes after transplant. We conducted an observational cohort study among our patient cohort >60 years old with a long follow up. (1). Patients and Methods: We used our database to study the results after transplant for 593 patients >60 years old who underwent a transplant between 2000–2017. The outcome was compared between live donor (LD; n = 257) recipients, an old-to-old (OTO, n = 215) group using an extended criteria donor (ECD) kidney, and a young-to-old (YTO, n = 123) group using a standard-criteria donor. The Kaplan–Meir method was used to calculate the patient and graft survival and Cox regression analysis in order to find risk factors associated with death. (2). Results: The 5- and 10-year patient survival was significantly better in the LD group (92.7% and 66.9%) compared with the OTO group (73.3% and 42.8%) and YTO group (70.9% and 40.6%) ($p < 0.0001$). The 5- and 10-year graft survival rates were 90.3% and 68.5% (LD), 61.7% and 30.9% (OTO), and 64.1% and 39.9%, respectively (YTO group; $p < 0.0001$ between the LD and the two DD groups). There was no difference in outcome between patients in their 60's and their 70's. Factors associated with mortality included: age (HR-1.060), DM (HR-1.773), IHD (HR-1.510), and LD/DD (HR-2.865). (3). Conclusions: Our 17-years of experience seems to justify the rational of an old-to-old allocation policy in the elderly population. Live-donor transplant should be encouraged whenever possible. Each individual decision of elderly candidates for transplant should be based on the patient's comorbidity and predicted life expectancy.

Keywords: dialysis; elderly; expanded criteria donor; kidney transplantation

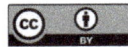

1. Introduction

Patients ≥60 years old are the largest growing age group in the end-stage renal disease (ESRD) population and comprise 40% of all patients with ESRD. About 20% of the candidates awaiting a transplant at any time in the given year are elderly patients [1]. The American Society of Transplantation evaluation guidelines state that there should be no absolute upper age limit for excluding patients whose overall health and life situation suggest that transplantation will be beneficial [2]. Kidney transplantation (KT) also offers a survival benefit in elderly patients, yet a subgroup analysis showed a diminished survival benefit in the 70–74 year-old age group [3]. Nevertheless, KT in the elderly population remains a controversial issue, especially among the age group of >70 years old. Rao et al. [4] showed the outcomes of 5667 elderly patients >70 years old waitlisted between the years 1990 and 2004. They found a 41% reduction in risk of death in patients transplanted versus patients who remained on the waiting list. They also showed that the recipients of expanded criteria donor kidneys had a 25% reduction in risk of death compared with patients who remained on the waiting list. The majority of patients in the elderly age group have associated comorbidities like diabetes, coronary artery disease, and peripheral vascular disease, which make them more frail and ineligible as transplant candidates [5,6]. However, certain elderly patients are good transplant candidates and have a significant survival benefit and improved quality of life after transplant. The question is what are the predictors of a good outcome, namely prolonged graft and patient survival, without associated posttransplant complications requiring readmissions? Previous reports have tried to delineate parameters that will help define this group of patients. In a report using decision analytic model comparing deceased donor KT to continued hemodialysis treatment, the authors concluded that if available within a timely period (<2 years), transplantation may offer substantial clinical benefits to older patients at a reasonable financial cost. Prolonged waiting times dramatically decrease the clinical benefits and economic attractiveness of transplantation [7]. In another large single center cohort study including 233 patients older than 65 years transplanted over a 15 year period, Heldal et al. showed that KT in these patients offered a survival advantage over dialysis treatment [8]. In their series of patients remaining on the transplantation waitlist, median survival from waitlisting was 3.4 (3.0–3.8) years compared with 4.8 (3.8–5.9) years in the transplant group. The 5-year survival of KT recipients was 66% compared with 33% among the waitlist patients. When looking at the scarce organ resource, the individual benefit of transplanting elderly patients has to be balanced against the corresponding increase in the number of patients awaiting grafts. In the above study from Finland, the median dialysis time for transplanted patients was only 12 months, reflecting a high organ donation rate, which justifies allocation of kidneys to elderly patients. This is not true however in many other parts of the world, where the median waiting time for transplant, such as in the US, can reach 4–5 years [1]. To overcome this limitation, several countries have created allocation policies that adjust the predicted recipient life expectancy with the projected graft survival by using extended criteria donor (ECD) in the elderly patients [9].

Eurotransplant Leiden started the Eurotransplant Senior Program "old for old" in 1999. Their allocation system placed a cut-off age of 65 for matching between donors and recipients. The kidneys are transplanted with a short cold ischemia time regardless of the human leukocyte antigen (HLA) compatibility [10]. In parallel, at also in 1999, the Israeli National Transplantation Center approved a similar "old-to-old" program for kidney transplantation using kidneys from donors >60 years old or ECD kidneys from donors >50 years old in patients older than 60 [11,12]. In the US, in order to implement a similar concept, a policy enabling the use of ECD kidneys was implemented in November 2000 [9,13]. In 2012, the US Organ Procurement and Transplantation Network (OPTN) replaced the ECD classification system with the Kidney Donor Profile Index (KDPI), which provided an estimate of the expected survival of a deceased donor kidney graft and a means to evaluate the suitability of deceased donor kidney possibilities. KDPI was calculated from donor variables including age, race, diabetes, hypertension, serum creatinine, height, weight, hepatitis C seropositivity, and cause of death, using the method described by the OPTN [14,15].

In this study, we report the long-term KT results at our center within the "old-to-old" program, and specifically analyze the outcomes in a subgroup of patients 70 years and older. A further analysis was done to define the risk factors associated with graft failure and patient death among our patient cohort older than 60 years old.

2. Patients and Methods

2.1. Patient Selection

This cohort study is based on a retrospective analysis of our center transplant database, including kidney transplants performed between 2000–2017. The study was approved by the Institutional Review Board of the Beilinson Medical Center. We used data of 593 kidney transplants in the elderly (aged >60 years) for the analysis.

First, we analyzed the long-term results of the subgroup of patients transplanted within the deceased donor old-to-old program (DD-OTO), including 213 patients, and compared them with two other groups, namely 123 patients who received a kidney from a deceased donor younger than 60 years old (DD-YTO) and another group of 257 patients who received a graft from a living donor (LD) during the same time interval. Then, we focused on the group of patients 70 and older and compared their graft and patient survival rates to that of patients in their 60s. Finally, we used a multifactorial regression analysis to find risk factors associated with graft loss and patient death in the elderly population.

Data were extracted from the medical records of the relevant hospital departments, including outpatient clinics, surgery, and anesthesia, and consisted of the recipient's and donor's age and sex, cause of ESRD (diabetic nephropathy, hypertensive disease, polycystic kidneys disease (PKD), focal and segmental glomerulosclerosis (FSGS), glomerulonephritis (GN), pyelonephritis, congenital, others, and unknown), preoperative weight and BMI (kg/m^2), comorbidities (diabetes mellitus (DM), ischemic heart disease (IHD), and hypertension (HTN)), dialysis duration before transplantation, graft from an LD or DD, panel reactive antibody (PRA), and human leukocyte antigen (HLA)-DR mismatch (MM). Outcomes and complications were determined by analyses of the patients, who all had their follow-ups at our transplant center.

2.2. Deceased Donor Kidney Allocation

In the deceased donor old-to-old (DD-OTO) group, kidneys from donors >60 or ECD donors >50 years (defined as donors with at least two risk factors: history of diabetes mellitus or hypertension, serum Cr. >1.5 mg/dL, and CVA as a cause of death) were allocated to patients older than 60 years with a PRA of 0% on three consecutive recent samples. PRA 0% was defined until 2008 by the classical PRA serological test against 20 healthy controls, while after 2008, class I and class II HLA Ab's was tested using Luminex technique (R&D System, Biotech Co., Minneapolis, MN, USA). In the deceased donor young-to-old (DD-YTO) group, allocation was based on the following four parameters: time on dialysis, degree of pre-sensitization according to percent PRA, B and DR-HLA matching, and age as a continuous variable. In 2012, two new parameters were added, namely (1) being a registered organ donor for over 3 years earned a patient two extra points, and (2) if a family member donated in the past, an extra nine points were added to the candidate's score.

2.3. Operative Management

Kidney transplantation was performed through an extraperitoneal approach in the iliac fossa. The renal vessels were anastomosed to the external iliac vessels, and the ureter was implanted into the bladder by an extravesical uretero-cystostomy using the anti-reflux technique. A double-J stent was routinely placed in the ureter and was removed 3 to 6 weeks after transplantation.

2.4. Perioperative Management

Maintenance immunosuppression included the calcineurin inhibitors tacrolimus (Prograf, Astellas Pharma, Middlesex, UK) starting on postoperative day 1 at a dose of 0.15 mg/kg, target 12-h trough levels of 8 to 12 ng/mL during the first 3 months and 5 to 8 ng/mL thereafter, or cyclosporine (Sandimmune Neoral, Novartis Pharmaceutical) starting on postoperative day 1 at a dose of 8 mg/kg, target 12-h trough levels of 150 to 300 ng/mL during the first 3 months and 100 to 200 ng/mL thereafter. Antiproliferative agents included 1000 mg mycophenolate mofetil (Cellcept, Roche Pharmaceuticals) twice daily for the first 2 weeks and 500 mg three times a day thereafter, or mycophenolic acid (Myfortic, Novartis Pharma) 720 mg twice daily for the first 2 weeks and 360 mg three times per day thereafter. All patients received perioperative intravenous corticosteroid therapy with methylprednisolone 500 mg on day 0, 250 mg on day 1, and 100 mg on day 2, after which they received oral prednisone 20 mg per day tapered to 5 mg per day within

3 months. Induction therapy consisted of one of the following: the anti–IL-2 receptor antagonist basiliximab (Simulect, Novartis Pharma) administered intravenously on days 0 and 4 at a dosage of 20 mg; daclizumab (Zenapax; Roche Pharmaceuticals, Basel, Switzerland) at a dosage of 1 mg/kg on days 0 and 14; or, in cases of immunologic high risk, rabbit antithymocyte globulin (ATG) (Thymoglobulin; Genzyme Corp) at an intravenous dosage of 1.0 mg/kg daily for 3 days starting intraoperatively. Part of the study population did not receive induction therapy. In January 2014, we changed our induction protocol for low risk (non-sensitized) deceased-donor patients and instead of Basilixumab, we used a single dose of Thymoglobulin in the OR.

2.5. Clinical Outcomes

The primary clinical outcomes of this study were graft failure (defined as death or return to dialysis), death-censored graft failure, and all-cause mortality. The outcome data of all recipients were censored in August 2019. Secondary outcomes were delayed graft function (DGF) defined as one or more dialysis after transplantation and primary non-function (PNF). Length of hospital stay after transplant and graft function were measured by Cr levels immediately and long-term after transplant.

2.6. Statistical Analysis

Mean values, standard deviations, and absolute and relative frequencies were calculated for the descriptive statistical analysis. Chi-squared tests were used to assess the difference in the frequencies between the four groups for categorical variables, and t-tests and analysis of variance (ANOVA) were applied for continuous variables. Variables that were significant on the univariate analysis were entered into a multivariate analysis. p values ≤ 0.05 were considered significant. Survival analysis was by the Kaplan–Meir Method, with the log rank test d for comparisons between groups and the Cox regression analysis applied for identifying risk factors for graft loss and demise. The results were expressed as hazard ratio (HR) with 95% confidence interval (CI). The covariates included in the logistic regression and Cox regression models were donor age and gender, recipient age and gender, diabetes, ischemic heart disease, graft type, dialysis (yes/no) prior to transplant, sensitization (PRA > 10%), and re-transplantation. Effect modification between donor types with covariates and outcomes were also examined. Variables that had an association with clinical outcomes with p-values of <0.10 in the unadjusted analyses were included in the multivariable-adjusted analyses. Statistical analyses were performed by IBM SPSS Statistics, software version 25.0 (IBM Corp., Armonk, NY, USA).

3. Results

3.1. Comparison between the Live Donor Group (LD) and the Two Deceased Donor Groups: Old-to-Old (DD-OTO) and Young-to-Old (DD-YTO) Recipients

In comparison between the three groups, the main differences were noted between the LD group and the two DD groups (Table 1). As part of the allocation, differences between these groups were that DD-OTO patients were non-sensitized with a lower level of HLA matching and a lower rate of re-transplantation. Their donor's mean age was significantly higher compared with the age of the donors in the two other groups. The LD patients had a shorter duration of dialysis before transplant, with 25% of them transplanted before the initiation of dialysis. The induction protocol was also different between the LD and the two DD groups, with a greater proportion of patients in the DD groups who received a single dose of ATG instead of IL-2 inhibitors as part of a new protocol introduced in 2013. The mean donor age of the LD and the DD-YTO groups was significantly lower compared to the mean donor age of the DD-OTO group. The above differences were translated into a better outcome in the LD group compared to that of the other two DD groups, including significantly lower DGF and PNF rates (Tables 2 and 3) as well as better graft and patient survival rates (Figures 1 and 2). The ten year uncensored patient survival rates were 42.8% in deceased donor old-to-old (DD-OTO), 40.6% in deceased donor young-to-old (DD-YTO), and 66.9% in live donor (LD), $p = 0.000$ LD compared to the two DD groups. The ten year uncensored graft survival rates were 30.9% in DD-OTO, 39.9% in DD-YTO, and 68.5% in LD, $p = 0.000$ LD, compared to the two DD groups (Figures 1 and 2). Graft and patient survival were similar in the two DD groups (Figures 1 and 2). Recipients in the LD and DD-YTO groups had a better death-censored graft survival (Figure 3), although graft and patient survivals were not different between the two DD groups. The estimated 10 year graft survival censored for death with a functioning graft was 65% in DD-OTO, 84.9% in DD-YTO, and 91.8% in LD, $p = 0.000$ LD, compared to the two DD groups and $p < 0.001$ DD-YTO vs. DD-OTO (Figure 3).

Table 1. Characteristics of patients in the three groups: living donor, deceased donor old-to-old (DD-OTO), and deceased donor young-to-old (DD-YTO).

	Living Donor $n = 257$	DD Old-to-Old $n = 213$	DD Young-to-Old $n = 123$	p Value LD vs. DD	p Value OTO vs. YTO
Mean follow-up (months)	63.0 ± 49.5	59.4 ± 47.4	60.6 ± 49.2	0.714	0.082
Recipient age (years)	64.9 ± 3.8	65.7 ± 5.0	64.5 ± 3.6	0.036	0.012
Recipient Gender M/F (%)	76.4/23.1	78.4/21.6	69.6/30.4	0.180	0.480
Primary Disease (%)				0.014	0.133
HTN	10.1	15.5	9.6		
DM	32.2	32.4	20.0		
PCKD	12.4	12.7	11.2		
GN	7.4	7.5	12.8		
Pyelonephritis	3.9	2.3	5.6		
FSGS	4.3	7.0	7.2		
IgA	5.4	2.8	2.8		
Other	10.5	6.1	14.4		
Unknown	13.8	13.7	16.4		
Diabetes (%)	49.6	45.1	34.2	0.020	0.093
IHD (%)	32.9	39.7	42.2	0.159	0.770
PRA class I (%)	8.3	0.0	11.4	0.001	0.015
PRA class II (%)	6.6	0.0	3.9	0.002	0.016
Time on dialysis (mo.)	21.5 ± 22.7	63.3 ± 28.8	61.9 ± 33.8	$p < 0.001$	0.486
HLA-B full-match (%)	6.7	1.2	4.2	$p < 0.001$	0.273
HLA-DR full-match (%)	6.7	2.9	10.3	$p < 0.001$	0.058
Re-transplantation (%)	8.1	3.8	9.6	0.205	0.086
Donor age (years)	45.9 ± 12.4	65.9 ± 4.4	47.1 ± 11.0	$p < 0.001$	$p < 0.001$
Donor gender M/F (%)	54.3/45.7	56.6/43.4	60.5/39.5	0.521	0.730
Induction (%)				$p < 0.001$	0.828
IL-2 inhibitor	75.3	46.4	48.8		
ATG	8.6	48.8	45.5		
Desensitization (IVIG + PP + Rituximab)	8.7	0.0	0.0		
Cold ischemia time (hours)	3.5 ± 1.8	10.1 ± 3.7	10.8 ± 3.8	$p < 0.001$	0.524

DD, deceased donor; LD, living donor; OTO, old-to-old; YTO, Young-to-Old; HTN, hypertension; DM, diabetes mellitus; PCKD, polycystic kidney disease; GN, glomerulonephritis; FSGS, focal segmental glomerulosclerosis; IgA, immunoglobulin A; IHD, ischemic heart disease; PRA, panel reactive antibody, class I and II; HLA-B/DR match, human leukocyte antigen; IL-2 inhibitor, interleukin 2 inhibitor; ATG, anti-thymocyte globulin; IVIG, intravenous immune globulin; PP, plasmapheresis.

Table 2. Kidney transplant outcomes.

	Living Donor $n = 257$	DD Old-to-Old $n = 213$	DD Young-to-Old $n = 123$	p Value LD vs. DD	p Value OTO vs. YTO
DGF (%)	9.7	41.3	47.2	$p < 0.001$	0.255
PNF (%)	0.4	2.3	1.6	0.001	0.366
Graft Failure (%)	4.7	18.8	11.2	$p < 0.001$	0.531
Death (%)	15.5	36.2	40.8	$p < 0.001$	0.395
Death with functioning graft (%)	11.6	25.8	33.6	$p < 0.001$	0.066
Length of stay (days)	12.5 ± 23.7	15.7 ± 11.6	15.9 ± 12.2	0.081	0.201
Cr 30 days (mg/dL)	1.36 ± 0.67	2.90 ± 1.29	1.91 ± 1.28	$p < 0.001$	0.668
Cr 1 year (mg/dL)	1.22 ± 0.37	1.74 ± 1.12	1.79 ± 1.49	$p < 0.001$	0.717
Cr 5 years (mg/dL)	1.35 ± 1.14	2.29 ± 2.19	1.79 ± 1.49	$p < 0.001$	0.124

DD, deceased donor; LD, living donor; OTO, old-to-old; YTO, Young-to-Old; DGF, delayed graft function; PNF, primary nonfunction; Cr, creatinine.

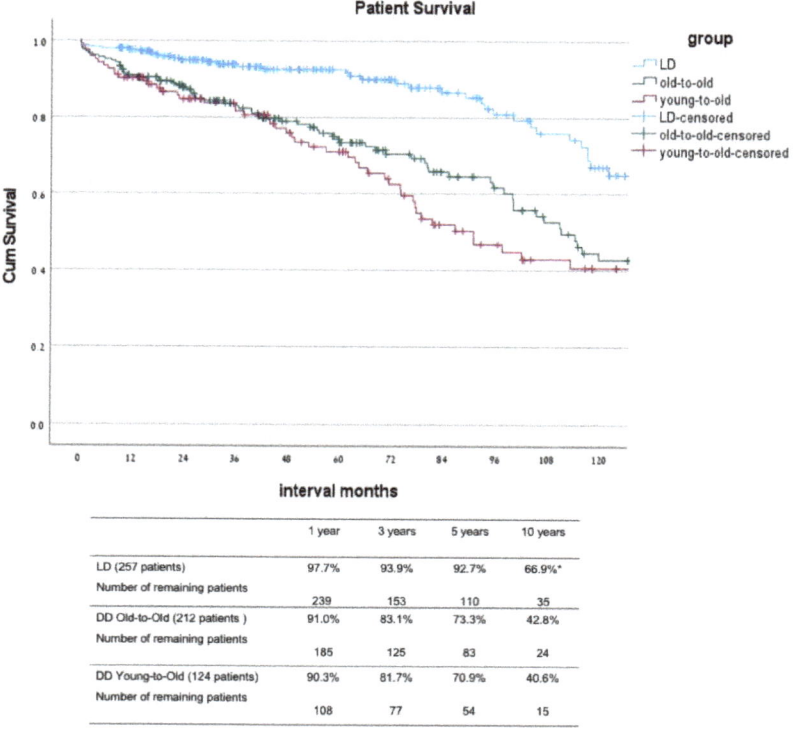

Figure 1. Kaplan–Meier patient survival of LD, DD-OTO, and DD-YTO. DD, deceased donor; LD, living donor; OTO, old-to-old; YTO, Young-to-Old.

Table 3. Cox regression multivariate analysis for death and graft loss.

Risk Factors for Death	Hazard Ratio	95% Confidence Interval	p Value
Age	1.060	1.019–1.101	0.004
DM	1.773	1.241–2.532	0.002
IHD	1.510	1.063–2.145	0.021
Donor type (DD/LD)	2.865	1.910–3.800	$p < 0.001$
Risk Factors for Graft Loss			
IHD	1.782	1.045–3.038	0.034
Donor age	1.025	1.000–1.051	0.050
Donor type DD/LD	6.064	2.315–15.881	$p < 0.001$

DM, diabetes mellitus; IHD, ischemic Heart disease; DD, deceased donor; LD, living donor.

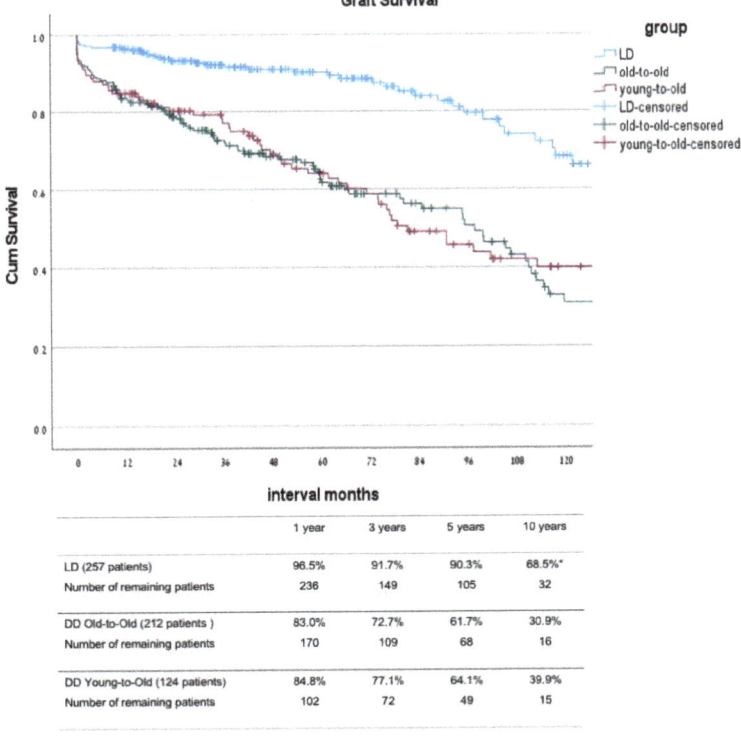

	1 year	3 years	5 years	10 years
LD (257 patients)	96.5%	91.7%	90.3%	68.5%*
Number of remaining patients	236	149	105	32
DD Old-to-Old (212 patients)	83.0%	72.7%	61.7%	30.9%
Number of remaining patients	170	109	68	16
DD Young-to-Old (124 patients)	84.8%	77.1%	64.1%	39.9%
Number of remaining patients	102	72	49	15

* $p < 0.001$ compared to the two DD groups (log rank test)

Figure 2. Kaplan–Meier graft survival of LD, DD-OTO, and DD-YTC. DD, deceased donor; LD, living donor; OTO, old-to-old; YTO, Young-to-Old.

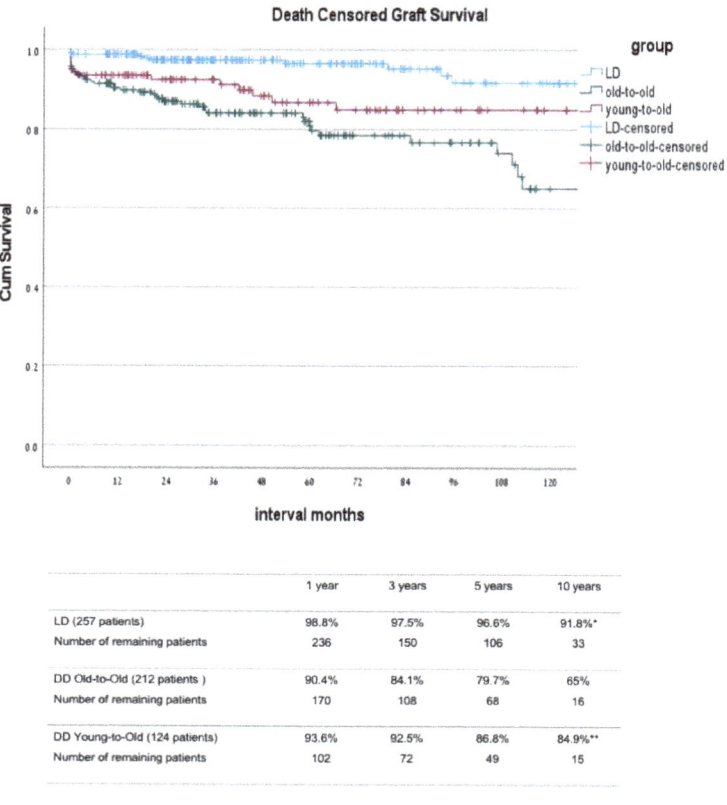

Figure 3. Kaplan–Meier death censored graft survival of LD, DD-OTO, and DD-YTO. DD, deceased donor; LD, Living donor; OTO, old-to-old; YTO, Young-to-Old.

In the Cox regression analysis (Table 3) looking for independent variables associated with risk of death after transplant, the following risk factors were found: age (HR 1.060), DM (HR 1.773), IHD (1.510), and donor type (DD vs. LD, HR 2.865). Variables associated with a risk of graft loss were IHD (HR 1.782), donor age (HR 1.025), and donor type (DD vs. LD, HR 6.064).

3.2. Comparison between Patients 70 and Older to Patients 60–69 Years

In the second part of our study, we compared the results after kidney transplantation in a subgroup of recipients 70 years and older ($n = 100$) to the remaining cohort of 60–69 year old patients ($n = 493$). Apart from the differences in mean age, the mean donor age and proportion of male to female were both higher in the patients $\geq$70 years old. Other parameters, including primary disease proportion of patients with DM and IHD, degree of sensitization, interval of dialysis pretransplant, HLA DR match, donor gender, induction type, and re-transplant rate, were not significantly different between the two groups. Living donor rates were lower in the $\geq$70 year old patient group with 12.8% compared to 19.8% in the 60–69 year old group ($p = 0.016$) (Table 4).

Table 4. Characteristics of patients in groups 60–69 and ≥70 years old.

	Patients 60–69 Years Old $n = 493$	Patients ≥ 70 Years Old $n = 100$	p Value
Recipient age (years)	63.7 ± 2.8	72.3 ± 2.4	$p < 0.001$
Recipient Gender M/F (%)	77.4/22.6	67/33	0.027
Primary Disease (%)			0.359
HTN	11.1	16.0	
DM	30.2	27.0	
PCKD	12.5	11.0	
GN	8.5	9.0	
Pyelonephritis	4.0	2.0	
FSGS	6.0	5.0	
IgA nephropathy	4.2	0.0	
Other	9.3	12.0	
Unknown	14.2	18.0	
Diabetes (%)	42.9	43.0	0.942
IHD (%)	38.0	33.3	0.392
PRA class I (%)	8.0	5.3	0.355
PRA class II (%)	3.7	3.7	1.000
Time on dialysis (mo.)	52.5 ± 31.3	46.4 ± 34.8	0.115
HLA-B full-match (%)	5.3	0.0	0.013
HLA-DR full-match (%)	7.0	2.6	0.108
Re-transplantation (%)	7.3	5.1	0.558
Donor age (years)	52.4 ± 13.8	57.8 ± 12.2	$p < 0.001$
Donor gender M/F (%)	55.2/44.8	63/37	0.230
Donor type LD (%)	19.8	12.8	0.016
Induction (%)			0.129
IL-2 inhibitor	59.2	61.0	
ATG	29.5	36.0	
Desensitization	4.3	1.0	
(PP ± Rituximab)	7.0	2.0	
Cold ischemia time (hours)	10.0 ± 3.5	10.7 ± 4.1	0.263

HTN, hypertension; DM, diabetes mellitus; PCKD, polycystic kidney disease; GN, glomerulonephritis; FSGS, focal segmental glomerulosclerosis; IgA, immunoglobulin A; IHD, ischemic heart disease; PRA, panel reactive antibody, class I and II; HLA-B/DR match, human leukocyte antigen; IL-2 inhibitor, interleukin 2 inhibitor; ATG, anti-thymocyte globulin; PP, plasmapheresis.

Graft survival rates (Figure 4) at 1, 3, 5, and 10 years after transplant in patients 70 and older were 90.9%, 83.3%, 74.9%, and 36.1%, respectively, while in patients 60–69 years old, the survival rates were 89.1%, 81.8%, 74.3%, and 49.2% ($p = 0.251$), respectively. Patient survival rates (Figure 5) at 1, 3, 5, and 10 years after transplant were 92.8%, 84.7%, 78.1%, and 36.7% in the 70 and older group, and 93.9%, 87.9%, 81.1%, and 53.9% in the 60–69 year old group, respectively ($p = 0.046$). Estimated graft survival censored in death with functioning graft (Figure 6) at 1, 3, 5, and 10 years after transplant were 98.0%, 96.6%, 93.5%, and 89.8% in the ≥70 year old group compared to 94.1%, 90.7%, 87.6%, and 79.7% in the 60–69 years old group, $p = 0.092$.

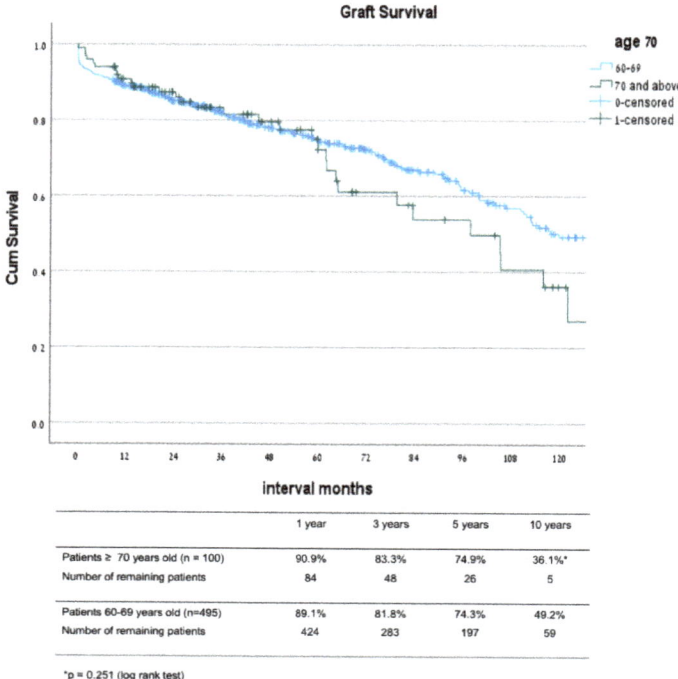

Figure 4. Graft survival: comparison between groups 60–69 and ≥70 years old.

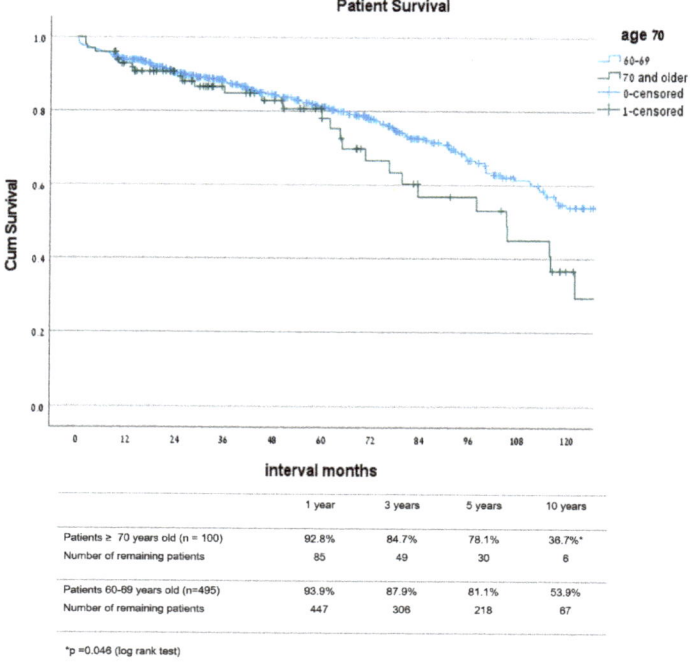

Figure 5. Patient survival: comparison between groups 60–69 and ≥70 years old.

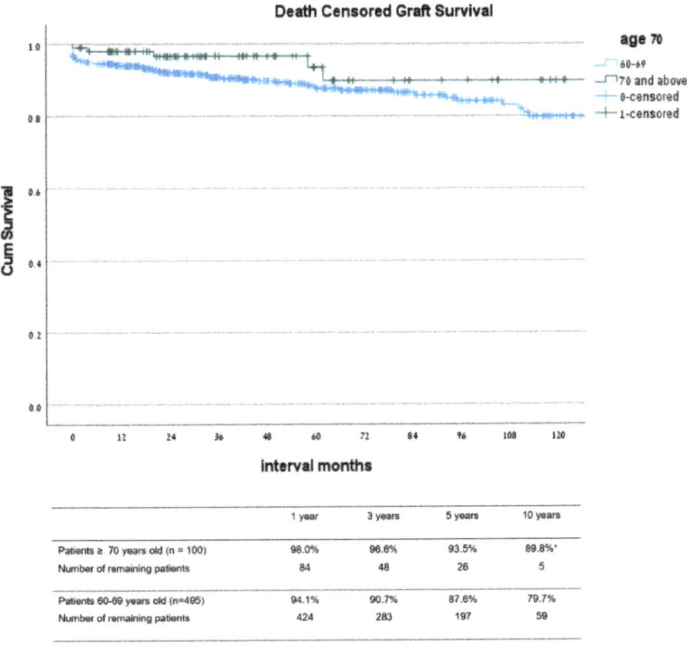

Figure 6. Estimated graft survival censored in death with functioning graft: comparison between groups 60–69 and ≥70 years old.

The rates of DGF, PNF, overall graft failure, death rates, length of hospital stay, and mean Cr levels at 1 month, 1 year, and 5 years after transplant were not different between the two groups (Table 5).

Table 5. Outcomes of patients in groups 60–69 and ≥70 years old.

	Patients 60–69 Years Old n = 493	Patients ≥ 70 Years Old n = 100	p Value
DGF (%)	28.5	32.0	0.746
PNF (%)	1.4	1.0	0.672
Graft failure (%)	32.5	32.0	0.929
Death (%)	27.6	31.0	0.493
Death with functioning graft (%)	17.9	26.0	0.054
Length of stay (days)	14.4 ± 19.4	14.0 ± 9.2	0.847
Cr 30 days (mg/dL)	1.76 ± 1.18	1.55 ± 0.67	0.084
Cr 1 year (mg/dL)	1.55 ± 1.09	1.38 ± 0.38	0.068
Cr 5 years (mg/dL)	1.77 ± 1.75	1.61 ± 0.78	0.668

DGF, delayed graft function; PNF, primary nonfunction; Cr, creatinine.

4. Discussion

It is well documented that kidney transplantation offers a survival benefit in the elderly population when compared to dialysis, and that chronological age should not be a barrier for access to transplant [16]. In our large cohort study with a long follow up, a median of 5 years, the 5-year survival rates for live donor recipients were of 92.7% and for deceased donor recipients >70%, which were better than the expected survival if remaining on dialysis. In our group of patients older than 70 years, the 3- and 5-survival rates were 84.7% and 78.1%, respectively, and were slightly lower than those for patients a decade younger. However, in our multivariate Cox regression analysis, age remained an important factor affecting survival, as expected with increased risk of death with a functioning graft in advanced age, as seen in our study. Kidney transplantation from deceased donors >65 or older is associated with suboptimal patient and graft survival. Nevertheless, when compared to patients remaining on dialysis there is reduced risk for death [17]. In a study published by Loveras et al., a paired survival analysis between recipients of kidneys from DD older than 65 with that of their paired patients on maintenance dialysis. They observed that patient and graft survival was reduced with the increasing age of the donor and recipient. Moreover, elderly recipients of these old kidneys had a reduced risk of death-censored graft failure compared to younger recipients of these grafts [18]. On the other hand, it has been reported that old recipients of young donor kidneys show graft survival exceeding patient survival, which means a significant graft-years loss [19].

Historically, there has been reluctance to use living donor transplants for older adults given their inherent limited life span. However, recent data suggest that living donor kidneys might be the best treatment option for elderly transplant recipients, just as it is for younger individuals [20]. Molnar et al. compared the association of ECD kidney and living kidney donation across different ages, including elderly recipients. They concluded that living donor kidney appears to be associated with greater survival across all age groups, including the elderly, although the significantly lower transplant loss rate is observed mainly in those younger than 70 years. Hence, they suggested that the elderly patients with ESRD gain years of life if they receive a kidney transplant, in particular from a living donor. Other data indicate that elderly transplant recipients have a 41% lower overall risk of death compared with wait-listed candidates [21]. Kidney donation from the patient's children in this age group may often be the only option, although it is not always accepted by the parent. Alternatively, a kidney donation from an older donor of the same age group should be considered. There are reports of good outcomes when using a graft from elderly living donors [22,23]. Given the relatively high probability of a poor outcome for older patients on the wait list, living donor transplantation, even with a donor 65 years or older, is preferable to waiting for a standard criteria deceased donor transplant [24]. Similar to previous reports in our study when comparing the outcome between three groups, live-donor and two groups of deceased donors also found a significant better patient and graft survival in the group of live donor recipients. These differences could be explained by the younger donor age, shorter duration of dialysis, and shorter cold ischemia in that group. Indeed, a Cox regression analysis including all these variables the type of donor remained the most significant variable affecting survival with HR of 2.865 (CI 1.910–4.297) for patient survival and 6.064 (CI 2.315–15.881) for graft survival. This finding reflects a better graft quality in the LD group when compared to the quality of grafts of the two DD groups associated with significantly lower rates of DGF and PNF after transplant, as well as lower creatinine levels along the follow up.

Differences between these two groups might also be contributed to by the selection bias of recipients with a better condition. In our study, 25% of patients in the LD group were transplanted before initiation of dialysis, whereas the mean dialysis span between initiation of dialysis to transplant in the two DD groups was >5 years. It is known that the longer elderly patients are on dialysis the worse is their general condition and frailty score, mainly because of the progression of cardiovascular and metabolic bone disease [5]. Schold et al. showed that when accepting an ECD for an elderly patient who is more than 2 years old on dialysis, the survival benefit of transplant over dialysis is markedly lower [25].

In our study, cardiovascular disease was found to be a significant risk factor affecting both patient and graft survival after transplant. The hazard ratio for death was 1.773 (CI

1.241–2.532) and for graft loss 1.782 (CI 1.045–3.038). Similar findings were reported in a series from Brazil including 366 patients older than 60, where diabetes mellitus as a cause of renal failure had a hazard ratio (HR) of 1.507 (CI 1.038 to 2.189) for death after transplant [26]. Patient and graft survivals at 5 years in this series were 76.6% and 72.2% similar to the results in our series. The incidence of major cardiac events is maximal during the first month after transplantation, associated with the stress of surgery, fluid resuscitation and infectious complications associated with hemodynamic instability. To address that problem and lower the cardiovascular risk, there is a need to prepare those candidates with known IHD and to manage them in collaboration with a cardiologist familiar with transplantation. Revascularization of asymptomatic IHD does not reduce risks of mortality for people with type 2 diabetes nor in those undergoing major vascular surgery [27,28]. There are no contemporary data in ESRD to determine whether revascularization is helpful or harmful overall; however, the risks of revascularization in ESRD are higher than for the general population. Given these uncertainties, there is a recommendation for screening candidates at high risk for IHD at time of evaluation, in order to guide medical management and inform risk [29,30].

In our series, 29.7% of the patients had diabetic nephropathy as the cause for ESRD and their overall death rate along the follow up was 32.4% compared to 21.8% in the remaining cohort. Moreover, DM was associated with HR of 1.773 for death after transplant. Indeed, previous studies have also shown that diabetes mellitus is associated with lower graft and patient survival after transplant in the elderly population. The rationale behind allocation programs based on age matching between donors and elderly recipients was based on utility considerations. Despite lower survival rates when using ECD donors for that population, the survival advantage benefit over wait-list patients has been shown in previous reports. In a report of 244 patients transplanted along the two decades of the ESP program, patient survival rates at 1, 5, and 10 years were 91.7%, 66.3% and 38%, respectively. Death censored graft survival for the same intervals were 93.3%, 82.6%, and 70.4%, respectively [31]. In the US, where allocation system is based on match between ECD kidneys having a high KDPI and patient risk score, a gain in survival over staying on dialysis is seen when ECD kidneys with high KDPI are transplanted in high-risk patients [32]. In a study to predict survival after transplant the authors combined two scores, the estimated patient post-transplant survival (EPTS) score and KDPI score. An Estimated Post Transplant Survival (EPTS) score is assigned to all adult candidates on the kidney waiting list and is based on four factors: time on dialysis, current diagnosis of diabetes, prior solid organ transplants, and age. The score is associated with how long the candidate will need a functioning kidney transplant when compared with other candidates [33]. As for candidates with an EPTS score of 80, 5-year waitlist survival was 47.6%, and 5-year post-KT survival was 78.9% after receiving kidneys with a KDPI of 20% and was 70.7% after receiving kidneys with a KDPI of 80%. The impact of KDPI on survival benefit varied greatly by EPTS score. For candidates with low EPTS scores (e.g, 40), survival benefit decreased with a higher KDPI but was still substantial even with a KDPI of 100% (>16 percentage points) [34].

In our study, the group of "old-to-old" had a patient survival of 1, 5, and 10 years of 91.0%, 73.3%, and 42.8%, respectively. Death censored graft survival rates in the same intervals were 90.4%, 79.7%, and 65.0%, reflecting comparable results of the ESP program. When evaluating the results in our patient population of 70 years and older, patient survival at 1- and 5- years were no different from the younger cohort, with the drop to 36.7% at 10 years, which is explained by their death for aging and associated comorbidities. No difference in graft survival was seen between these two groups. This is despite a younger donor age and in the 60–69 year old group (52.4 ± 13.8 and 57.8 ± 12.2, respectively, $p < 0.0001$) and a lower proportion of live donor. Yet, on the long term, about 30% of these patients are dying with a functioning graft, a death that is associated mostly with their cardiovascular comorbidities [29].

In a study calculating the costs of transplant in the elderly population assuming a 2-year wait-listed time, transplantation remained economically attractive for 70 years old patients incremental cost effectiveness (ICE), $79,359 per quality-adjusted life years (QALY), but was less economically attractive for those over 75 years of age (ICE, $99,553) or for 70 years old with either cardiovascular disease or diabetes (ICE, $126,751 and $161,090 per QALY, respectively) [7]. The authors concluded that transplantation compared with dialysis continues to increase life expectancy at an advanced age, but it does so at an increased cost. The data also show that for the older patients, the attractiveness of transplantation is highly sensitive to the time spent waiting for the transplant.

In our series, elderly patients who received DD kidney had a high rate of delayed graft function (~40%) requiring dialysis and a long mean hospital stay (16 days). Although the DGF rate was significantly lower in the LD group (9.7%), the length of mean hospital stay was still relatively long (12.5 days), which explains the higher costs associated of transplantation in that age group. Nevertheless, LD kidney transplantation even when using a match-age donor in our study, as well as in other previous reports, has shown favorable outcomes associated with prolonged survival and therefore should be advocated whenever possible.

The strength of our study is its large cohort of elderly patients with a long follow-up with a mean duration of 68 months. Moreover, this is a single center study with a uniform recipient and immunosuppressive protocol with minimal changes overtime and a steady donor screening. In addition, all patients had their follow-up throughout the whole period at our nephrology clinic.

However, our study has several limitations that bear mention. First, it is retrospective in design. Second, there are some missing data parameters such as dialysis interval prior to transplant and rejection episodes. There is a selection bias with living donor candidates being carefully selected immediately before their elective transplant, while DD transplants are urgent procedures. Annual evaluation of DD KT candidates enables the deterioration of existing comorbidities or the increase of new medical problems. As a consequence, some of the urgent DD KT are done under sub optimal conditions rather than aborting after years on the waitlist. The differences between LD and DD transplants makes them unmatched. Lastly, we did not use a frailty score in our study, a factor that is well known to influence outcome after transplant in the elderly population [5].

In summary, in our study of KT in elderly patients >60 years with a mean follow up of 5.6 years, we showed comparable results of the "old-to-old" program to those reported in the literature. In the whole patient cohort, patient survival was independent of donor age, while recipient age and comorbidities were significant factors affecting outcome in that age group. Donor age was a risk factor of graft loss with HR of 1.025 (1.00–1.051) in that age group, reflecting the importance of graft quality within the high-risk population. The results after LD transplantation were significantly better, a finding that is explained by favorable donor and recipient factors, such as shorter dialysis duration and cold ischemia, as well as younger donor age. Risk factors for death are donor type, recipient age, and presence of DM and IHD. Whereas risk factors for graft loss are IHD, donor type (DD/LD), and donor age. Finally, age was found to be a significant factor affecting graft and patient survivals in multifactorial regression analysis, within the older group of patients $\geq$70 years results after transplant were acceptable and not different to those of patients in the former decade of life.

5. Conclusions

Our results support continuous practice of the old-to old allocation policy based on utility considerations. However, whenever live donor transplantation is available, it should be encouraged. Transplant candidacy of elderly patients should be based on the patient's general condition, performance, and cognitive status, as well as their predicted life expectancy.

Author Contributions: Conceptualization, R.Y. and E.M.; methodology, E.M. and R.R; software, E.M.; validation, R.R., E.M. and R.Y.; formal analysis, R.Y., E.M. and R.G.; investigation, R.R. and R.Y.; resources, R.G.; data curation, E.M.; writing—original draft preparation, R.Y. and E.M.; writing—review and editing, E.M., R.R., and R.G.; visualization, R.G.; supervision, E.M.; project administration, R.Y. All authors have read and agreed to the published version of the manuscript.

Funding: This research received no external funding.

Institutional Review Board Statement: The study was conducted according to the guidelines of the Declaration of Helsinki, and approved by the Institutional Review Board of Beilinson Medical Center (0606-18/08.2018).

Informed Consent Statement: Patient consent was waived due to the retrospective and non-interventional design of the study.

Data Availability Statement: The datasets used and/or analyzed during the current study are available from the corresponding author upon reasonable request.

Conflicts of Interest: The authors declare no conflict of interest.

References

1. Hart, A.; Smith, J.M.; Skeans, M.A.; Gustafson, S.K.; Wilk, A.R.; Castro, S.; Foutz, J.; Wainright, J.L.; Snyder, J.J.; Kasiske, B.L.; et al. OPTN/SRTR 2018 annual data report: Kidney. *Am. J. Transplant.* **2020**, *20*, 20–130. [CrossRef] [PubMed]
2. Kasiske, B.L.; Cangro, C.B.; Hariharan, S.; Hricik, D.E.; Kerman, R.H.; Roth, D.; Rush, D.N.; Vazquez, M.A.; Weir, M.R.; American Society of Transplantation. The evaluation of renal transplantation candidates—Clinical practice guidelines. *Am. J. Transplant.* **2001**, *1*, 3–95. [PubMed]
3. Wolfe, R.A.; Ashby, V.B.; Milford, E.L.; Ojo, A.O.; Ettenger, R.E.; Agodoa, L.Y.C.; Held, P.J.; Port, F.K. Comparison of mortality in all patients on dialysis, patients on dialysis awaiting transplantation, and recipients of a first cadaveric transplant. *N. Engl. J. Med.* **1999**, *341*, 1725–1730. [CrossRef]
4. Rao, P.S.; Merion, R.M.; Ashby, V.B.; Port, F.K.; Wolfe, R.A.; Kayler, L.K. Renal transplantation in elderly patients older than 70 years of age: Results from the scientific registry of transplant recipients. *Transplantation* **2007**, *83*, 1069–1074. [CrossRef] [PubMed]
5. Harhay, M.N.; Rao, M.K.; Woodside, K.J.; Johansen, K.L.; Lentine, K.L.; Tullius, S.G.; Parsons, R.F.; Alhamad, T.; Berger, J.; Cheng, X.S.; et al. An overview of frailty in kidney transplantation: Measurement, management and future considerations. *Nephrol. Dial. Transpl.* **2020**, *35*, 1099–1112. [CrossRef]
6. Dolla, C.; Naso, E.; Mella, A. Impact of type 2 diabetes mellitus on kidney transplant rates and clinical outcomes among waitlisted candidates in a single center European experience. *Sci. Rep.* **2020**, *10*, 1–7. [CrossRef]
7. Jassal, S.V.; Krahn, M.; Naglie, G.; Zaltzman, J.S.; Roscoe, J.M.; Cole, E.H.; Redelmeier, D.A. Kidney transplantation in the elderly: A decision analysis. *J. Am. Soc. Nephrol.* **2003**, *14*, 187–196. [CrossRef]
8. Heldal, K.; Hartmann, A.; Grootendorst, D.C.; de Jager, D.J.; Leivestad, T.; Foss, A.; Midtvedt, K. Benefit of kidney transplantation beyond 70 years of age. *Nephrol. Dial. Transpl.* **2009**, *25*, 1680–1687. [CrossRef]
9. Rosengard, B.R.; Feng, S.; Alfrey, E.J.; Zaroff, J.G.; Emond, J.C.; Henry, M.L.; Garrity, E.R.; Roberts, J.P.; Wynn, J.; Metzger, R.A.; et al. Report of the Crystal City meeting to maximize the use of organs recovered from the cadaver donor. *Am. J. Transplant.* **2002**, *2*, 701–711. [CrossRef]
10. Schlieper, G.; Ivens, K.; Voiculescu, A.; Luther, B.; Sandmann, W.; Grabensee, B. Eurotransplant senior program 'old for old': Results from 10 patients. *Clin. Transpl.* **2001**, *15*, 100–105. [CrossRef]
11. Weiss-Salz, I.; Mandel, M.; Galai, N.; Boner, G.; Mor, E.; Nakache, R.; Simchen, E.; Israeli Transplantation Consortium. Negative impact of "old-to-old" donations on success of cadaveric renal transplants. *Clin. Transpl.* **2005**, *19*, 372–376. [CrossRef] [PubMed]
12. Lavee, J.; Ashkenazi, T.; Gurman, G.; Steinberg, D. A new law for allocation of donor organs in Israel. *Lancet* **2010**, *375*, 1131–1133. [CrossRef]
13. Port, F.K.; Bragg-Gresham, J.L.; Metzger, R.A.; Dykstra, D.M.; Gillespie, B.W.; Young, E.W.; Delmonico, F.L.; Wynn, J.J.; Merion, R.M.; Wolfe, R.A.; et al. Donor characteristics associated with reduced graft survival: An approach to expanding the pool of kidney donors. *Transplantation* **2002**, *74*, 1281–1286. [CrossRef] [PubMed]
14. Tanriover, B.; Mohan, S.; Cohen, D.J. Kidneys at higher risk of discard: Expanding the role of dual kidney transplantation. *Am. J. Transplant.* **2014**, *14*, 404–415. [CrossRef] [PubMed]
15. A Guide to Calculating and Interpreting the Kidney Donor Profile Index (KDPI). 2020. Available online: https://optn.transplant.hrsa.gov/media/1512/guide_to_calculating_interpreting_kdpi.pdf (accessed on 23 March 2020).
16. Ojo, A.O.; Hanson, J.A.; Meier-Kriesche, H.-U.; Okechukwu, C.N.; Wolfe, R.A.; Leichtman, A.B.; Agodoa, L.Y.; Kaplan, B.; Port, F.K. Survival in recipients of marginal cadaveric donor kidneys compared with other recipients and wait-listed transplant candidates. *J. Am. Soc. Nephrol.* **2001**, *12*, 589–597. [CrossRef]
17. Crespo, M.; Pascual, J. Strategies for an expanded use of kidneys from elderly donors. *Transplantation* **2017**, *101*, 727–745. [CrossRef]

18. Lloveras, J.; Arcos, E.; Comas, J.; Crespo, M.; Pascual, J. A paired survival analysis comparing hemodialysis and kidney transplantation from deceased elderly donors older than 65 years. *Transplantation* **2015**, *99*, 991–996. [CrossRef] [PubMed]
19. Meier-Kriesche, H.-U.; Schold, J.D.; Gaston, R.S.; Wadstrom, J.; Kaplan, B. Kidneys from deceased donors: Maximizing the value of a scarce resource. *Am. J. Transpl.* **2005**, *5*, 1725–1730. [CrossRef]
20. Gill, J.; Bunnapradist, S.; Danovitch, G.M.; Gjertson, D.; Gill, J.S.; Cecka, M. Outcomes of kidney transplantation from older living donors. *Am. J. Kidney Dis.* **2008**, *52*, 541–552. [CrossRef]
21. Molnar, M.Z.; Streja, E.; Kovesdy, C.P.; Shah, A.; Huang, E.; Bunnapradist, S.; Krishnan, M.; Kopple, J.D.; Kalantar-Zadeh, K. Age and the associations of living donor and expanded criteria donor kidneys with kidney transplant outcomes. *Am. J. Kidney Dis.* **2012**, *59*, 841–848. [CrossRef] [PubMed]
22. Berger, J.C.; Muzaale, A.D.; James, N.; Hoque, M.O.; Wang, J.M.G.; Montgomery, R.A.; Massie, A.B.; Hall, E.C.; Segev, D.L. Living kidney donors ages 70 and older: Recipient and donor outcomes. *Clin. J. Am. Soc. Nephrol.* **2011**, *6*, 2887–2893. [CrossRef]
23. Young, A.; Kim, S.J.; Speechley, M.R.; Huang, A.; Knoll, G.; Prasad, G.V.R.; Treleaven, D.; Diamant, M.; Garg, A.X.; for the Donor Nephrectomy Outcomes Research (DONOR) Network. Accepting kidneys from older living donors: Impact on transplant recipient outcomes. *Am. J. Transplant.* **2011**, *11*, 743–750. [CrossRef]
24. Chang, P.; Gill, J.; Dong, J.; Rose, C.; Yan, H.; Landsberg, D.; Cole, E.H.; Gill, J.S. Article living donor age and kidney allograft half-life: Implications for living donor paired exchange programs. *Clin. J. Am. Soc. Nephrol.* **2012**, *7*, 835–841. [CrossRef] [PubMed]
25. Schold, J.D.; Meier-Kriesche, H.-U. Which renal transplant candidates should accept marginal kidneys in exchange for a shorter waiting time on dialysis? *Clin. J. Am. Soc. Nephrol.* **2006**, *1*, 532–538. [CrossRef]
26. Orlandi, P.F.; Cristelli, M.P.; Aldworth, C.A.R.; Freitas, T.V.D.S.; Felipe, C.R.; Júnior, H.T.S.; Pestana, J.O.M.D.A. Long-term outcomes of elderly kidney transplant recipients. *J. Bras. Nefrol.* **2015**, *37*, 212–220. [CrossRef] [PubMed]
27. Kidney Disease: Improving Global Outcomes (KDIGO) Kidney Transplant Candidate Work Group. KDIGO Clinical Practice Guideline on the Evaluation and Management of Candidates for Kidney Transplantation. *Transplantation* **2020**, *104*, S11–S103. [CrossRef] [PubMed]
28. McFalls, E.O.; Ward, H.B.; Moritz, T.E.; Goldman, S.; Krupski, W.C.; Littooy, F.; Pierpont, G.; Santilli, S.; Rapp, J.; Hattler, B.; et al. Coronary-artery revascularization before elective major vascular surgery. *N. Engl. J. Med.* **2004**, *351*, 2795–2804. [CrossRef]
29. Chadban, S.J.; Ahn, C.; Axelrod, D.A.; Foster, B.J.; Kasiske, B.L.; Kher, V.; Kumar, D.; Oberbauer, R.; Pascual, J.; Pilmore, H.L.; et al. Summary of the Kidney Disease: Improving Global Outcomes (KDIGO) clinical practice guideline on the evaluation and management of candidates for kidney transplantation. *Transplantation* **2020**, *104*, 708–714. [CrossRef]
30. Ibrahim, H.N.; Murad, D.N.; Knoll, G.A. Thinking Outside the Box: Novel Kidney Protective Strategies in Kidney Transplantation. *Clin. J. Am. Soc. Nephrol.* **2021**, *16*, 1–8. [CrossRef]
31. Schachtner, T.; Otto, N.M.; Reinke, P. Two decades of the Eurotransplant Senior Program: The gender gap in mortality impacts patient survival after kidney transplantation. *Clin. Kidney J.* **2020**, *13*, 1091–1100. [CrossRef]
32. Jay, C.L.; Washburn, K.; Dean, P.G.; Helmick, R.A.; Pugh, J.; Stegall, M.D. Survival benefit in older patients associated with earlier transplant with high KDPI kidneys. *Transplantation* **2017**, *101*, 867–872. [CrossRef] [PubMed]
33. UNOS. Questions and Answers for Transplant Candidates about the Kidney Allocation System How Are Kidneys Classified? What Goes into a KDPI Score? Available online: www.unos.org (accessed on 13 October 2021).
34. Bae, S.; Massie, A.B.; Thomas, A.G.; Bahn, G.; Luo, X.; Jackson, K.; Ottmann, S.E.; Brennan, D.C.; Desai, N.M.; Coresh, J.; et al. Who can tolerate a marginal kidney? Predicting survival after deceased-donor kidney transplantation by donor-recipient combination. *Am. J. Transpl.* **2019**, *19*, 425–433. [CrossRef] [PubMed]

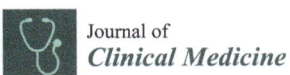 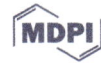

Article

Intraoperative Near-Infrared Spectroscopy Monitoring of Renal Allograft Reperfusion in Kidney Transplant Recipients: A Feasibility and Proof-of-Concept Study

Hien Lau [1], Alberto Jarrin Lopez [1], Natsuki Eguchi [1], Akihiro Shimomura [1], Antoney Ferrey [2], Ekamol Tantisattamo [2], Uttam Reddy [2], Donald Dafoe [1] and Hirohito Ichii [1,*]

Citation: Lau, H.; Lopez, A.J.; Eguchi, N.; Shimomura, A.; Ferrey, A.; Tantisattamo, E.; Reddy, U.; Dafoe, D.; Ichii, H. Intraoperative Near-Infrared Spectroscopy Monitoring of Renal Allograft Reperfusion in Kidney Transplant Recipients: A Feasibility and Proof-of-Concept Study. *J. Clin. Med.* **2021**, *10*, 4292. https://doi.org/10.3390/jcm10194292

Academic Editor: Eytan Mor

Received: 25 August 2021
Accepted: 19 September 2021
Published: 22 September 2021

Publisher's Note: MDPI stays neutral with regard to jurisdictional claims in published maps and institutional affiliations.

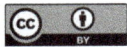

Copyright: © 2021 by the authors. Licensee MDPI, Basel, Switzerland. This article is an open access article distributed under the terms and conditions of the Creative Commons Attribution (CC BY) license (https://creativecommons.org/licenses/by/4.0/).

[1] Division of Transplantation, Department of Surgery, University of California, Irvine, CA 92868, USA; hlau3@hs.uci.edu (H.L.); ajarrinl@hs.uci.edu (A.J.L.); neguchi@hs.uci.edu (N.E.); shimo-mu@kid.med.osaka-u.ac.jp (A.S.); ddafoe@hs.uci.edu (D.D.)
[2] Division of Nephrology, Hypertension and Kidney Transplantation, Department of Medicine, University of California, Irvine, CA 92868, USA; ferreya@hs.uci.edu (A.F.); etantisa@hs.uci.edu (E.T.); ureddy@hs.uci.edu (U.R.)
*   Correspondence: hichii@hs.uci.edu

Abstract: Conventional renal function markers are unable to measure renal allograft perfusion intraoperatively, leading to delayed recognition of initial allograft function. A handheld near-infrared spectroscopy (NIRS) device that can provide real-time assessment of renal allograft perfusion by quantifying regional tissue oxygen saturation levels (rSO_2) was approved by the FDA. This pilot study evaluated the feasibility of intraoperative NIRS monitoring of allograft reperfusion in renal transplant recipients (RTR). Intraoperative renal allograft rSO_2 and perfusion rates were measured in living (LDRT, $n = 3$) and deceased donor RTR (DDRT, $n = 4$) during the first 50 min post-reperfusion and correlated with renal function markers 30 days post-transplantation. Intraoperative renal allograft rSO_2 for the DDRT group remained significantly lower than the LDRT group throughout the 50 min. Reperfusion rates were significantly faster in the LDRT group during the first 5 min post-reperfusion but remained stable thereafter in both groups. Intraoperative rSO_2 were similar among the upper pole, renal hilum, and lower pole, and strongly correlated with allograft function and hemodynamic parameters up to 14 days post-transplantation. NIRS successfully detected differences in intraoperative renal allograft rSO_2, warranting future studies to evaluate it as an objective method to measure ischemic injury and perfusion for the optimization of preservation/reperfusion protocols and early prediction of allograft function.

Keywords: clinical research practice; near-infrared spectroscopy; kidney transplantation; initial allograft function; intraoperative; tissue oxygen saturation

1. Introduction

Kidney transplantation (KT) is the treatment of choice for patients with end-stage renal disease due to the improved prognosis and quality of life compared to maintenance dialysis [1]. The current supply of donor kidneys has not met the demand for KT [2]. While living donor renal transplants (LDRT) generally have better outcomes, deceased donor kidneys have been the majority organs supplied for transplant in the United States [3]. In comparison to LDRT, deceased donor renal transplants (DDRT) generally have worse allograft function, a higher rate of complications, and longer hospital stay during the early post-transplant period [4,5]. Moreover, slow initial allograft function has been correlated with an increased risk of acute rejection, higher incidence of long-term allograft loss, and worse patient survival [4,6–8]. Therefore, prompt evaluation and treatment are crucial to optimize allograft perfusion and minimize ischemic insult, leading to better allograft function.

Up to now, conventional laboratory markers, such as serum creatinine, urine output in donors and cold ischemic time (CIT) are widely used to predict initial allograft function [9]. However, there are very limited reliable intraoperative methods to assess real-time allograft condition, resulting in late detection of slow allograft function and injury during the early post-transplant period [10]. Furthermore, transplant surgeons currently evaluate and predict initial allograft function in the critical early post-transplantation period through the assessment of color, texture, and capillary refill after reperfusion of the allograft, which is highly subjective and varies greatly based on the surgeons' experience. Due to the severe shortage of organs, marginal kidneys, which are defined as having a higher percent kidney-donor profile index, are increasingly being transplanted. For this reason, the development of a marker for the early evaluation of allograft quality, which can reliably predict slow allograft function, will assist physicians in the adjustment of therapeutic management, and improve allograft function, thus limiting further allograft injury during the immediate posttransplant period [3,11].

Near-infrared spectroscopy (NIRS) devices can measure regional tissue oxygen saturation levels (rSO_2) and provide real-time assessment of tissue perfusion based on differences in light-absorbing properties of oxygenated and deoxygenated hemoglobin [12]. The perfusion of kidney allografts measured by a NIRS monitor following pediatric KT has recently been shown to be significantly correlated to the current gold standard, Doppler ultrasound [13]. During the 72-h posttransplantation period, continuous renal NIRS measurements were strongly correlated with serum creatinine and eGFR in pediatric KT recipients [14]. Despite the proven benefits, the utilization of NIRS devices to monitor allograft perfusion has not been investigated intraoperatively because of their inconveniently bulky size and in adult KT due to the large skin-to-kidney distance [15]. A wireless, non-invasive, and handheld NIRS device was recently developed and approved by the FDA; however, its use has only been studied in porcine skin flap and bowel models [16–18] to our knowledge.

As measuring renal allograft rSO_2 levels intraoperatively with a handheld NIRS device can circumvent the distance limitation and offer an objective method for the early assessment of allograft reperfusion, this pilot study examined the feasibility of intraoperative NIRS monitoring in KT recipients by comparing intraoperative allograft rSO_2 levels between LDRT and DDRT and correlating these levels to conventional markers of renal function during the first 30 days after KT.

2. Materials and Methods

2.1. Patients Eligibility and Study Design

In this prospective study, adults >18 years of age undergoing either LDRT or DDRT were randomly recruited between September 2018 and March 2020 at the University of California, Irvine Medical Center. The study was approved by the research ethics committee at the University of California Irvine Institutional Review Board (protocol # 2018-4395). Written informed consent was obtained from all participants prior to participation. All methods were carried out in accordance with relevant guidelines and regulations. The study was conducted according to the principles of the Declaration of Helsinki and Istanbul.

2.2. Near-Infrared Spectroscopy Measurements

Intraoperative monitoring of renal allograft reperfusion was performed using a handheld, non-invasive, and FDA-approved NIRS tissue oximetry sensor device (Intra.Ox, ViOptix, Inc. Newark, CA, USA) that can provide real-time and instantaneous rSO_2 measurements [16,18]. During the surgical procedure, rSO_2 levels were measured pre- and post-reperfusion (i.e., removal of vascular clamps) at 3, 5, 10, and 20 min by placing the device directly over three regions of the allograft: upper pole (UP), renal hilum (RH), and lower pole (LP). NIRS measurements were also taken at 30 and 50 min. The mean arterial pressure of all participants was adjusted to approximately 80–90 mmHg. To optimize the accuracy of rSO_2 measurements and minimize external light interference, bloodstains on the allograft were cleaned with laparotomy sponges, and surgical lights were moved away before each measurement.

2.3. Laboratory Measurements

Serum creatinine, blood urea nitrogen (BUN), urine output, systolic blood pressure (BP), and mean arterial pressure (MAP) were measured preoperatively (pre-op) and on postoperative days (POD) 1, 3, 7, 14 and 30 as part of their standard-of-care clinic visits. The estimated glomerular filtration rate (eGFR) was calculated as previously described [19].

2.4. Statistical Analysis

Data normality was analyzed using a Shapiro–Wilk test. Normally distributed continuous variables, including age, weight, height, CIT, length of hospital stay, rSO_2 levels, systolic BP, and MAP, are expressed as mean ± standard error of the mean (SEM). Median and range are used to present continuous variables with a non-normal distribution. The categorical variable, gender, was described as percentages and analyzed using a chi-square test. An unpaired two-tailed t-test was used to compare continuous variables with a normal distribution, while non-normally distributed continuous variables were compared using a two-sided Mann-Whitney U test. The differences in rSO_2 levels among three regions were analyzed in both groups using a one-way analysis of variance (ANOVA) with Bonferroni correction for multiple comparisons. Linear regression analysis was performed to construct trend lines and estimate the rates of change in rSO_2 levels from pre-reperfusion to 5 min post-reperfusion and from 20 to 50 min post-reperfusion. Comparisons of rates of change in rSO_2 levels per minute between two groups were conducted using an analysis of covariance (ANCOVA). The average rSO_2 levels post-reperfusion at 3, 5, 10, and 20 min were correlated to conventional markers of renal function, including serum creatinine, eGFR, BUN, and urine output, using a non-parametric Spearman's correlation coefficient test and to hemodynamic parameters related to allograft perfusion, including systolic BP and MAP, using a parametric Pearson's correlation coefficient test. A $p < 0.05$ was defined as statistically significant. All statistical analyses were performed using SPSS Statistics 25 (IBM SPSS, Chicago, IL, USA).

3. Results

3.1. Characteristics of Living and Deceased Renal Transplant Recipients

Of the seven KT recipients randomly recruited, three recipients underwent LDRT and four recipients received DDRT. Both groups had no differences in age, gender, weight, and height (Table 1). There was no significant difference in the length of hospital stay between the two groups (LDRT: 6.3 ± 1.3 days vs. DDRT: 7.5 ± 1.2 days; $p = 0.545$) (Table 1). The average CIT were 2.2 ± 0.1 h in LDRT and 25.3 ± 1.4 h in DDRT ($p = 0.057$) (Table 1).

Table 1. Characteristics of living and deceased donor renal transplant recipients.

	LDRT ($n = 3$)	DDRT ($n = 4$)	p-Value
Age (years)	38.0 ± 9.2	59.5 ± 3.5	0.057
Female, n (%)	1 (33.3%)	1 (25.0%)	0.999
Weight (kg)	69.2 ± 9.5	87.2 ± 7.2	0.183
Height (m)	1.6 ± 0.06	1.7 ± 0.01	0.761
Cold ischemic time (hours)	2.2 ± 0.1	25.3 ± 1.4	0.057
Hospital stay (days)	6.3 ± 1.3	7.5 ± 1.2	0.545

Data are expressed as mean ± standard error of the mean. LDRT: living donor renal transplant. DDRT: deceased donor renal transplant. ICU: intensive care unit.

3.2. Tissue Oxygen Saturation (rSO_2) Level at the UP, RH, and LP of the Kidney Allograft in Living and Deceased Donor Renal Transplants after Reperfusion

Allograft rSO_2 levels pre-reperfusion in two groups were not different at UP, RH, and LP (LDRT: 30.0 ± 4.2%, 30.0 ± 5.5%, 29.0 ± 1.5% vs. DDRT: 30.0 ± 2.3%, 35.8 ± 5.6%,

30.0 ± 2.8%, respectively) (Figure 1A–C). After the removal of vascular clamps, rSO$_2$ levels at UP of the allograft in LDRT group were significantly higher than DDRT group at 10 min, but not at 3, 5, or 20 min (LDRT: 61.3 ± 5.7%, 55.7 ± 3.4%, 61.7 ± 4.4%, 60.3 ± 5.0% vs. DDRT: 43.5 ± 3.6%, 41.3 ± 5.0%, 46.3 ± 5.3%, 47.0 ± 4.1%, respectively) (Figure 1A–C). At RH, rSO$_2$ levels in LDRT group were significantly higher than DDRT group at 3, 5, and 10 min after reperfusion, but not at 20 min (LDRT: 54.0 ± 2.0%, 60.0 ± 2.5%, 58.3 ± 4.2%, 59.3 ± 5.9% vs. DDRT: 37.5 ± 4.2%, 43.0 ± 3.2%, 44.3 ± 3.0%, 46.5 ± 3.2, respectively) (Figure 1A–C). When rSO$_2$ levels was measured at LP, LDRT group had significantly greater measurements than DDRT group at 5 and 10 min, but not at 3 and 20 min (LDRT: 55.7 ± 5.7%, 58.0 ± 2.5%, 55.0 ± 3.0%, 57.7 ± 5.2% vs. DDRT: 37.0 ± 2.5%, 41.0 ± 1.7%, 39.5 ± 5.4%, 43.3 ± 5.3%, respectively) (Figure 1A–C). Although the average rSO$_2$ levels at three regions were similar between two groups pre-reperfusion, these levels became significantly higher in LDRT group at 3-, 5-, 10-, and 20-min post-reperfusion (LDRT: 29.7 ± 2.1%, 54.9 ± 1.5%, 59.1 ± 2.4%, 59.2 ± 2.2%, 59.1 ± 2.7% vs. DDRT: 32.0 ± 2.2%, 39.4 ± 2.6%, 42.1 ± 2.3%, 42.9 ± 1.6%, 45.6 ± 2.3%, respectively) (Figure 1D). Even after 30- and 50-min post-reperfusion, LDRT group had significantly greater average rSO$_2$ levels at three regions (LDRT: 66.3 ± 2.0%, 63.2 ± 3.2% vs. DDRT: 46.0 ± 3.2%, 43.0 ± 4.6%, respectively) (Supplementary Figure S1A).

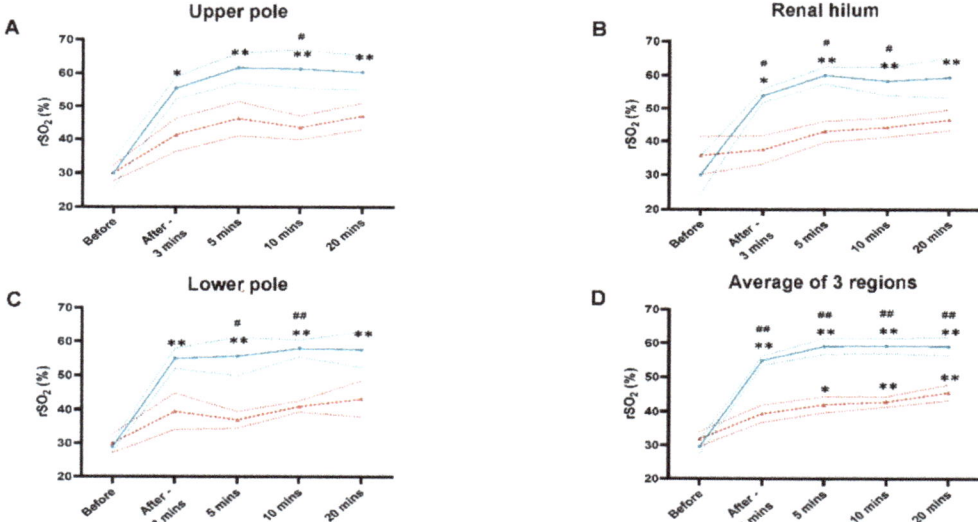

Figure 1. Tissue oxygen saturation (rSO$_2$) level curves of the kidney allograft in living ($n = 3$, solid turquoise line and closed circles) and deceased donor renal transplants ($n = 4$, dash red line and closed triangles) before and after 20 min (mins) of reperfusion. Tissue oxygen saturation levels of the kidney allograft in living and deceased donor renal transplants were measured at three regions (upper pole, renal hilum, and lower pole) using a handheld tissue oximetry sensor device before and after reperfusion at 3, 5, 10 and 20 min. (**A**) Tissue oxygen saturation level curves measured at the upper pole of the kidney allograft. (**B**) Tissue oxygen saturation level curves measured at the renal hilum of the kidney allograft. (**C**) Tissue oxygen saturation level curves measured at the lower pole of the kidney allograft. (**D**) Average tissue oxygen saturation level curves measured at three regions of the kidney allograft. * $p < 0.05$ vs. before reperfusion. ** $p < 0.01$ vs. before reperfusion. # $p < 0.05$ vs. deceased donor kidney allografts. ## $p < 0.01$ vs. deceased donor kidney allografts. Data are expressed as mean ± SEM.

In the LDRT group, rSO$_2$ levels measured at 3-, 5-, 10-, and 20-min post-reperfusion were significantly increased compared to the levels pre-reperfusion at all three regions (Figure 1A–C). However, these differences were not observed in the DDRT group as changes in rSO$_2$ levels at all three regions from pre-reperfusion to post-reperfusion at 3, 5, 10, and 20 min were not significant (Figure 1A–C). The average rSO$_2$ levels at three regions in the LDRT group were significantly greater post-reperfusion at 3, 5, 10, and 20 min compared to pre-reperfusion (Figure 1D). In the DDRT group, changes in rSO$_2$ levels from pre-reperfusion to post-reperfusion only reached statistical significance at 5, 10, and 20 min, but not at 3 min (Figure 1D). Moreover, the average rSO$_2$ levels at three regions in both groups had no significant changes from 5 to 50 min post-reperfusion (Supplementary Figure S1A).

To determine whether rSO$_2$ levels were higher at a particular region of the allograft, a comparison of measurements among three regions was performed and showed no significant differences at all-time points in both groups (Table 2)

Table 2. Comparison of tissue oxygen saturation (rSO$_2$) levels measured at three regions (upper pole, renal hilum, and lower pole) of the kidney allograft in either living or deceased donor renal transplants before and after reperfusion at 3, 5, 10 and 20 min.

	LDRT (n = 3)					DDRT (n = 4)				
	Before	After-3 min	5 min	10 min	20 min	Before	After-3 min	5 min	10 min	20 min
Upper pole (%)	30.0 ± 4.2	55.7 ± 3.4	61.7 ± 4.4	61.3 ± 5.7	60.3 ± 5.0	30.0 ± 2.3	41.3 ± 5.0	46.3 ± 5.3	43.5 ± 3.6	47.0 ± 4.1
Renal hilum (%)	30.0 ± 5.5	54.0 ± 2.0	60.0 ± 2.5	58.3 ± 4.2	59.3 ± 5.9	35.8 ± 5.6	37.5 ± 4.2	43.0 ± 3.2	44.3 ± 3.0	46.5 ± 3.2
Lower pole (%)	29.0 ± 1.5	55.0 ± 3.0	55.7 ± 5.7	58.0 ± 2.5	57.7 ± 5.2	30.0 ± 2.8	39.5 ± 5.4	37.0 ± 2.5	41.0 ± 1.7	43.3 ± 5.3
p-value	0.980	0.918	0.631	0.840	0.940	0.503	0.865	0.275	0.711	0.801

Data are expressed as mean ± SEM. LDRT: living donor renal transplant. DDRT: deceased donor renal transplant. mins: minutes.

3.3. Linear Regression Analysis of Tissue Oxygen Saturation (rSO$_2$) Levels of the Kidney Allograft in Living and Deceased Donor Renal Transplant after Reperfusion

In the DDRT group, the increase in average rSO$_2$ levels at three regions only achieved statistical significance after 5 min of reperfusion compared to 3 min in the LDRT group (Figure 1D). This indicated a slower reperfusion rate in the DDRT group; therefore, linear regression analysis of the increase in rSO$_2$ levels over 5 min of reperfusion was performed to compare the rates of increase in rSO$_2$ levels between two groups at all three regions (Figure 2A–D). While all trend lines of the increase in rSO$_2$ levels with time were positive, only three regions of the kidney allograft in LDRT group and UP of the allograft in DDRT group reached statistical significance (UP: $p < 0.001$, =0.019; RH: $p < 0.001$, =0.275; LP: $p = 0.004$, 0.187, respectively) (Figure 2A–C). Significantly positive trend lines of the increase in average rSO$_2$ levels at three regions over 5 min of reperfusion were observed in both groups ($p < 0.001$, = 0.003, respectively) (Figure 2D). A comparison of slopes of the trend lines revealed that the LDRT group had 1.98, 4.46-, and 3.63-times higher rates of increase in rSO$_2$ levels with time at UP, RH, and LP compared to the DDRT group, respectively (Table 3). Moreover, the rate of increase in the average rSO$_2$ levels at three regions in the LDRT group was 2.94 times higher than the DDRT group after 5 min of reperfusion (Table 3). Linear regression analysis further revealed that rates of change in average rSO$_2$ levels at three regions from 5 to 50 min post-reperfusion did not significantly differ from zero in both groups and were similar between these two groups (0.126%·min^{-1}, 0.034%·min^{-1}; $p = 0.103$, 0.673, 0.431, respectively) (Supplementary Figure S1B).

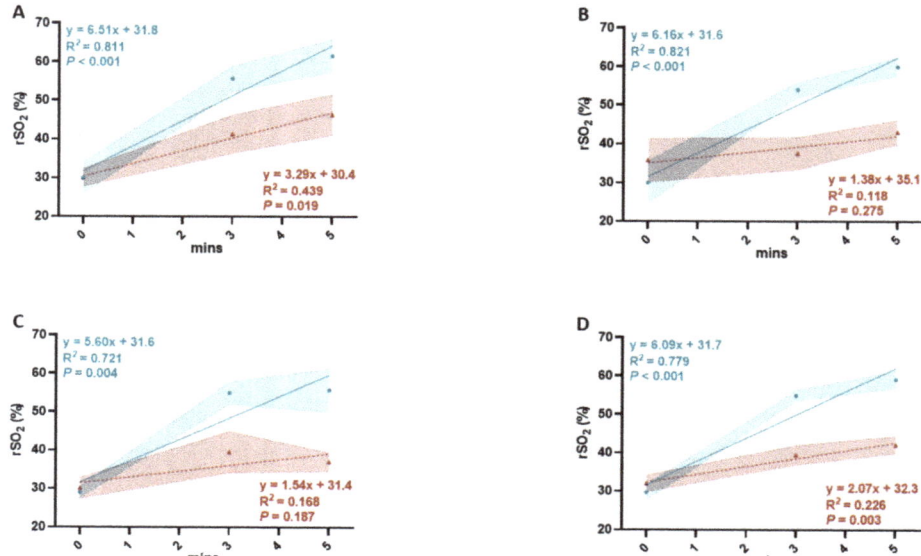

Figure 2. Linear regression analysis of tissue oxygen saturation (rSO$_2$) levels of the kidney allograft in living ($n = 3$, solid turquoise line and closed circles) and deceased donor renal transplants ($n = 4$, dash red line and closed triangles) over 5 min (mins) after reperfusion. Trend lines and R^2 coefficients of tissue oxygen saturation levels measured at three regions (upper pole, renal hilum, and lower pole) of the kidney allograft over 5 min of reperfusion in living and deceased donor renal transplants were calculated using linear regression analysis. (**A**) Trend lines and R^2 coefficients of tissue oxygen saturation levels measured at the upper pole of the kidney allograft. (**B**) Trend lines and R^2 coefficients of tissue oxygen saturation levels measured at the renal hilum of the kidney allograft. (**C**) Trend lines and R^2 coefficients of tissue oxygen saturation levels measured at the lower pole of the kidney allograft. (**D**) Trend lines and R^2 coefficients of average tissue oxygen saturation levels measured at three regions of the kidney allograft. Trend line equations, R^2 coefficients, and p-values for living and deceased donor renal transplants are displayed in matching colors. Data are expressed as mean ± SEM.

Table 3. Comparison of the rates of change in tissue oxygen saturation (rSO$_2$) levels per minute at three regions (upper pole, renal hilum, and lower pole) of the kidney allograft calculated from linear regression analysis over 5 min of reperfusion in living and deceased donor renal transplants.

	LDRT [95% CI]	DDRT [95% CI]	p-Value
Upper pole (%·min^{-1})	6.51 [3.70, 9.32]	3.29 [0.668, 5.91]	0.077
Renal hilum (%·min^{-1})	6.16 [3.58, 8.73]	1.38 [−1.29, 4.05]	0.011
Lower pole (%·min^{-1})	5.60 [2.49, 8.71]	1.54 [−0.879, 3.96]	0.028
Average of three regions (%·min^{-1})	6.09 [4.75, 7.42]	2.07 [0.734, 3.41]	<0.001

LDRT: living donor renal transplant. DDRT: deceased donor renal transplant. CI: confidence interval. %·min^{-1}: the change in the percentage of tissue oxygen saturation levels per minute.

3.4. Correlation of Averaged Tissue Oxygen Saturation (rSO$_2$) Levels Measured at UP, RH, LP of Kidney Allograft with Renal Function and Hemodynamic Parameters of Living and Deceased Donor Renal Transplants before and after Transplantation

A comparison of conventional markers related to renal function, including serum creatinine, eGFR, BUN, and urine output, on the pre-op day and POD 1, 3, 7, 14, and 30 indicated no significant differences between the two groups (Figure 3A–D). Hemodynamic parameters, including systolic BP and MAP, of the LDRT group, only became significantly higher than the DDRT group on POD 3 and were similar on the pre-op day as well as POD 1, 7, 14, and 30 (Figure 3E,F). Correlation analysis showed average rSO$_2$ levels at three regions correlated well with markers of renal function from POD 1 to 14 (Table 4). At 5 min post-reperfusion, average rSO$_2$ levels were significantly associated with a decrease in serum creatinine on POD 1 and 3 ($r = -0.93, -0.96$, respectively), an increase in eGFR on POD 1, 3, and 7 ($r = 0.93, 0.96, 0.89$, respectively), a decrease in BUN on POD 3 and 7 ($r = -0.86, -0.93$, respectively), and an increase in urine output on POD 1 ($r = 0.82$) (Table 4). Average rSO$_2$ levels at 10 min also showed a strong negative correlation with serum creatinine on POD 3 ($r = -0.89$), positive correlation with eGFR on POD 3 ($r = 0.89$), and negative correlation with BUN on POD 7 ($r = -0.86$). After 20 min of reperfusion, average rSO$_2$ levels were significantly correlated with a decrease in serum creatinine on POD 3 ($r = -0.86$), an increase in eGFR on POD 3, 7, and 14 ($r = 0.86, 0.86, 0.89$, respectively), a decrease in BUN on POD 3 and 7 ($r = -0.96, -0.93$, respectively), and an increase in urine output on POD 14 ($r = 0.79$). When correlated to hemodynamic parameters, average rSO$_2$ levels at three regions over 20 min of reperfusion showed a strong association from POD 1 to 14 (Table 4). At 3 min of reperfusion, average rSO$_2$ levels were significantly correlated with the increases in systolic BP and MAP on POD 1 ($r = 0.88, 0.83$) (Table 4). After 5 and 10 min of reperfusion, average rSO$_2$ levels were strongly associated with the increases in systolic BP and MAP on POD 3 ($r = 0.84, 0.84, 0.87, 0.76$, respectively) (Table 4). Moreover, average rSO$_2$ levels at 5- and 10-min post-reperfusion showed a strong negative correlation with systolic BP on POD 14 (5 min: $r = -0.79, -0.79$, respectively) (Table 4). At 20 min post-reperfusion, average rSO$_2$ levels were significantly associated with the increase in MAP on POD 3 ($r = 0.85$). After 30 days of KT, rSO$_2$ levels at all-time points were not significantly associated with any markers of renal function or hemodynamic parameters measured in the current study (Table 4).

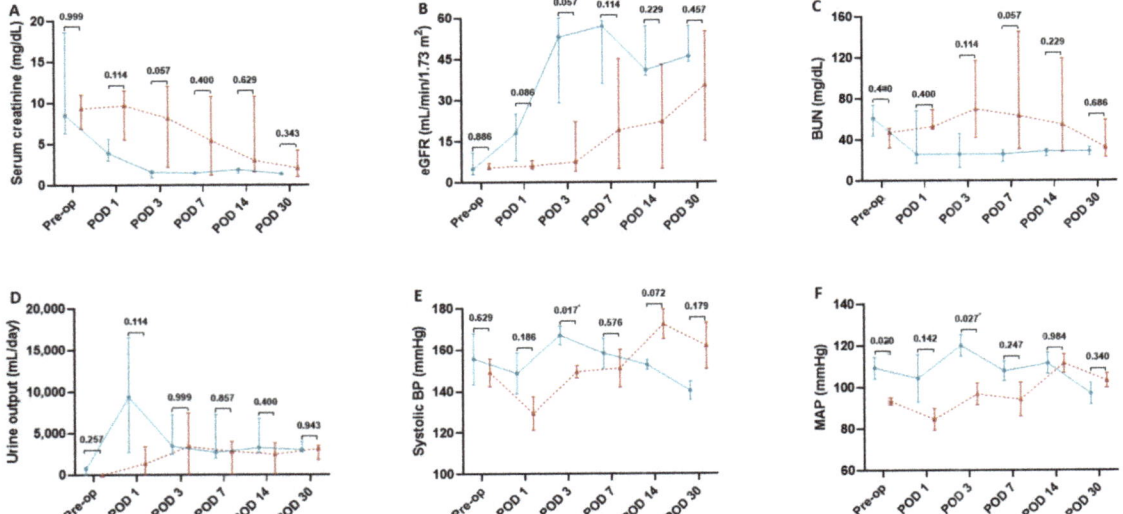

Figure 3. Renal function and hemodynamic parameters of living ($n = 3$, solid turquoise line and closed circles) and deceased donor renal transplants ($n = 4$, dash red line and closed triangles) before and after transplantation. Renal function and hemodynamic parameters of living and deceased donor renal transplants were measured preoperatively (pre-op) and on postoperative day (POD) 1, 3, 7, 14 and 30. (**A**) Serum creatinine levels. (**B**) Estimated glomerular filtration rate (eGFR). (**C**) Blood urea nitrogen levels (BUN). (**D**) Urine output. (**E**) Systolic blood pressure (BP). (**F**) Mean arterial pressure (MAP). The number above each time point represents the *p*-value of living vs. deceased donor renal transplants. * $p < 0.05$. Serum creatinine levels, eGFR, and BUN levels are expressed as median and range. Systolic BP and MAP are expressed as mean ± SEM.

Table 4. Correlation of averaged tissue oxygen saturation (rSO$_2$) levels measured at three regions (upper pole, renal hilum, and lower pole) of the kidney allograft with renal function and hemodynamic parameters before and after renal transplants.

		Average rSO$_2$ of 3 Regions After							
		3 min		5 min		10 min		20 min	
		r	p-Value	r	p-Value	r	p-Value	r	p-Value
Serum Creatinine (mg/dL)	POD 1	−0.57	0.180	−0.93 **	0.003	−0.71	0.071	−0.64	0.119
	POD 3	−0.71	0.071	−0.96 **	<0.001	−0.89 **	0.007	−0.86 *	0.014
	POD 7	−0.37	0.413	−0.70	0.077	−0.70	0.077	−0.52	0.233
	POD 14	−0.14	0.760	−0.39	0.383	−0.68	0.094	−0.36	0.432
	POD 30	−0.31	0.504	−0.63	0.129	−0.74	0.058	−0.41	0.355
eGFR (mL/min/1.73 m^2)	POD 1	0.66	0.111	0.93 **	0.003	0.75	0.054	0.63	0.139
	POD 3	0.71	0.071	0.96 **	<0.001	0.89 **	0.007	0.86 *	0.014
	POD 7	0.71	0.071	0.89 **	0.007	0.75	0.052	0.86 *	0.014
	POD 14	0.71	0.071	0.75	0.052	0.54	0.215	0.89 **	0.007
	POD 30	0.43	0.333	0.69	0.090	0.51	0.248	0.52	0.229
BUN (mg/dL)	POD 1	−0.29	0.535	−0.64	0.119	−0.36	0.432	−0.54	0.215
	POD 3	−0.68	0.094	−0.86 *	0.014	−0.71	0.071	−0.96 **	<0.001
	POD 7	−0.75	0.052	−0.93 **	0.003	−0.86 *	0.014	−0.93 **	0.003
	POD 14	−0.43	0.337	−0.61	0.148	−0.75	0.052	−0.61	0.148
	POD 30	−0.52	0.229	−0.22	0.641	−0.11	0.818	−0.51	0.248
Urine Output (mL/day)	POD 1	0.75	0.052	0.82 *	0.023	0.68	0.094	0.75	0.052
	POD 3	0.21	0.645	0.29	0.535	0.14	0.760	0.68	0.094
	POD 7	0.29	0.535	0.43	0.337	0.29	0.535	0.68	0.094
	POD 14	0.75	0.052	0.50	0.253	0.21	0.645	0.79 *	0.036
	POD 30	0.36	0.427	0.02	0.969	−0.23	0.613	0.16	0.728
Systolic BP (mmHg)	POD 1	0.88 **	0.009	0.49	0.261	0.24	0.611	0.53	0.218
	POD 3	0.42	0.343	0.84 *	0.018	0.87 *	0.011	0.47	0.288
	POD 7	0.50	0.259	0.15	0.743	0.18	0.704	0.12	0.805
	POD 14	−0.26	0.569	−0.79 *	0.034	−0.79 *	0.034	−0.65	0.115
	POD 30	−0.54	0.209	−0.52	0.229	−0.50	0.256	−0.45	0.317
MAP (mmHg)	POD 1	0.83 *	0.020	0.57	0.181	0.36	0.425	0.68	0.094
	POD 3	0.65	0.117	0.84 *	0.019	0.76 *	0.046	0.85 *	0.015
	POD 7	0.65	0.114	0.42	0.350	0.47	0.290	0.47	0.286
	POD 14	0.33	0.468	0.07	0.887	−0.11	0.815	0.47	0.289
	POD 30	−0.23	0.615	−0.37	0.411	−0.30	0.510	0.08	0.858

eGFR: estimated glomerular filtration rate. BUN: blood urea nitrogen. BP: blood pressure. MAP: mean arterial pressure. POD: postoperative day. * $p < 0.05$. ** $p < 0.01$.

4. Discussion

Current clinical and laboratory indices are inadequate for the early detection of slow kidney allograft function and injury during the immediate post-transplant period [20]. NIRS monitoring has been demonstrated to be an earlier predictor of acute kidney injury (AKI) after cardiac surgery, and, recently, used to measure the early postoperative allograft perfusion status in pediatric KT recipients [13,14,21]. However, no studies have explored the intraoperative application of NIRS monitoring in KT. The current pilot study examined the feasibility of intraoperative NIRS monitoring of kidney allografts by comparing intraoperative rSO$_2$ levels between LDRT and DDRT and correlating these levels to conventional markers of renal function in the first 30 days after KT. The major finding was that allografts from the LDRT recipients had significantly higher rSO$_2$ levels and faster rates of increase in rSO$_2$ levels than the DDRT recipients after reperfusion. Moreover, intraoperative rSO$_2$ levels were strongly correlated with renal function and hemodynamic parameters up until POD 14.

To our knowledge, this is the first study to establish a baseline renal allograft rSO$_2$ level measured intraoperatively with a handheld NIRS device, which was approximately 30% pre-reperfusion in both the LDRT and the DDRT recipients. This baseline value agrees with previous studies, concluding that a rSO$_2$ level of 30% or less represents significant free flap ischemia and requires operative correction [16,22]. The validity of this baseline value was further confirmed by the similarity between rSO$_2$ levels before reperfusion of KT recipients. Our results of the increase in rSO$_2$ levels post-reperfusion in both groups support others' observation that rSO$_2$ levels of rat kidneys with short and long CIT rose immediately post-reperfusion [23]. The novel findings that kidney allografts from LDRT had significantly higher intraoperative rSO$_2$ levels than DDRT post-reperfusion was expected since deceased donor kidney allografts generally suffered from prolonged ischemic injury and decreased microvascular flow [24]. This impairment in microvascular perfusion has been attributed to a 42% and 16% reduction of total blood flow volume and endothelial glycocalyx thickness in the peritubular capillary network [25]. Our data are in accordance with previous findings that kidneys with acute injury had significantly worse rSO$_2$ levels during cardiac surgery than those without acute injury [26]. Interestingly, Vidal et al. have shown renal allograft rSO$_2$ levels from POD 1 to 3 were comparable between pediatric LDRT and DDRT [14]. Furthermore, the increase in rSO$_2$ levels from POD 1 to 3 was not significantly different in recipients with or without delayed allograft function (DGF), indicating that the renal perfusion status was similar between two groups during the early postoperative course despite differences in kidney function [14]. These results suggest the slow initial allograft function is most likely due to the ischemic damage that occurred during organ preservation and reperfusion. As a recent study has reported a 20% decline in kidney rSO$_2$ levels from the baseline could predict hypoperfusion and AKI, a more than 20% difference in rSO$_2$ levels between LDRT and DDRT groups from 30 to 50 min post-reperfusion indicated that allografts in DDRT recipients were markedly under perfused [21]. Additionally, the immediate postoperative rSO$_2$ level has previously been demonstrated to be approximately 70% in kidney allografts of both pediatric LDRT and DDRT, including recipients with DGF [14]. Using this value as the baseline, the rSO$_2$ level of approximately 45% at 50 min after reperfusion in DDRT recipients represents substantial hypoperfusion and inadequate reperfusion capacity. This could explain why half of DDRT recipients in the current study experienced slow allograft function (serum creatinine > 1.5 mg/dL and creatinine reduction ratio < 20% between POD 1 and 3) while all LDRT recipients had immediate allograft function [7]. Intraoperative assessment of allograft reperfusion may offer a better objective method to evaluate the extent of ischemic injury and initial allograft function.

Allografts from LDRT recipients were observed to have faster rates of increase in rSO$_2$ levels up until 5 min post-reperfusion compared to DDRT recipients. This finding supports our observation that allografts in DDRT recipients required more time to reach higher rSO$_2$ levels post-reperfusion. In accordance with these results, rat kidneys with a longer CIT have been shown to have a slower rate of reperfusion compared to a shorter CIT [23]. Our findings that rSO$_2$ levels did not change significantly from 5 to 50 min and the rates of change in rSO$_2$ levels remained stable after 5 min of reperfusion is in line with previous studies [23,27]. Vaughan et al. has demonstrated that a sharp increase in rSO$_2$ levels during the first 10 min post-reperfusion in rats with a 45-min ischemia was followed by a flat rate of change in rSO$_2$ levels from 10 min to 4.5 h post-reperfusion [23]. Grosenick et al. have reported that rSO$_2$ levels in rat kidneys rose quickly within 3 min post-reperfusion and stayed unchanged until the end of the experiment [27]. The decrease in perfusion rates after the first few minutes of reperfusion could be because allografts from the LDRT recipients had significantly larger blood vessel diameter and higher microvascular blood flow velocity than the DDRT recipients at 5 min but not at 30 min after reperfusion [25]. As the reproducibility of NIRS monitoring has been proposed to be improved by at least two simultaneous measurements, our study found no differences in rSO$_2$ levels between the three regions in both groups [28]. Similarly, a previous study has shown postoperative rSO$_2$ levels of pediatric KT recipients were similar at the upper and lower poles [13]. Taken together, these findings confirm the responsiveness and validity of intraoperative NIRS monitoring to quantify changes in allograft reperfusion during the early reperfusion period.

In various clinical studies, NIRS monitoring has been reported to be an earlier indicator of renal hypoperfusion and acute injury compared to conventional makers of renal function [21,26,29]. Our findings of no significant differences in renal function measured between the LDRT and the DDRT recipients, except for higher intraoperative rSO$_2$ levels in the former group, are consistent with previous evidence, showing that infants who developed AKI from day 2 to 7 of life had significantly higher rSO$_2$ levels, but not serum creatinine and urine output, during the first 24 h of life compared to those without AKI [29]. Another study has reported intraoperative NIRS monitoring was an earlier predictor of AKI after pediatric cardiopulmonary bypass surgery than cystatin C and neutrophil gelatinase-associated lipocalin, which have been demonstrated to increase before significant changes in serum creatinine can be detected [26,30,31]. These findings are plausible as serum creatinine remains within the normal range until 50% of renal function is lost [32]. In concordance with the current results that indicated a strong association of intraoperative rSO$_2$ levels with renal function and hemodynamic indices, allograft rSO$_2$ levels have been correlated with serum creatinine, eGFR, urine output, and systolic BP during the early postoperative period [13,14,29,33]. As a recent study has utilized renal NIRS measurements to adjust fluid therapy in neonatal digestive surgeries, our findings strengthen the growing evidence that NIRS monitoring of allograft perfusion will assist to improve the current initial post-transplant management [34]. Although our pilot study demonstrated several significant correlations between intraoperative rSO$_2$ level with conventional markers of renal function, post-transplant urine output remains the most common biomarker that indicates improvement in allograft function at the immediate post-transplant period. Therefore, intraoperative rSO$_2$ level at 5 min post-reperfusion may assist clinicians to predict the signs of regaining early allograft function and appropriately modify volume management.

The limitation of our study is its small sample size, which did not allow sensitivity analysis by stratifying DDRT recipients based on CIT, warm ischemic time, the status of initial allograft function, death status, and preservation with or without machine perfusion because all these factors can impact reperfusion capacity and allograft outcomes [6,35–38]. Even though differences in intraoperative rSO$_2$ levels and reperfusion rates between two groups were statistically significant, evaluating intraoperative rSO$_2$ levels of allografts with varying severity of the ischemic injury will further validate intraoperative NIRS monitoring and identify cutoff values for the earlier prediction of initial allograft function. Since it is not yet feasible to reliably assess renal allograft rSO$_2$ levels in adult recipients after closure due to the large skin-to-kidney distance, the time required for rSO$_2$ levels of allografts from DDRT recipients to return to levels that are comparable to those of LDRT recipients could not be determined [15]. As variations in fluid therapy strategies have been shown to affect renal rSO$_2$ levels, changes in intraoperative rSO$_2$ levels due to different fluid and pharmacologic treatments were also not recorded [34].

In conclusion, this pilot study, to our best knowledge, is the first to show the feasibility of measuring renal allograft rSO$_2$ levels intraoperatively in KT recipients with a handheld NIRS device. Intraoperative NIRS monitoring was capable of detecting higher rSO$_2$ levels throughout 50 min of reperfusion and faster perfusion rates during the early reperfusion phase in kidney allografts of LDRT recipients compared to those of DDRT recipients. These values were similar between the three regions and strongly associated with conventional markers of renal function up to 14 days after transplantation. Since utilizing a handheld NIRS device offers the advantage of being able to measure renal allograft perfusion by direct contact immediately after reperfusion, future studies will evaluate its intraoperative use as an objective method to assess the ischemic injury and reperfusion capacity for the optimization of preservation/reperfusion protocols and early prediction of initial allograft function.

Supplementary Materials: The following are available online at https://www.mdpi.com/2077-0383/10/19/4292/s1, Figure S1: Curves and linear regression analysis of average tissue oxygen saturation (rSO$_2$) levels measured at three regions (upper pole, renal hilum, and lower pole) of the kidney allograft in living (solid turquoise line and closed circles, LDRT) and deceased donor renal transplants (dash red line and closed triangles, DDRT) from 5 min to 50 min (mins) after reperfusion.

Author Contributions: H.L. participated in research design, the performance of the research, writing the paper, and data analysis. A.J.L. participated in the writing of the article. N.E. participated in the writing of the article. A.S. participated in the research design and writing of the article. A.F. participated in the research design and writing of the article. E.T. participated in the research design and writing of the article. U.R. participated in the research design and writing of the article. D.D. participated in the research design and writing of the article. H.I. participated in the performance of research, research design, data analysis, and oversaw the project. All authors have read and agreed to the published version of the manuscript.

Funding: The authors declare no funding was received for this study.

Institutional Review Board Statement: This study was approved by the research ethics committee at the Institutional Review Board of University of California Irvine (protocol # 2018-4395 and the date of approval: 21 June 2018).

Informed Consent Statement: Informed consent was obtained from all subjects involved in the study.

Data Availability Statement: The data that support the findings of this study are available from the corresponding author upon request.

Acknowledgments: A handheld near-infrared spectroscopy (NIRS) device was provided from ViOptix, Inc. (Newark, CA, USA). The company did not have any control over the data or editing of the article.

Conflicts of Interest: The authors declare no conflict of interest.

Abbreviations

Abbreviations
AKI	acute kidney injury
BP	blood pressure
BUN	blood urea nitrogen
CIT	cold ischemic time
DDRT	deceased donor renal transplant
eGFR	estimated glomerular filtration rate
KT	kidney transplant
LDRT	living donor renal transplant
LP	lower pole
MAP	mean arterial pressure
NIRS	near-infrared spectroscopy
POD	postoperative day
RH	renal hilum
rSO$_2$	regional tissue oxygen saturation
UP	upper pole

References

1. Tonelli, M.; Wiebe, N.; Knoll, G.; Bello, A.; Browne, S.; Jadhav, D.; Klarenbach, S.; Gill, J. Systematic review: Kidney transplantation compared with dialysis in clinically relevant outcomes. *Am. J. Transplant.* **2011**, *11*, 2093–2109. [CrossRef]
2. Matas, A.J.; Smith, J.M.; Skeans, M.A.; Thompson, B.; Gustafson, S.K.; Schnitzler, M.A.; Stewart, D.E.; Cherikh, W.S.; Wainright, J.L.; Snyder, J.J.; et al. OPTN/SRTR 2012 Annual Data Report: Kidney. *Am. J. Transplant.* **2014**, *14* (Suppl. 1), 11–44. [CrossRef] [PubMed]
3. Heilman, R.L.; Mathur, A.; Smith, M.L.; Kaplan, B.; Reddy, K.S. Increasing the Use of Kidneys from Unconventional and High-Risk Deceased Donors. *Am. J. Transplant.* **2016**, *16*, 3086–3092. [CrossRef] [PubMed]
4. Zeraati, A.A.; Naghibi, M.; Kianoush, S.; Ashraf, H. Impact of slow and delayed graft function on kidney graft survival between various subgroups among renal transplant patients. *Transplant. Proc.* **2009**, *41*, 2777–2780. [CrossRef]
5. Guimarães, J.; Araújo, A.M.; Santos, F.; Nunes, C.S.; Casal, M. Living-donor and Deceased-donor Renal Transplantation: Differences in Early Outcome—A Single-center Experience. *Transplant. Proc.* **2015**, *47*, 958–962. [CrossRef]

6. Najarian, J.S.; Gillingham, K.J.; Sutherland, D.E.; Reinsmoen, N.L.; Payne, W.D.; Matas, A.J. The impact of the quality of initial graft function on cadaver kidney transplants. *Transplantation* **1994**, *57*, 812–816. [CrossRef]
7. Wang, C.J.; Tuffaha, A.; Phadnis, M.A.; Mahnken, J.D.; Wetmore, J.B. Association of Slow Graft Function with Long-Term Outcomes in Kidney Transplant Recipients. *Ann. Transplant.* **2018**, *23*, 224–231. [CrossRef]
8. Humar, A.; Ramcharan, T.; Kandaswamy, R.; Gillingham, K.; Payne, W.D.; Matas, A.J. Risk factors for slow graft function after kidney transplants: A multivariate analysis. *Clin. Transplant.* **2002**, *16*, 425–429. [CrossRef] [PubMed]
9. Bagshaw, S.M.; Gibney, R.T. Conventional markers of kidney function. *Crit. Care Med.* **2008**, *36* (Suppl. 4), S152–S158. [CrossRef] [PubMed]
10. Lohkamp, L.N.; Öllinger, R.; Chatzigeorgiou, A.; Illigens, B.M.; Siepmann, T. Intraoperative biomarkers in renal transplantation. *Nephrology* **2016**, *21*, 188–199. [CrossRef]
11. Keitel, E.; Michelon, T.; dos Santos, A.F.; Bittar, A.E.; Goldani, J.C.; D'Almeida Bianco, P.; Bruno, R.M.; Losekann, A.; Messias, A.A.; Bender, D.; et al. Renal transplants using expanded cadaver donor criteria. *Ann. Transplant.* **2004**, *9*, 23–24. [PubMed]
12. Murkin, J.M.; Arango, M. Near-infrared spectroscopy as an index of brain and tissue oxygenation. *Br. J. Anaesth* **2009**, *103* (Suppl. 1), i3–i13. [CrossRef] [PubMed]
13. Malakasioti, G.; Marks, S.D.; Watson, T.; Williams, F.; Taylor-Allkins, M.; Mamode, N.; Morgan, J.; Hayes, W.N. Continuous monitoring of kidney transplant perfusion with near-infrared spectroscopy. *Nephrol. Dial. Transplant.* **2018**, *33*, 1863–1869. [CrossRef] [PubMed]
14. Vidal, E.; Amigoni, A.; Brugnolaro, V.; Ghirardo, G.; Gamba, P.; Pettenazzo, A.; Zanon, G.F.; Cosma, C.; Plebani, M.; Murer, L. Near-infrared spectroscopy as continuous real-time monitoring for kidney graft perfusion. *Pediatr. Nephrol.* **2014**, *29*, 909–914. [CrossRef] [PubMed]
15. Scheeren, T.W.; Schober, P.; Schwarte, L.A. Monitoring tissue oxygenation by near infrared spectroscopy (NIRS): Background and current applications. *J. Clin. Monit. Comput.* **2012**, *26*, 279–287. [CrossRef]
16. Lohman, R.F.; Ozturk, C.N.; Djohan, R.; Tang, H.R.; Chen, H.; Bechtel, K.L. Predicting skin flap viability using a new intraoperative tissue oximetry sensor: A feasibility study in pigs. *J. Reconstr. Microsurg.* **2014**, *30*, 405–412.
17. Khavanin, N.; Qiu, C.; Darrach, H.; Kraenzlin, F.; Kokosis, G.; Han, T.; Sacks, J.M. Intraoperative Perfusion Assessment in Mastectomy Skin Flaps: How Close are We to Preventing Complications? *J. Reconstr. Microsurg.* **2019**, *35*, 471–478. [CrossRef]
18. Khavanin, N.; Almaazmi, H.; Darrach, H.; Kraenzlin, F.; Safar, B.; Sacks, J.M. Comparison of the ViOptix Intra.Ox Near Infrared Tissue Spectrometer and Indocyanine Green Angiography in a Porcine Bowel Model. *J. Reconstr. Microsurg.* **2020**, *36*, 426–431. [CrossRef] [PubMed]
19. Hameed, A.M.; Pleass, H.C.; Wong, G.; Hawthorne, W.J. Maximizing kidneys for transplantation using machine perfusion: From the past to the future: A comprehensive systematic review and meta-analysis. *Medicine* **2016**, *95*, e5083. [CrossRef] [PubMed]
20. Levey, A.S.; Stevens, L.A.; Schmid, C.H.; Zhang, Y.L.; Castro, A.F., III; Feldman, H.I.; Kusek, J.W.; Eggers, P.; van Lente, F.; Greene, T.; et al. A new equation to estimate glomerular filtration rate. *Ann. Intern. Med.* **2009**, *150*, 604–612. [CrossRef]
21. Malyszko, J.; Lukaszyk, E.; Glowinska, I.; Durlik, M. Biomarkers of delayed graft function as a form of acute kidney injury in kidney transplantation. *Sci. Rep.* **2015**, *5*, 11684. [CrossRef]
22. Ortega-Loubon, C.; Fernández-Molina, M.; Fierro, I.; Jorge-Monjas, P.; Carrascal, Y.; Gómez-Herreras, J.I.; Tamayo, E. Postoperative kidney oxygen saturation as a novel marker for acute kidney injury after adult cardiac surgery. *J. Thorac. Cardiovasc. Surg.* **2019**, *157*, 2340–2351.e3. [CrossRef]
23. Keller, A. Noninvasive tissue oximetry for flap monitoring: An initial study. *J. Reconstr. Microsurg.* **2007**, *23*, 189–197. [CrossRef]
24. Vaughan, D.L.; Wickramasinghe, Y.A.B.D.; Russell, G.I.; Thorniley, M.S.; Houston, R.F.; Ruban, E.; Rolfe, P. Near infrared spectroscopy: Blood and tissue oxygenation in renal ischemia-reperfusion injury in rats. *Int. J. Angiol.* **1995**, *4*, 25–30. [CrossRef]
25. Ponticelli, C.E. The impact of cold ischemia time on renal transplant outcome. *Kidney Int.* **2015**, *87*, 272–275. [CrossRef] [PubMed]
26. Snoeijs, M.G.; Vink, H.; Voesten, N.; Christiaans, M.H.; Daemen, J.W.; Peppelenbosch, A.G.; Tordoir, J.H.; Peutz-Kootstra, C.J.; Buurman, W.A.; Schurink, G.W.; et al. Acute ischemic injury to the renal microvasculature in human kidney transplantation. *Am. J. Physiol.-Ren. Physiol.* **2010**, *299*, F1134–F1140. [CrossRef]
27. Ruf, B.; Bonelli, V.; Balling, G.; Hörer, J.; Nagdyman, N.; Braun, S.L.; Ewert, P.; Reiter, K. Intraoperative renal near-infrared spectroscopy indicates developing acute kidney injury in infants undergoing cardiac surgery with cardiopulmonary bypass: A case-control study. *Crit. Care* **2015**, *19*, 27. [CrossRef] [PubMed]
28. Grosenick, D.; Cantow, K.; Arakelyan, K.; Wabnitz, H.; Flemming, B.; Skalweit, A.; Ladwig, M.; Macdonald, R.; Niendorf, T.; Seeliger, E. Detailing renal hemodynamics and oxygenation in rats by a combined near-infrared spectroscopy and invasive probe approach. *Biomed. Opt. Express* **2015**, *6*, 309–323. [CrossRef] [PubMed]
29. Hyttel-Sorensen, S.; Sorensen, L.C.; Riera, J.; Greisen, G. Tissue oximetry: A comparison of mean values of regional tissue saturation, reproducibility and dynamic range of four NIRS-instruments on the human forearm. *Biomed. Opt. Express* **2011**, *2*, 3047–3057. [CrossRef] [PubMed]
30. Bonsante, F.; Ramful, D.; Binquet, C.; Samperiz, S.; Daniel, S.; Gouyon, J.B.; Iacobelli, S. Low Renal Oxygen Saturation at Near-Infrared Spectroscopy on the First Day of Life Is Associated with Developing Acute Kidney Injury in Very Preterm Infants. *Neonatology* **2019**, *115*, 198–204. [CrossRef]
31. Herget-Rosenthal, S.; Marggraf, G.; Hüsing, J.; Göring, F.; Pietruck, F.; Janssen, O.; Philipp, T.; Kribben, A. Early detection of acute renal failure by serum cystatin C. *Kidney Int.* **2004**, *66*, 1115–1122. [CrossRef]

32. Haase-Fielitz, A.; Bellomo, R.; Devarajan, P.; Story, D.; Matalanis, G.; Dragun, D.; Haase, M. Novel and conventional serum biomarkers predicting acute kidney injury in adult cardiac surgery–a prospective cohort study. *Crit. Care Med.* **2009**, *37*, 553–560. [CrossRef]
33. Najafi, M. Serum creatinine role in predicting outcome after cardiac surgery beyond acute kidney injury. *World J. Cardiol.* **2014**, *6*, 1006–1021. [CrossRef] [PubMed]
34. Lau, P.E.; Cruz, S.; Garcia-Prats, J.; Cuevas, M.; Rhee, C.; Cass, D.L.; Horne, S.E.; Lee, T.C.; Welty, S.E.; Olutoye, O.O. Use of renal near-infrared spectroscopy measurements in congenital diaphragmatic hernia patients on ECMO. *J. Pediatr. Surg.* **2017**, *52*, 689–692. [CrossRef] [PubMed]
35. Beck, J.; Loron, G.; Masson, C.; Poli-Merol, M.L.; Guyot, E.; Guillot, C.; Bednarek, N.; François, C. Monitoring Cerebral and Renal Oxygenation Status during Neonatal Digestive Surgeries Using Near Infrared Spectroscopy. *Front. Pediatr.* **2017**, *5*, 140. [CrossRef] [PubMed]
36. Debout, A.; Foucher, Y.; Trébern-Launay, K.; Legendre, C.; Kreis, H.; Mourad, G.; Garrigue, V.; Morelon, E.; Buron, F.; Rostaing, L.; et al. Each additional hour of cold ischemia time significantly increases the risk of graft failure and mortality following renal transplantation. *Kidney Int.* **2015**, *87*, 343–349. [CrossRef] [PubMed]
37. Tennankore, K.K.; Kim, S.J.; Alwayn, I.P.; Kiberd, B.A. Prolonged warm ischemia time is associated with graft failure and mortality after kidney transplantation. *Kidney Int.* **2016**, *89*, 648–658. [CrossRef]
38. Gill, J.; Rose, C.; Lesage, J.; Joffres, Y.; Gill, J.; O'Connor, K. Use and Outcomes of Kidneys from Donation after Circulatory Death Donors in the United States. *J. Am. Soc. Nephrol.* **2017**, *28*, 3647–3657. [CrossRef]

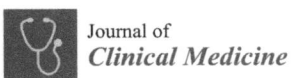

Article

Pretransplant Serum Uromodulin and Its Association with Delayed Graft Function Following Kidney Transplantation—A Prospective Cohort Study

Stephan Kemmner [1,2,*,†], Christopher Holzmann-Littig [1,†], Helene Sandberger [1], Quirin Bachmann [1], Flora Haberfellner [1], Carlos Torrez [1], Christoph Schmaderer [1], Uwe Heemann [1], Lutz Renders [1], Volker Assfalg [3], Tarek M. El-Achkar [4], Pranav S. Garimella [5], Jürgen Scherberich [6] and Dominik Steubl [1]

1 Department of Nephrology, Klinikum rechts der Isar, Technical University of Munich, 81675 Munich, Germany; christopher.holzmann-littig2@mri.tum.de (C.H.-L.); h.sandberger@gmx.net (H.S.); quirin.bachmann@tum.de (Q.B.); flora.haberfellner@tum.de (F.H.); carlos.at@live.de (C.T.); Christoph.Schmaderer@mri.tum.de (C.S.); Uwe.Heemann@mri.tum.de (U.H.); lutz.renders@tum.de (L.R.); dominik.steubl@gmx.de (D.S.)
2 Transplant Center, University Hospital Munich, Ludwig-Maximilians-University (LMU), 81377 Munich, Germany
3 Department of Surgery, Klinikum rechts der Isar, Technical University of Munich, 81675 Munich, Germany; Volker.assfalg@tum.de
4 Department of Medicine, Division of Nephrology, Indiana University School of Medicine, Indianapolis, IN 46202-5188, USA; telachka@iu.edu
5 Division of Nephrology-Hypertension, University of California San Diego, San Diego, CA 92093-9111, USA; pgarimella@health.ucsd.edu
6 Department of Nephrology and Clinical Immunology, Klinikum München-Harlaching, Teaching Hospital of the Ludwig-Maximilians-University, 81545 Munich, Germany; j.scherberich@web.de
* Correspondence: stephan.kemmner@tum.de
† These authors contributed equally to this work.

Abstract: Delayed graft function (DGF) following kidney transplantation is associated with increased risk of graft failure, but biomarkers to predict DGF are scarce. We evaluated serum uromodulin (sUMOD), a potential marker for tubular integrity with immunomodulatory capacities, in kidney transplant recipients and its association with DGF. We included 239 kidney transplant recipients and measured sUMOD pretransplant and on postoperative Day 1 (POD1) as independent variables. The primary outcome was DGF, defined as need for dialysis within one week after transplantation. In total, 64 patients (27%) experienced DGF. In multivariable logistic regression analysis adjusting for recipient, donor and transplant associated risk factors each 10 ng/mL higher pretransplant sUMOD was associated with 47% lower odds for DGF (odds ratio (OR) 0.53, 95% confidence interval (95%-CI) 0.30–0.82). When categorizing pretransplant sUMOD into quartiles, the quartile with the lowest values had 4.4-fold higher odds for DGF compared to the highest quartile (OR 4.41, 95%-CI 1.54–13.93). Adding pretransplant sUMOD to a model containing established risk factors for DGF in multivariable receiver-operating-characteristics (ROC) curve analysis, the area-under-the-curve improved from 0.786 [95%-CI 0.723–0.848] to 0.813 [95%-CI 0.755–0.871, $p = 0.05$]. SUMOD on POD1 was not associated with DGF. In conclusion, higher pretransplant sUMOD was independently associated with lower odds for DGF, potentially serving as a non-invasive marker to stratify patients according to their risk for developing DGF early in the setting of kidney transplantation.

Keywords: uromodulin; Tamm-Horsfall-protein; kidney transplantation; delayed graft function; ischemia-reperfusion injury

1. Introduction

Delayed graft function (DGF), commonly defined as need for dialysis within the first week after kidney transplantation, affects around 25–50% of patients, and is associated with a higher risk for acute rejection episodes and reduced long-term graft survival [1–4]. DGF presents histologically mainly as severe ischemia-reperfusion injury (IRI) with inflammatory tubular damage [5]. IRI triggers a long-term inflammation leading to interstitial fibrosis and tubular atrophy and reduces overall graft survival [6–8]. Therefore, understanding and potentially targeting the pathophysiology of IRI might improve long-term kidney graft survival [9]. However, measures to ameliorate IRI and markers predicting DGF before transplantation are scarce and still have limited diagnostic value [10].

Uromodulin (also known as Tamm-Horsfall protein), is a kidney derived glycoprotein with a molecular weight of around 100 kDa, exclusively expressed by epithelial cells of the thick ascending limb of the loop of Henle and the distal tubule [11–13]. The molecule is secreted both into the urine as well as the interstitium and circulation [14–16]. Thereby, interstitial uromodulin largely corresponds to serum concentrations in different forms of kidney disease [16]. Uromodulin is encoded by the UMOD gene, and mice lacking the UMOD gene showed more inflammation and tubular injury compared to wild type following renal IRI. In addition, they also demonstrate a greater necrotic and inflammatory phenotype of cell death rather than apoptotic, suggesting that interstitial uromodulin may have immunomodulating and anti-inflammatory capacities [17–19]. Uromodulin deficiency is also associated with delayed and in part incomplete kidney recovery following renal IRI in mice [14]. These data suggest that higher serum uromodulin (sUMOD) in the acute phase of kidney transplantation may be protective against IRI. Furthermore, higher sUMOD posttransplant is associated with lower risk for long-term kidney transplant failure [20,21]. However, the role of sUMOD in the early setting of transplantation and IRI remains to be investigated.

Here, we propose that recipient's sUMOD plays an important role in the recovery from IRI after kidney transplantation, and thus sUMOD might be of predictive value for the incidence of DGF after kidney transplantation. In this study we evaluated recipient's sUMOD pretransplant and on postoperative Day 1 (POD1) as a marker for prediction/early detection of DGF in kidney transplant recipients.

2. Materials and Methods

2.1. Study Participants and Study Design

In this single-center prospective observational cohort study, we recruited 239 patients undergoing kidney or combined kidney-pancreas transplantation following deceased or living donation in our tertiary care hospital. All patients who were able to provide informed consent were included in the study. Local institutional review boards of the Technical University of Munich, Germany approved the study methods. The study adheres to the declaration of Helsinki and the declaration of Istanbul.

2.2. Exposure

Serum samples for measuring sUMOD in the recipients were obtained 24 h prior to kidney transplantation in living organ donations and up to 5 h pretransplant in deceased donations, again on the first postoperative day (POD1) and subsequent time points later. Since all patients were hospitalized during the sample collection and no patient withdrew from the study, no patients were lost to follow-up for the primary endpoint (see below).

The samples were stored at −80 °C until they were thawed. sUMOD analyses were performed in singlicate using a commercial enzyme-linked immunosorbent assay (ELISA, Euroimmun, Medizinische Labordiagnostika AG, Lübeck, Germany) based on the manufacturer's instructions. This assay is based on a colorimetric sandwich immunoassay using a polyclonal antibody against human uromodulin as the capture antibody and a biotinylated polyclonal antibody against human uromodulin as the detection antibody. Quality characteristics of the ELISA are as follows: intra-assay coefficient of variation 1.8–3.2%, inter-assay coefficient of variation 6.6–7.8%, mean linearity recovery 97%, and lower limit of detection 2.0 ng/mL.

2.3. Outcomes

The primary outcome was DGF, defined as the need for more than one dialysis within one week after transplantation as has been defined in prior clinical studies [22,23]. For example, one dialysis due to potassium lowering was not considered as DGF. Notably, in our tertiary center we avoid pretransplant dialysis to reduce cold ischemia time whenever reasonable, which leads to postoperative dialysis for hyperkalemia in some cases.

2.4. Statistical Analysis

We describe the population using mean ($\pm$ standard deviation) for continuous variables and number with percentages for binary and categorical variables.

Multivariable logistic regression models were used to evaluate the association of sUMOD pretransplant and on POD1 as independent variables and DGF as the dependent variable. We applied a series of nested models: (i) unadjusted; (ii) adjusted for age, body-mass index (BMI) and dialysis vintage; (iii) Model 1 plus serum creatinine on POD1 ("Model 2"; we adjusted serum creatinine on POD1 as it appears to be an important variable for the decision to apply kidney replacement therapy postoperatively); (iv) Model 2 plus cold ischemia time (CIT), living vs. deceased donor transplantation, and expanded criteria donors (ECD) vs. standard criteria donors ("Model 3"). ECD are donors that are either older than 60 years, or 50–59 years old and meet at least two of the following criteria: cerebrovascular death, history of hypertension, and/or last serum creatinine greater than 1.5 mg/dL [24]. Due to the number of endpoints, we limited the analysis to these co-variables. Of note, we use the ECD classification for the adjustment because it covers donor age, donor serum creatinine and the donor cardiovascular cause of death. All variables were selected based on their clinical relevance for the outcomes of interest and are known risk factors for the primary endpoint DGF [2,5,25]. We performed multivariable receiver-operating-characteristic (ROC) curve analyses to evaluate the diagnostic value of preoperative sUMOD in addition to established risk factors (recipient age and BMI, dialysis vintage, CIT, deceased vs. living donation, ECD, "Model A") for the prediction of DGF ("Model B"). All analyses were conducted using R, version 3.5.1 (R Core Team (2018), Vienna, Austria).

3. Results

3.1. Population Characteristics

The mean age of the cohort was 51 ± 14 years, 31.4% were female, 90 (37.7%) received an organ from a living donor, 79 (33.1%) had cardiovascular disease at baseline. Mean serum creatinine concentration was 6.0 ± 2.3 mg/dL on POD1. Demographics of the entire cohort and stratified by preoperative sUMOD quartiles are shown in Table 1.

A total of 64 (26.8%) renal allograft recipients experienced DGF. Patients who experienced DGF were older, more often male, had a higher BMI and a greater prevalence of cardiovascular disease (Table 2). The time on dialysis before transplantation (dialysis vintage) was significantly longer in recipients who developed DGF (2208 ± 1456 days vs. 1321 ± 1331, $p < 0.001$). The mean serum creatinine on POD1 was significantly higher in patients with DGF (7.1 ± 2.4 mg/dL vs. 5.6 ± 2.1 mg/dL, $p < 0.001$). Referring to donor characteristics, kidney transplants with subsequent DGF were derived from donors who were more often male, had a higher BMI, a higher prevalence of diabetes and had a significantly higher serum creatinine before donation. Furthermore, cold and warm ischemia time were significantly longer for donor kidneys who developed DGF. Further information on DGF vs. non-DGF patients can be found in Table 2.

Table 1. Overall baseline characteristics (n = 239) and baseline characteristics of participants stratified by quartiles distributed according to pretransplant serum uromodulin (sUMOD).

Characteristics	Total	Quartile 1 sUMOD: <2.59 ng/mL	Quartile 2 sUMOD: 2.59–7.04 ng/mL	Quartile 3 sUMOD: >7.04–14.66 ng/mL	Quartile 4 sUMOD: >14.66 ng/mL	p-Value
Number (no.) of patients	239	60	60	59	60	
Recipient demographics						
Age [years]	51 ± 14	50 ± 14	54 ± 13	52 ± 14	49 ± 16	0.185
Female, no. (%)	75 (31.4)	17 (28.3)	20 (33.3)	15 (25.4)	23 (38.3)	0.443
Body-mass index [kg/m^2]	25.3 ± 4.8	25.0 ± 5.1	25.6 ± 5.1	26.0 ± 4.8	24.8 ± 4.3	0.525
Diabetes, no. (%)	48 (20.1)	4 (6.7)	18 (30.0)	15 (25.4)	11 (18.3)	0.009
Hypertension, no. (%)	194 (81.2)	46 (76.7)	51 (85.0)	50 (84.7)	47 (78.3)	0.536
Cardiovascular disease, no. (%)	79 (33.1)	18 (30.0)	25 (41.7)	22 (37.3)	14 (23.3)	0.151
Dialysis vintage [days]	1559 ± 1418	2137 (1469)	1921 ± 1392	1220 ± 1267	953 ± 1215	<0.001
Preemptive transplant, no. (%)	29 (12.1)	3 (5.0)	1 (1.7)	7 (11.9)	18 (30.0)	<0.001
Pretransplant sUMOD [ng/mL]	14.9 ± 23.8	0.9 ± 0.8	4.5 ± 1.3	10.1 ± 2.0	44.2 ± 32.8	<0.001
Recipient laboratory measures on postoperative Day 1 (POD1)						
sUMOD [ng/mL]	52.3 ± 50.2	56.0 ± 65.1	50.6 ± 51.1	36.4 ± 24.5	65.3 ± 48.7	0.014
Serum creatinine [mg/dL]	6.0 ± 2.3	6.0 ± 2.1	6.7 ± 2.4	6.1 ± 2.4	5.2 ± 2.2	0.004
Hemoglobin [g/dL]	10.3 ± 1.6	10.3 ± 1.8	10.6 ± 1.6)	10.5 ± 1.4	10.0 ± 1.6	0.223
Leucocyte count [G/L]	11.6 ± 4.2	10.6 ± 3.8	11.7 ± 3.8	11.6 ± 4.5	12.6 ± 4.5	0.095
C-reactive protein [mg/dL]	3.4 ± 2.3	2.6 ± 1.4	6.0 ± 3.6	3.2 ± 1.7	2.8 ± 1.6	<0.001
Sodium [mmol/L]	141 ± 4	140 ± 4	141 ± 4	141 ± 5	141 ± 4	0.093
Potassium [mmol/L]	4.9 ± 0.8	5.1 ± 0.7	5.0 ± 0.8	4.7 ± 0.7	4.6 ± 0.8	<0.001
Donor characteristics						
Age [years]	54.4 ± 15.5	51 ± 16	55 ± 16	55 ± 15	52 ± 15	0.256
Female, no. (%)	118 (49.4)	25 (41.7)	32 (53.3)	29 (49.2)	32 (53.3)	0.536
Body-mass index [kg/m^2]	26.4 ± 4.4	27.0 ± 5.2	26.0 ± 3.7	26.5 ± 4.5	26.1 ± 3.8	0.574
Diabetes, no. (%)						0.131
No	166 (69.5)	37 (61.7)	46 (76.7)	35 (59.3)	48 (80.0)	
Yes	15 (6.3)	4 (6.7)	4 (6.7)	5 (8.5)	2 (3.3)	
Unknown	58 (24.3)	19 (31.7)	10 (16.7)	19 (32.2)	10 (16.7)	
Hypertension, no. (%)						0.071
No	119 (49.8)	29 (48.3)	30 (50.0)	23 (39.0)	37 (61.7)	
Yes	79 (33.1)	16 (26.7)	22 (36.7)	27 (45.8)	14 (23.3)	
Unknown	41 (17.2)	15 (25.0)	8 (13.3)	9 (15.3)	9 (15.0)	
Serum creatinine [mg/dL]	1.0 ± 0.7	1.0 ± 0.8	0.9 ± 0.5)	1.1 ± 0.8	1.0 ± 0.7	0.740
Expanded criteria donor, no (%)	97 (40.6)	20 (33.3)	28 (46.7)	28 (47.5)	21 (35.0)	0.245
Transplant related variables						
Living donation, no. (%)	90 (37.7)	14 (23.3)	14 (23.3)	27 (45.8)	35 (58.3)	<0.001
Cold ischemic time [hours]	8 ± 6	10 ± 6	10 ± 6	7 ± 5	6 ± 6	<0.001
Warm ischemic time [minutes]	25 ± 13	26 ± 12	27 ± 13	27 ± 16	23 ± 7	0.313
Primary non-function, no. (%)	8 (3.3)	1 (1.7)	2 (3.3)	3 (5.1)	2 (3.3)	0.783
No. of HLA-mismatches	4 ± 2	4 ± 2	4 ± 2	3 ± 2	3 ± 2	0.410

Continuous variables presented as mean ± standard deviation, categorical variables presented in percentage of referring population. The p-value will compare variables between quartiles calculated by parametric testing. sUMOD, serum uromodulin.

Table 2. Baseline characteristics of participants stratified by status regarding delayed graft function (DGF).

Characteristics	Without DGF	With DGF	p-Value
Number (no.) of patients	175	64	
Recipient demographics			
Age [years]	50 ± 14	56 ± 13	0.003
Female, no. (%)	61 (34.9)	14 (21.9)	0.079
Body-mass index [kg/m^2]	24.5 ± 4.4	27.8 ± 5.2	<0.001
Diabetes, no. (%)	30 (17.1)	18 (28.1)	0.090
Hypertension, no. (%)	141 (80.6)	53 (82.8)	0.837

Table 2. Cont.

Characteristics	Without DGF	With DGF	p-Value
Cardiovascular disease, no. (%)	45 (25.7)	34 (53.1)	<0.001
Dialysis vintage [days]	1321 ± 1331	2208 ± 1456	<0.001
Preemptive transplant, no. (%)	28 (16.0)	1 (1.6)	<0.001
Pretransplant sUMOD [ng/mL]	18.3 ± 26.8	5.9 ± 6.4	<0.001
Recipient laboratory measures on postoperative Day 1 (POD1)			
sUMOD [ng/mL]	51.7 ± 50.3	54.0 ± 50.4	0.747
Serum creatinine [mg/dL]	5.6 ± 2.2	7.1 ± 2.4	<0.001
Hemoglobin [g/dL]	10.3 ± 1.6	10.4 ± 1.8	0.687
Leucocyte count [G/L]	11.5 ± 4.2	12.0 ± 4.2	0.479
C-reactive protein [mg/dL]	3.5 ± 2.6	3.2 ± 1.3	0.585
Sodium [mmol/L]	141 ± 4	139 ± 5	0.005
Potassium [mmol/L]	4.7 ± 0.7	5.4 ± 0.6	<0.001
Donor characteristics			
Age [years]	52 ± 15	57 ± 15	0.021
Female, no. (%)	96 (54.9)	22 (34.4)	0.008
Body-mass index [kg/m^2]	25.8 ± 3.7	28.1 ± 5.5	<0.001
Diabetes, no. (%)			<0.001
No	131 (74.9)	35 (54.7)	
Yes	5 (2.9)	10 (15.6)	
Unknown	39 (22.3)	19 (29.7)	
Hypertension, no. (%)			0.209
No	93 (53.1)	26 (40.6)	
Yes	55 (31.4)	24 (37.5)	
Unknown	27 (15.4)	14 (21.9)	
Serum creatinine [mg/dL]	1.0 ± 0.6	1.1 ± 0.9	0.057
Expanded criteria donor, no (%)	64 (36.6)	33 (51.6)	0.052
Transplant related variables			
Living donation, no. (%)	79 (45.1)	11 (17.2)	<0.001
Cold ischemic time [hours]	7.2 ± 6.0	9.9 ± 5.5	0.002
Warm ischemic time [minutes]	24 ± 12	29 ± 14	0.006
Primary non-function, no. (%)	0 (0)	8 (12.5)	<0.001
No. of HLA-mismatches	3 ± 2	3 ± 2	0.650

Continuous variables presented as means ± standard deviation, categorical variables presented in percentage of referring population. The p-value will compare recipients with DGF and without DGF calculated by parametric testing. sUMOD, serum uromodulin.

3.2. Course of sUMOD during the Transplant Process and Short Term Follow Up

The mean sUMOD levels in the total cohort was 14.9 ± 23.8 ng/mL preoperatively, 52.3 ± 50.2 ng/mL on POD1 and remained stable after this up to 31–120 days after transplantation (Figure 1). Patients with DGF had significantly lower pretransplant sUMOD levels compared to patients without DGF (5.9 ± 6.4 ng/mL vs. 18.3 ± 26.8 ng/mL, $p < 0.001$). There was no significant difference in sUMOD levels on POD1 between patients with and without DGF (54.0 ± 50.4 ng/mL vs. 51.7 ± 50.3 ng/mL, $p = 0.888$; Table 1). However, while sUMOD levels decreased again in patients with DGF in the postoperative period, we did see a further increase in patients without DGF (Figure 1). In contrast, serum creatinine levels were higher in the DGF subgroup pretransplant and remained higher over the whole postoperative period compared to the non-DGF subgroup (Figure 1).

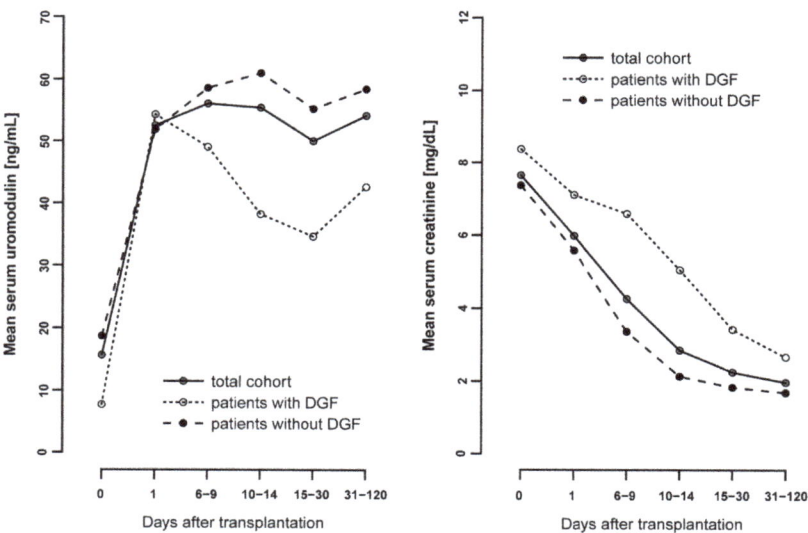

Figure 1. Mean serum uromodulin values [ng/mL] from pretransplant to follow-up (up to 120 days after transplantation) compared to the mean serum creatinine [mg/dL] in the total cohort and in patients with and without delayed graft function (DGF).

3.3. Pretransplant sUMOD and DGF

In univariable analysis, each 10 ng/mL higher preoperative sUMOD was associated with 49% lower odds for DGF (OR 0.51, 95%-CI 0.32–0.73, Table 3). This association remained statistically significant after multivariable adjustment (OR 0.53, 95%-CI 0.30–0.82). When categorized into quartiles, the quartile with the lowest preoperative sUMOD levels had 4.4-fold higher odds for DGF compared to the highest quartile in multivariable analysis (OR 4.41, 95%-CI 1.54–13.93, Table 3).

Table 3. Associations of serum uromodulin (sUMOD) pretransplant and on postoperative Day 1 with delayed graft function (DGF) in the kidney transplant.

	Events	Unadjusted	Model 1 [a]	Model 2 [b]	Model 3 [c]
Pretransplant sUMOD					
Per 10 ng/mL higher sUMOD	64/239	0.51 (0.32–0.73)	0.54 (0.31–0.81)	0.55 (0.31–0.83)	0.53 (0.30–0.82)
Q1	25/60	5.41 (2.21–14.80)	4.47 (1.62–13.61)	4.30 (1.53–13.31)	4.41 (1.54–13.93)
Q2	20/60	3.79 (1.52–10.46)	2.55 (0.93–7.61)	1.94 (0.68–5.93)	1.95 (0.67–6.08)
Q3	12/59	1.93 (0.72–5.58)	1.52 (0.52–4.70)	1.28 (0.42–4.06)	1.29 (0.42–4.14)
Q4	7/60	1 (ref.)	1 (ref.)	1 (ref.)	1 (ref.)
sUMOD on postoperative Day 1					
Per 10 ng/mL higher sUMOD	63/237 *	1.01 (0.95–1.07)	1.01 (0.95–1.07)	1.03 (0.96–1.09)	1.03 (0.96–1.09)
Q1	16/60	0.90 (0.40–2.01)	0.71 (0.28–1.75)	0.70 (0.27–1.78)	0.71 (0.27–1.86)
Q2	14/59	0.77 (0.33–1.74)	0.72 (0.27–1.85)	0.77 (0.29–2.03)	0.79 (0.29–2.14)
Q3	16/59	0.92 (0.41–2.06)	0.84 (0.34–2.07)	0.88 (0.35–2.22)	0.86 (0.34–2.17)
Q4	17/59	1 (ref.)	1 (ref.)	1 (ref.)	1 (ref.)

Results are presented as odds ratios with 95%-confidence intervals given in parentheses. Delayed graft function is defined as the requirement of >1 dialysis treatment within the first week after transplantation. Quartile distribution according to preoperative serum uromodulin (sUMOD): Quartile 1 (Q1) ≤ 2.59 ng/mL, Quartile 2 (Q2) > 2.59–7.04 ng/mL, Quartile 3 (Q3) > 7.04–14.66 ng/mL, Quartile 4 (Q4) > 14.66 ng/mL. Quartile distribution according to postoperative Day 1 serum uromodulin (sUMOD): Quartile 1 (Q1) ≤ 22.00 ng/mL, Quartile 2 (Q2) > 22.00–36.97 ng/mL, Quartile 3 (Q3) > 36.97–68.44 ng/mL, Quartile 4 (Q4) > 68.44 ng/mL. * Two patients missing due to missing sUMOD values on postoperative Day 1. [a] Adjusted for recipients age, recipients body-mass-index and dialysis vintage. [b] Model 1 + serum creatinine on postoperative Day 1. [c] Model 2 + cold-ischemia time, living vs. deceased donor transplantation, expanded criteria donors (ECD).

In order to rule out potential confounding through preemptive transplantation we performed a sensitivity analysis in which we adjusted our multivariable logistic regression Model 1 for preemptive transplantation (categorical variable yes vs. no) instead of dialysis vintage. We did not add preemptive transplantation as another covariable in order to avoid overfitting of the model. In this additional analysis with pretransplant sUMOD as a continuous variable, we identified a similar OR for the association of sUMOD with DGF (OR 0.50 (95%-CI 0.28–0.79) per 10 ng/mL higher sUMOD).

sUMOD on POD1 was not significantly associated with DGF, neither as a continuous nor a categorical variable (Table 3).

3.4. ROC-Analysis to Evaluate Preoperative sUMOD as a Predictor for DGF

In multivariable ROC curve analysis, Model A (including risk factors for DGF without preoperative sUMOD) worked moderately well to predict DGF (area under the curve (AUC) 0.786 [95%-CI 0.723–0.848], Figure 2). Model B (i.e., adding sUMOD to Model A) increased the predictive accuracy at borderline statistical significance (AUC 0.813 [95%-CI 0.755–0.871], p = 0.05) as presented in Figure 2.

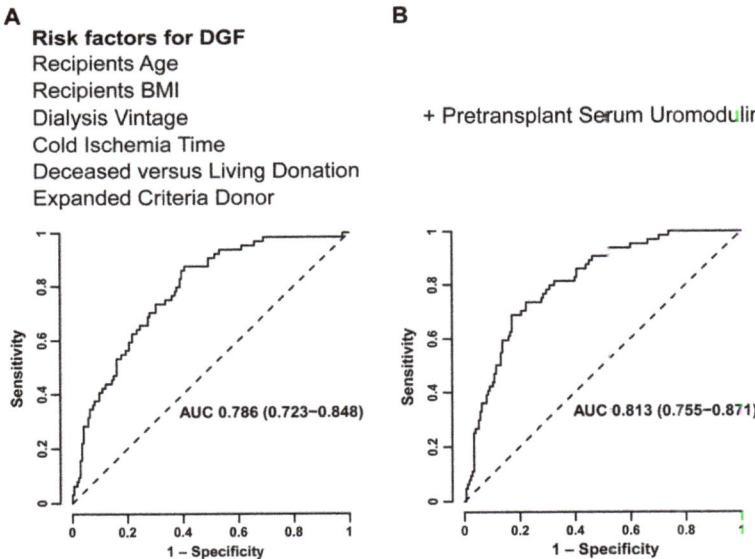

Figure 2. Multivariable receiver-operating-characteristic (ROC) curve analysis evaluating models including established risk factors (recipient age and body-mass-index (BMI), dialysis vintage, cold ischemia time, deceased vs. living donation, expanded criteria donors) for the prediction of delayed graft function (DGF) without (**A**) and with preoperative serum uromodulin (**B**).

4. Discussion

In the current study, we demonstrate that a higher pretransplant sUMOD in kidney transplant recipients is independently associated with a lower risk for DGF. Furthermore, preoperative sUMOD was of additional predictive value when added to a model of established risk factors for DGF. Surprisingly, we detected no association between sUMOD on POD1 and DGF.

We further mapped the course of sUMOD before, during and in the early phase after transplantation (up to 120 days following kidney transplantation) with and without the occurrence of DGF. We demonstrated that over the longer course after transplantation patients without DGF maintained higher sUMOD levels, while in patients with DGF we detected a subsequent decline in sUMOD in the postoperative period. The subsequent decrease in sUMOD is consistent with a recent study showing decrease in circulating uromodulin following AKI in a cohort of liver transplant patients undergoing surgery [26], reflecting tubular mass and function in the longer-term, non-acute setting.

sUMOD has been positively associated with reduced risk for kidney failure, cardiovascular events and mortality in geriatric and chronic kidney disease populations [27,28]. In kidney transplant setting, higher sUMOD in the first year after transplantation has also been associated with better long-term allograft survival in kidney transplant recipients [20,21]. Further, decreased concentrations of sUMOD can be observed in the early course of tubulointerstitial injury in the kidney transplant [29]. This is in line with our observations, that a higher pretransplant sUMOD is associated with lower risk for DGF due to IRI and subsequently higher sUMOD levels over the longer-term course following renal transplantation. None of the previous studies performed uromodulin measurements just before and after kidney transplantation.

Higher pretransplant sUMOD could represent the anti-inflammatory capacity of the recipient towards the following inflammation due to IRI. Interstitial or sUMOD has been shown to downregulate proinflammatory signaling in the kidney, reflecting its immunomodulatory and reno-protective capacity [30]. Recently, it was demonstrated that uromodulin inhibits the generation of reactive oxygen species both in the kidney and systemically [26]. In line with this, UMOD deficient mice experiencing IRI are at higher risk for acute kidney injury with higher interstitial inflammation and cell infiltration [17,19]. Furthermore, UMOD deficient mice showed delayed and incomplete recovery from acute kidney injury after IRI, which is explained by a lack of upregulation of uromodulin expression after IRI [14].

Although it is challenging to directly extrapolate results from murine models of IRI to human transplantation, results from these models support our observations, that a higher sUMOD in the recipient just before transplantation is associated with lower risk for DGF [31]. SUMOD is hypothesized to be a molecule with abilities in modulating inflammation against an evolving IRI, which in turn is thought to be one of the main mechanisms predisposing to DGF [32]. The findings that higher levels of preoperative sUMOD are associated with less risk of DGF leads to the hypothesis that there is a "high uromodulin" state before transplantation may be beneficial. However, given the observational nature of this data, we cannot conclude on whether sUMOD has a causal role to play in the development of DGF. Despite we detected significant differences in sUMOD levels between patients with and without DGF, absolute differences appear to be small compared to differences in sUMOD levels between healthy individuals and patients at different CKD stages [16]. Therefore, it remains to be validated that the differences we detected between DGF and non-DGF translate into physiologically relevant differences in uromodulin activity.

It is interesting that sUMOD increases initially in patients with or without DGF, which might reflect the release of "donor" sUMOD from the transplanted kidney. Patients with DGF have a subsequent profound and persistent decrease in sUMOD. The fact that we do not see an association between sUMOD on POD1 and delayed graft function could reflect the dynamic pathophysiological process occurring during this early time period in the transplanted kidney, which may be critical to the subsequent course of injury or recovery. The initial increase could represent general reactive reno-protection-intended induction of uromodulin production in the setting of renal IRI, which is related to its immune-modulatory capacities in the interstitium [14,17].

While sUMOD on POD1 might be influenced by acute inflammation and hypoxic stress, long-term sUMOD should reflect tubular function/mass [20,21]. However, as the primary aim of our study was to evaluate sUMOD as a predictive marker or a marker for early detection of DGF, sUMOD pre-transplant and on POD1 was the focus of our statistical analysis.

One strength of our study is the use of both pre- as well as the post-transplant period. While we did not directly adjust for residual kidney function in the multivariable approach, we propose that with adjusting for dialysis vintage and kidney transplantation after living donation we also captured residual kidney function to some extent, as it is well known that residual kidney function decreases along with the time spent of dialysis. In general, due to its molecular mass of 95 kDa sUMOD is highly unlikely to be removed by both hemo- and peritoneal dialysis.

A major limitation in the present study is that patients without DGF received kidneys from "healthier" donors with shorter ischemia time (see Table 2), that are less vulnerable to tubular injury. Although, we tried to account for this difference by adjusting for a number of covariables, which are supposed to be relevant risk factors for DGF (i.e., ECD, deceased vs. living donation, CIT) [2,5,25] there remains the potential residual confounding. Furthermore, DGF due to renal IRI is a common problem after deceased donation [2], but the proportion of patients after living donation in the present cohort is relatively high at almost 38%. We included transplant patients both after deceased as well as after living donation due to the otherwise small number of patients in a single center analysis. Further, we adjusted for living donation in statistical analysis as mentioned above. However, even after adjustment for deceased vs. living donation as well as dialysis vintage with expected shorter dialysis time before transplantation after living donation due to the large proportion of preemptive transplantations, recipients pretransplant sUMOD was independently associated with lower risk for DGF following transplantation. Finally, we lack data on single nucleotide polymorphisms (SNPs) that are known to influence uromodulin concentrations [33,34], and therefore, cannot comment on how these SNPs may affect our findings.

5. Conclusions

In conclusion, lower pretransplant sUMOD is independently associated with DGF after kidney transplantation and might therefore function as an early non-invasive marker to identify patients at increased risk for DGF following IRI and subsequent complicated course after kidney transplantation.

Author Contributions: D.S. designed the study. S.K., D.S. and C.H.-L. performed analysis of the study and wrote the manuscript. S.K., H.S., V.A., L.R. and D.S. were involved in collecting the blood samples. S.K., C.H.-L., H.S., F.H., C.T., Q.B. and C.S. collected data. P.S.G and D.S. critically discussed statistical analysis. U.H., T.M.E.-A., P.S.G. and J.S. oversaw the study and critically discussed the manuscript. All co-authors have contributed substantially to the final version of the manuscript. All authors have read and agreed to the published version of the manuscript.

Funding: There are no funding sources.

Institutional Review Board Statement: The study was conducted according to the guidelines of the Declaration of Helsinki and approved by the ethics committee of the Technical University of Munich (No: 246/14).

Informed Consent Statement: Informed consent to participate and to publish was obtained from all individual participants included in the study.

Data Availability Statement: The dataset generated during the current study is available from corresponding author upon reasonable request.

Acknowledgments: The authors are grateful to the study participants and to the residents on the transplant ward for drawing blood from study participants.

Conflicts of Interest: The authors declare that they have no conflict of interest.

Abbreviations

List of Abbreviations
AUC   Area under the curve
BMI   Body-mass index
CIT   Cold ischemia time
ECD   Expanded criteria donor
eGFR   Estimated glomerular filtration rate
ELISA   Enzyme-linked immunosorbent assay
DGF   Delayed graft function
IRI   Ischemia-reperfusion injury
95%-CI   95% confidence interval
OR   Odds ratio
POD1   Postoperative Day 1
ROC   Receiver-operating-characteristics
sUMOD   Serum uromodulin.

References

1. Perico, N.; Cattaneo, D.; Sayegh, M.H.; Remuzzi, G. Delayed graft function in kidney transplantation. *Lancet* **2004**, *364*, 1814–1827. [CrossRef]
2. Siedlecki, A.; Irish, W.; Brennan, D.C. Delayed graft function in the kidney transplant. *Am. J. Transpl.* **2011**, *112*, 2279–2296. [CrossRef]
3. Yarlagadda, S.G.; Coca, S.G.; Garg, A.X.; Doshi, M.; Poggio, E.; Marcus, R.J.; Parikh, C.R. Marked variation in the definition and diagnosis of delayed graft function: A systematic review. *Nephrol. Dial. Transpl.* **2008**, *23*, 2995–3003. [CrossRef]
4. Bahl, D.; Haddad, Z.; Datoo, A.; Qazi, Y.A. Delayed graft function in kidney transplantation. *Curr. Opin. Organ Transpl.* **2019**, *24*, 82–86. [CrossRef]
5. Schroppel, B.; Legendre, C. Delayed kidney graft function: From mechanism to translation. *Kidney Int.* **2014**, *86*, 251–258. [CrossRef]
6. Linkermann, A.; Stockwell, B.R.; Krautwald, S.; Anders, H.J. Regulated cell death and inflammation: An auto-amplification loop causes organ failure. *Nat. Rev. Immunol.* **2014**, *14*, 759–767. [CrossRef]
7. Chawla, L.S.; Eggers, P.W.; Star, R.A.; Kimmel, P.L. Acute kidney injury and chronic kidney disease as interconnected syndromes. *N. Engl. J. Med.* **2014**, *371*, 58–66. [CrossRef] [PubMed]
8. Venkatachalam, M.A.; Weinberg, J.M.; Kriz, W.; Bidani, A.K. Failed Tubule Recovery, AKI-CKD Transition, and Kidney Disease Progression. *J. Am. Soc. Nephrol.* **2015**, *26*, 1765–1776. [CrossRef] [PubMed]
9. Chapman, J.R. Progress in Transplantation: Will It Be Achieved in Big Steps or by Marginal Gains? *Am. J. Kidney Dis.* **2017**, *69*, 287–295. [CrossRef] [PubMed]
10. Lohkamp, L.N.; Ollinger, R.; Chatzigeorgiou, A.; Illigens, B.M.; Siepmann, T. Intraoperative biomarkers in renal transplantation. *Nephrology* **2016**, *21*, 188–199. [CrossRef] [PubMed]
11. Pennica, D.; Kohr, W.J.; Kuang, W.J.; Glaister, D.; Aggarwal, B.B.; Chen, E.Y.; Goeddel, D.V. Identification of human uromodulin as the Tamm-Horsfall urinary glycoprotein. *Science* **1987**, *236*, 83–88. [CrossRef]
12. Zhu, X.; Cheng, J.; Gao, J.; Lepor, H.; Zhang, Z.T.; Pak, J.; Wu, X.R. Isolation of mouse THP gene promoter and demonstration of its kidney-specific activity in transgenic mice. *Am. J. Physiol. Ren. Physiol.* **2002**, *282*, F608–F617. [CrossRef]
13. Serafini-Cessi, F.; Malagolini, N.; Cavallone, D. Tamm-Horsfall glycoprotein: Biology and clinical relevance. *Am. J. Kidney Dis.* **2003**, *42*, 658–676. [CrossRef]
14. El-Achkar, T.M.; McCracken, R.; Liu, Y.; Heitmeier, M.R.; Bourgeois, S.; Ryerse, J.; Wu, X.R. Tamm-Horsfall protein translocates to the basolateral domain of thick ascending limbs, interstitium, and circulation during recovery from acute kidney injury. *Am. J. Physiol. Ren. Physiol.* **2013**, *304*, F1066–F1075. [CrossRef] [PubMed]
15. El-Achkar, T.M.; Wu, X.R. Uromodulin in kidney injury: An instigator, bystander, or protector? *Am. J. Kidney Dis* **2012**, *59*, 452–461. [CrossRef] [PubMed]
16. Scherberich, J.E.; Gruber, R.; Nockher, W.A.; Christensen, E.I.; Schmitt, H.; Herbst, V.; Block, M.; Kaden, J.; Schlumberger, W. Serum uromodulin-a marker of kidney function and renal parenchymal integrity. *Nephrol. Dial. Transpl.* **2018**, *33*, 284–295. [CrossRef] [PubMed]
17. El-Achkar, T.M.; Wu, X.R.; Rauchman, M.; McCracken, R.; Kiefer, S.; Dagher, P.C. Tamm-Horsfall protein protects the kidney from ischemic injury by decreasing inflammation and altering TLR4 expression. *Am. J. Physiol. Ren. Physiol.* **2008**, *295*, F534–F544. [CrossRef] [PubMed]
18. Micanovic, R.; Khan, S.; Janosevic, D.; Lee, M.E.; Hato, T.; Srour, E.F.; Winfree, S.; Ghosh, J.; Tong, Y.; Rice, S.E.; et al. Tamm-Horsfall Protein Regulates Mononuclear Phagocytes in the Kidney. *J. Am. Soc. Nephrol.* **2018**, *29*, 841–856. [CrossRef] [PubMed]

19. El-Achkar, T.M.; McCracken, R.; Rauchman, M.; Heitmeier, M.R.; Al-Aly, Z.; Dagher, P.C.; Wu, X.R. Tamm-Horsfall protein-deficient thick ascending limbs promote injury to neighboring S3 segments in an MIP-2-dependent mechanism. *Am. J. Physiol. Ren. Physiol.* **2011**, *300*, F999–F1007. [CrossRef] [PubMed]
20. Steubl, D.; Block, M.; Herbst, V.; Schlumberger, W.; Nockher, A.; Angermann, S.; Schmaderer, C.; Heemann, U.; Renders, L.; Scherberich, J. Serum uromodulin predicts graft failure in renal transplant recipients. *Biomarkers* **2017**, *22*, 171–177. [CrossRef]
21. Bostom, A.; Steubl, D.; Garimella, P.S.; Franceschini, N.; Roberts, M.B.; Pasch, A.; Ix, J.H.; Tuttle, K.R.; Ivanova, A.; Shireman, T.; et al. Serum Uromodulin: A Biomarker of Long-Term Kidney Allograft Failure. *Am. J. Nephrol.* **2018**, *47*, 275–282. [CrossRef]
22. Hall, I.E.; Reese, P.P.; Doshi, M.D.; Weng, F.L.; Schroppel, B.; Asch, W.S.; Ficek, J.; Thiessen-Philbrook, H.; Parikh, C.R. Delayed Graft Function Phenotypes and 12-Month Kidney Transplant Outcomes. *Transplantation* **2017**, *101*, 1913–1923. [CrossRef]
23. Wu, W.K.; Famure, O.; Li, Y.; Kim, S.J. Delayed graft function and the risk of acute rejection in the modern era of kidney transplantation. *Kidney Int.* **2015**, *88*, 851–858. [CrossRef]
24. Querard, A.H.; Le Borgne, F.; Dion, A.; Giral, M.; Mourad, G.; Garrigue, V.; Rostaing, L.; Kamar, N.; Loupy, A.; Legendre, C.; et al. Propensity score-based comparison of the graft failure risk between kidney transplant recipients of standard and expanded criteria donor grafts: Toward increasing the pool of marginal donors. *Am. J. Transpl.* **2018**, *18*, 1151–1157. [CrossRef]
25. Sharif, A.; Borrows, R. Delayed graft function after kidney transplantation: The clinical perspective. *Am. J. Kidney Dis.* **2013**, *62*, 150–158. [CrossRef]
26. LaFavers, K.A.; Macedo, E.; Garimella, P.S.; Lima, C.; Khan, S.; Myslinski, J.; McClintick, J.; Witzmann, F.A.; Winfree, S.; Phillips, C.L.; et al. Circulating uromodulin inhibits systemic oxidative stress by inactivating the TRPM2 channel. *Sci. Transl. Med.* **2019**, *11*, eaaw3639. [CrossRef] [PubMed]
27. Steubl, D.; Buzkova, P.; Garimella, P.S.; Ix, J.H.; Devarajan, P.; Bennett, M.R.; Chaves, P.H.M.; Shlipak, M.G.; Bansal, N.; Sarnak, M.J. Association of Serum Uromodulin with ESKD and Kidney Function Decline in the Elderly: The Cardiovascular Health Study. *Am. J. Kidney Dis.* **2019**, *74*, 501–509. [CrossRef] [PubMed]
28. Steubl, D.; Buzkova, P.; Garimella, P.S.; Ix, J.H.; Devarajan, P.; Bennett, M.R.; Chaves, P.H.M.; Shlipak, M.G.; Bansal, N.; Sarnak, M.J. Association of serum uromodulin with mortality and cardiovascular disease in the elderly-the Cardiovascular Health Study. *Nephrol. Dial. Transpl.* **2020**, *35*, 1399–1405. [CrossRef]
29. Borstnar, S.; Veceric-Haler, Z.; Bostjancic, E.; Pipan Tkalec, Z.; Kovac, D.; Lindic, J.; Kojc, N. Uromodulin and microRNAs in Kidney Transplantation-Association with Kidney Graft Function. *Int. J. Mol. Sci.* **2020**, *21*, 5592. [CrossRef] [PubMed]
30. Micanovic, R.; Chitteti, B.R.; Dagher, P.C.; Srour, E.F.; Khan, S.; Hato, T.; Lyle, A.; Tong, Y.; Wu, X.R.; El-Achkar, T.M. Tamm-Horsfall Protein Regulates Granulopoiesis and Systemic Neutrophil Homeostasis. *J. Am. Soc. Nephrol.* **2015**, *26*, 2172–2182. [CrossRef] [PubMed]
31. Chen, C.-C.; Chapman, W.C.; Hanto, D.W. Ischemia-Reperfusion injury in kidney transplantation. *Front. Biosci.* **2015**, *7*, 117–134.
32. Grenda, R. Delayed graft function and its management in children. *Pediatric Nephrol.* **2017**, *32*, 1157–1167. [CrossRef]
33. Kottgen, A.; Hwang, S.J.; Larson, M.G.; Van Eyk, J.E.; Fu, Q.; Benjamin, E.J.; Dehghan, A.; Glazer, N.L.; Kao, W.H.; Harris, T.B.; et al. Uromodulin levels associate with a common UMOD variant and risk for incident CKD. *J. Am. Soc. Nephrol.* **2010**, *21*, 337–344. [CrossRef] [PubMed]
34. Delgado, G.E.; Kleber, M.E.; Scharnagl, H.; Kramer, B.K.; Marz, W.; Scherberich, J.E. Serum Uromodulin and Mortality Risk in Patients Undergoing Coronary Angiography. *J. Am. Soc. Nephrol.* **2017**, *28*, 2201–2210. [CrossRef] [PubMed]

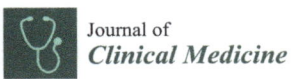

Article

Apheresis Efficacy and Tolerance in the Setting of HLA-Incompatible Kidney Transplantation

Johan Noble [1,2,†], Antoine Metzger [1,†], Hamza Naciri Bennani [1], Melanie Daligault [1], Dominique Masson [3], Florian Terrec [1], Farida Imerzoukene [1], Beatrice Bardy [3], Gaelle Fiard [4,5], Raphael Marlu [6], Eloi Chevallier [1], Benedicte Janbon [1], Paolo Malvezzi [1], Lionel Rostaing [1,2,*] and Thomas Jouve [1,2]

1. Nephrology, Hemodialysis, Apheresis and Kidney Transplantation Department, University Hospital Grenoble, 38000 Grenoble, France; jnoble@chu-grenoble.fr (J.N.); ametzger@ch-annecygenevois.fr (A.M.); hnaciribennani@chu-grenoble.fr (H.N.B.); mdailgault@chu-grenoble.fr (M.D.); fterrec@chu-grenoble.fr (F.T.); fimerzoukene@chu-grenoble.fr (F.I.); echevallier1@chu-grenoble.fr (E.C.); bjanbon@chu-grenoble.fr (B.J.); pmalvezzi@chu-grenoble.fr (P.M.); tjouve@chu-grenoble.fr (T.J.)
2. University Grenoble Alpes, 38000 Grenoble, France
3. HLA Laboratory—Établissement Français du Sang-EFS-, 38000 Grenoble, France; dominique.masson@efs.sante.fr (D.M.); beatrice.bardy@efs.sante.fr (B.B.)
4. Urology Department, University Hospital Grenoble, 38000 Grenoble, France; gfiard@chu-grenoble.fr
5. TIMC-IMAG, Grenoble INP, CNRS, University Grenoble Alpes, F-38000 Grenoble, France
6. Haemostasis Laboratory, University Hospital Grenoble, 38000 Grenoble, France; rmarlu@chu-grenoble.fr
* Correspondence: lrostaing@chu-grenoble.fr; Tel.: +33-476768945; Fax: +33-476765263
† These authors contributed equally to the paper.

Abstract: Nearly 18% of patients on a waiting list for kidney transplantation (KT) are highly sensitized, which make access to KT more difficult. We assessed the efficacy and tolerance of different techniques (plasma exchanges [PE], double-filtration plasmapheresis [DFPP], and immunoadsorption [IA]) to remove donor specific antibodies (DSA) in the setting of HLA-incompatible (HLAi) KT. All patients that underwent apheresis for HLAi KT within a single center were included. Intra-session and inter-session Mean Fluorescence Intensity (MFI) decrease in DSA, clinical and biological tolerances were assessed. A total of 881 sessions were performed for 45 patients: 107 DFPP, 54 PE, 720 IA. The procedures led to HLAi KT in 39 patients (87%) after 29 (15–51) days. A higher volume of treated plasma was associated with a greater decrease of inter-session class I and II DSA ($p = 0.04$, $p = 0.02$). IA, PE, and a lower maximal DSA MFI were associated with a greater decrease in intra-session class II DSA ($p < 0.01$). Safety was good: severe adverse events occurred in 17 sessions (1.9%), more frequently with DFPP (6.5%) $p < 0.01$. Hypotension occurred in 154 sessions (17.5%), more frequently with DFPP ($p < 0.01$). Apheresis is well tolerated (IA and PE > DFPP) and effective at removing HLA antibodies and allows HLAi KT for sensitized patients.

Keywords: plasmapheresis; kidney transplantation; desensitization; donor specific antibody

1. Introduction

Chronic kidney disease (CKD) and end-stage kidney disease (ESKD) are global public health problems. Kidney transplantation (KT) provides the best results in terms of survival, quality of life, and health-care savings compared to hemodialysis (HD) when kidney replacement is necessary [1].

Currently, the major causes of restricting access to KT are graft shortage and a recipient's sensitization to anti-human leukocyte antigens (HLA) In France, about 30% of patients on waiting lists for a KT are sensitized [2]. The number of newly listed patients has increased by 35% over the past 10 years and the number of patients on waiting lists has increased by 82% within 10 years. Pre-existing donor-specific alloantibodies (DSA), defining HLA-incompatible (HLAi) KT, may restrict access to a living-donor transplant or delay access to a deceased-donor KT. Highly sensitized patients remain on a waiting list for two to three times longer than non-sensitized candidates [3].

Options to enable access to KT for sensitized patients include acceptable mismatch programs, paired donation, or desensitization [4]. HLA desensitization significantly improves access to a deceased- or living-donor KT [5]. In 2016, Orandi et al. reported a survival benefit in the USA for sensitized patients undergoing desensitization for HLAi living-donor KT compared to those remaining on a waiting list [6].

The goal of desensitization is to reduce DSA mean fluorescence intensity (MFI) as much as possible to obtain a negative cytotoxic crossmatch at the time of KT. Various desensitization protocols have been used in the setting of HLAi KT: most involve plasmapheresis, but also intravenous immunoglobulins and B-cell depleting agents [7]. Plasmapheresis includes several types of extracorporeal therapies that can be used to remove antibodies (anti-HLA antibodies and DSA): plasma exchange (PE), double-filtration plasmapheresis (DFPP), and semi specific immunoadsorption (IA). To date, there is no evidence for superiority of one technique over another and no study has compared the different apheresis techniques in connection to HLA desensitization. The aim of this study was to assess the efficacy, safety and tolerance of each apheresis technique in the setting of desensitization for HLAi KT.

2. Materials and Methods

2.1. Study Population

In this single-center study, all adult patients that had undergone desensitization for HLAi KT in the University Hospital of Grenoble, since January 2016, were included. Inclusion into the desensitization protocol required being on the KT waiting list for >3 years, having no infectious or neoplastic co-morbidities, and having optimal results from a cardiac check-up within the previous three months. For living-donor KT, patients were included in case of pre-existing DSA of >1500 MFI. MFI assessment was performed using a bead assay (Luminex Single Antigen assay, Immucor, Norcross, GA, USA). For deceased donors, recipients had to be highly sensitized (i.e., to have a historical calculated panel-reactive alloantibody (cPRA) of $\geq$80%). The cPRA is calculated as the percentage of HLA antigens out of a panel reacting with the serum of a patient. It represents the percentage of donors expected to react with the serum of the patient. The screening for pretransplant HLA sensitization was also performed by Luminex assay. There were 22 living-kidney and 28 deceased-donor kidney-transplant candidates in this study.

All patients signed an informed consent form. All medical data were collected from our database (CNIL (French National committee for data protection) approval number 1987785v0).

2.2. Endpoints

The primary outcome was the efficacy of performing HLAi KT after desensitization and to compare the efficacy to remove HLA antibodies and DSAs between the three apheresis techniques. DSAs were monitored at least once a week during the desensitization period until KT.

"Intra-session DSA reduction" was defined as the percentage reduction in the immunodominant DSA MFI between pre- and post-apheresis session.

"Inter-session DSA reduction" was defined as the percentage reduction within two consecutive immunodominant DSA MFIs measured before an apheresis session and performed using the same apheresis technique (IA, DFPP, or PE). The number of sessions between two consecutives MFI measures varied but was taken into account within the analyses.

The secondary endpoints were the safety of the apheresis techniques, based on the number of severe adverse events, hemodynamic tolerance, and the evolution of biological parameters (platelet, hemoglobin, leukocytes, fibrinogen). Severe adverse events were defined in this study as occurring during an apheresis session and that led to discontinuing a session or that needed hospitalization. Hypotension was defined as a nadir systolic blood pressure of ≤90 mmHg during apheresis. Technical issues were defined as the need for a nurse's intervention.

2.3. Procedures

Desensitization and immunosuppression protocols are summarized in Figure 1A for living donors and Figure 1B for deceased donors and was realize in one center. Patients received two rituximab injections (375 mg/m^2 each). The immunosuppressive regimen consisted of prednisone (0.5 mg/kg), mycophenolate mofetil (500 mg × 2 per day), and tacrolimus (initial dose 0.1 mg/kg/day, with a target trough concentration of between 8 and 10 ng/mL).

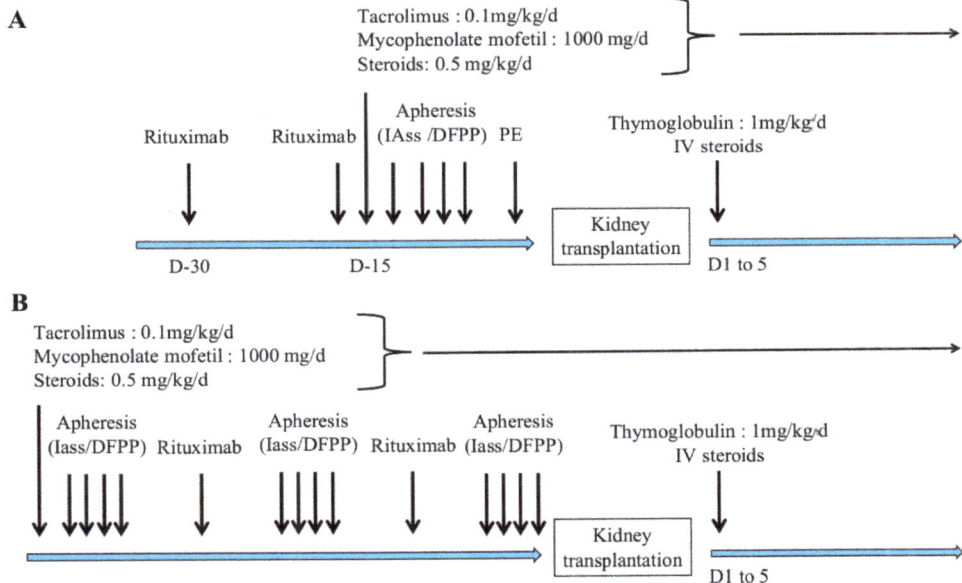

Figure 1. Desensitization and immunosuppression protocol for HLA-incompatible kidney transplantation. Panel (**A**) shows the protocol for living donors HLAi kidney transplantation. Panel (**B**) shows the protocol for deceased donors HLAi kidney transplantation. IAss: semi-specific immunoadsorption; DFPP: double-filtration plasmapheresis; PE: plasma exchange.

Apheresis sessions were performed by IA, PE, or DFPP according to the initial MFI (s) of DSA (s) for living-donor kidney-recipient KT or according to the immunodominant anti-HLA alloantibody for a deceased donor's KT. PE or DFPP was performed if MFI was <6000 and IA was performed if MFI was >6000.

PE was performed by centrifugation using a Spectra Optia® (BCT Lakewood, Terumo, CO, USA) or Comtec® (Fresenius Kabi, France). Filtration was carried out with a Plasmaflo™ OP-08W (Asahi Kasei Medical, Tokyo, Japan). DFPP was equipped with two filters in series. A primary filter with large pores (Plasmaflo™ OP-08W) separated cells and plasma, followed by a specific secondary filter (Cascadeflo™ EC-20W) for immunoglobulin filtration. IA was performed after plasma centrifugation on two adsorber Globaffin® columns (Fresenius Medical Care, St. Wendel, Germany) working in tandem. IA could be coupled with membrane filtration (Monet®). Monet® filter was used to enhance the removal of molecules possibly involved in the post-transplantation rejection risk such as IgM, C1q, properdin, mannose-binding lectin [8]. It was associated with IA when HLA antibody titer was high (i.e., >12,000). All patients received prophylactic antibiotherapy with phenoxymethylpenicillin and sulfamethoxazole-trimethoprim. Apheresis sessions were carried out in parallel with the hemodialysis sessions. Intravenous Immunoglobulins (IVIg) were given at low dose (1.5 g) in case of low IgG level (<4 g/L) before the apheresis session for substitution purposes.

2.4. Desensitization Protocol

For living-donor KT, the protocol consisted of four or five apheresis sessions per week for 2 weeks prior to KT. If the DSA MFI was >12,000, IA was performed daily. If DSA MFI was <6000, IA could be replaced by DFPP or PE to achieve a threshold MFI of < 3000 before KT. KT was performed when DSAs had an MFI of <3000, i.e., a negative-flow cytometric crossmatch in our center on the day before KT. A systematic graft biopsy was performed at 1, 3 and 12 months.

For deceased-donor KT, three to five apheresis sessions per week were carried out until a compatible kidney graft was available. If no nationally available graft was proposed within 45 days after starting desensitization, the first local ABO-compatible graft, matched for age and weight, was proposed. To facilitate the purification of high MFIs HLA antibodies, some patients with high level of antibodies (MFI > 12000) and waiting for a deceased donor were primed by receiving tocilizumab injections before the start of apheresis [9].

2.5. Statistical Analyses

Quantitative data are presented as means ± standard deviations (SD), or as medians with quartiles (Q1–Q3). Qualitative data are presented as the numbers of patients and percentages. The chi-squared test was used for categorical variables; the Wilcoxon or the Kruskal—Wallis test was used for continuous variables. Multiple linear-regression analysis was performed to identify the independent factors associated with inter-session and intra-session immunodominant DSA evolution. All parameters significantly associated with immunodominant DSA inter-session and intra-session decrease were included in the multivariate analyses except for the number of sessions that was closely correlated to the total volume of treated plasma and did not provide additional relevant data. Data adjusted in the multivariate inter-session model were the total volume of treated plasma and the type of apheresis technique (ie PE, DFPP and IA). Data adjusted in the multivariate intra-session model were the total volume of treated plasma, the type of apheresis technique and the initial MFI of the immunodominant DSA. In order to assess the impact of patient's variability on DSA reduction, we used a mixed model that allowed to predict the fixed effect and variability of the apheresis. A two-sided p-value of < 0.05 was considered statistically significant. Statistical analyses were conducted using R statistical software.

3. Results

3.1. Study Population

Between August 2016 and November 2020, 45 patients were desensitized in the setting of HLAi KT at Grenoble University Hospital (Table 1). Patients were aged 53 ± 13 years, and 25 (55.6%) were women. Mean body-mass index was 24 ± 4 kg/m^2. Seventeen patients (44%) were desensitized in the setting of a living-donor HLAi KT. Among these, eight were also ABO incompatible. Mean cPRA was 84.6 ± 26.3% (96 ± 5% for deceased donors and 65 ± 35% for living donors). A total of twenty-three (59%) had undergone a previous KT and median time on dialysis before desensitization was 65 (16.5–110) months.

At the beginning of desensitization, for living donors, the median immunodominant class I DSA MFI was 6195 (2458–11,347) and was 2191 (1180–7238) for class II DSAs. The deceased-donor median for immunodominant class I DSA MFIs was 13,929 (5237–18,606) and was 5508 (2079–10,872) for class II DSA. Retrospectively, 27 (60%) patients had more than one DSA. Regarding class I DSAs, anti HLA-A was present in 77.7% of patients, anti HLA-B in 63% of patients, and anti HLA-C in 15%. Regarding class II DSAs, anti HLA-DP was present in 28% of patients, anti-HLA-DQ in 36%, and anti HLA-DR in 44%.

Table 1. Baseline characteristics of patients according to kidney transplant donor type.

	Desensitization with Living Donors	Desensitization with a Total of Deceased Donors	Total	p-Value
	N = 18	N = 27	N = 45	
Age at inclusion (years)	53.6 ± 15	51.9 ± 12	52.6 ± 13	0.84
Male/Female gender ratio	7/11	13/14	20/25	0.54
Body Mass index (Kg/m^2)	24.5 ± 3	24.2 ± 4	24.3 ± 4	0.54
History of previous transplantation—N (%)	6 (35.3)	17 (77.3)	23 (59)	0.02
Pre-emptive kidney trans—N (%)	1 (5.9)	0 (0)	1 (2.6)	0.25
Time on dialysis (months)	17 ± 15	150 ± 114	92 ± 108	<0.001
cPRA (%)	65 ± 35	96 ± 5	84 ± 26	<0.001
>1 class I DSA—N (%)	11 (65)	16 (59)	27 (60)	0.09
>1 class II DSA—N (%)	12 (66.6)	13 (48)	25 (55.5)	0.01
Number of class I Missmatch—N (%)	17 KT	22 KT	39 KT	
1	1 (5.8)	0 (0)	1 (2.5)	
2	7 (41)	6 (27)	13 (33.3)	0.31
3	8 (47)	9 (41)	17 (43.5)	
4	1 (5.8)	5 (22.7)	6 (15.3)	
Number of class II Missmatch—N (%)				
0	3 (17.6)	3 (13.6)	6 (15.3)	
1	3 (17.6)	5 (22.7)	8 (20.5)	0.93
2	7 (41)	8 (36.3)	15 (38.4)	
3	2 (11.7)	3 (13.6)	5 (12.8)	
4	2 (11.7)	1 (4.5)	3 (7.7)	
Mean number of PE sessions	2 ± 1	1 ± 1	1 ± 1	0.04
Mean number of DFPP sessions	3 ± 3	2 ± 3	2 ± 3	0.61
Mean number of IA sessions	6 ± 7	22 ± 17	16 ± 15	<0.001
Trough tacrolimus level (ng/mL) at inclusion	4.9 ± 0.5	9.8 ± 5.8	8.5 ± 5.5	0.02

cPRA: calculated Panel Reative Antigen, DSA: Donor specific antibody, DFPP: double-filtration plasmapheresis; PE: plasmatic exchange; IA: immunoadsorption.

3.2. Characteristics of Apheresis for HLAi Kidney Transplantation

Between January 2016 and January 2020, 881 apheresis sessions were carried out for the 45 patients in the setting of HLA-incompatible KT. The characteristics of all apheresis sessions are summarized in Table 2. The number of sessions per patient was 15 [10–24]. IA was the most performed technique with 720 (81.7%) sessions. The median duration between the first and last session for each patient was 29 (15–51) days. The median duration of one session was 3.2 h (2.6–3.9): IA sessions took significantly longer (3.5 ± 0.8 h) compared to DFPP (2.1 ± 0.6 h) and PE (1.9 ± 0.6 h) ($p < 0.001$). Each patient had 9 ± 6 IA sessions, 2 ± 1 PE sessions, and 3 ± 2 DFPP sessions. The Monet® filter was added in 340 IA sessions (47.2%). A total of thirteen patients (28.9%) had received at least one injection of tocilizumab prior to apheresis desensitization at a dose of 8 mg/kg. A total of nineteen (42.2%) patients received IVIg injections in 47 IA sessions (6.5%) at the dose of 140 mg/kg, i.e., a mean dose of 9.5 ± 7 g Fibrinogen was infused after 51 sessions at a mean dose of 1.8 ± 0.8 g.

Table 2. Characteristics of sessions according to apheresis technique.

	DFPP (N = 107)	PE (N = 54)	IA (N = 720)	Total (N = 881)	p-Value
Duration of session (hours). Median [IQ]	2 (1.8–2.3)	1.7 (1.5–2.0)	3.5 (2.9–4.0)	3.2 (2.6–3.9)	<0.01
Treated plasma volume (L). Median [IQ]	3675 (3000–4200)	4200 (2564–3685)	6641 (5520–7523)	6035 (4803–7286)	<0.01
Blood flow (mL/min) Mean ± SD	146 ± 14	63 ± 38	54 ± 7	65 ± 32	<0.01
Substitution volume (L) Mean ± SD	259 ± 224	2857 ± 750	104 ± 53	295 ± 717	<0.01
Substitution fluid N (%)					
– Albumin 20%	10 (9.3%)	0 (0%)	720 (100%)	730 (83%)	
– Albumin 20% + saline serum	88 (82.2%)	0 (0%)	0 (0%)	88 (10%)	<0.01
– Albumin 4%	9 (8.4%)	20 (37%)	0 (0%)	29 (3.2%)	
– FFP	0 (0%)	34 (63.0%)	0 (0%)	34 (3.9%)	

DFPP: double-filtration plasmapheresis; PE: plasmatic exchange; IA: immunoadsorption; FFP: fresh frozen plasma.

3.3. Efficacy of Apheresis and Access to Kidney Transplantation

Regarding assess to KT, 39 (87%) patients received an HLAi KT at post-desensitization. A total of six desensitized patients did not receive a transplant: this was because of failure to remove HLA antibodies from three patients (6.6%) or intercurrent events occurring during the desensitization period for the other three patients (6.6%). The intercurrent events were one myocardial infarction (with death), a pulmonary infection (pneumocystis), and a digestive perforation. One patient died during the desensitization protocol period from acute coronary syndrome. The number of sessions was associated with the MFI level of the immunodominant DSA before the desensitization. An MFI increase of 276 of the DSA before the desensitization procedure was associated with an additional session needed to access to KT (p < 0.001).

We then assessed factors associated with intra- and inter-session DSA evolution.

Intra-session analyses: For class I DSAs, the mean decrease of MFI was 13 ± 4%. In univariate and multivariate analyses, the volume of purified plasma was significantly associated with a higher decrease in intra-session MFI (p = 0.03). For class II DSAs, the mean decrease in MFIs was 83 ± 22%. In univariate and multivariate analyses, IA and PE, and a lower initial DSA MFI were significantly associated with a higher decrease in intra-session MFI (p < 0.01) (Table 3). The mixed model used to predict patient variability impact on the apheresis effect showed similar results to the previous model meaning that the patient variability did not significantly impacted the antibodies removal (Tables S1 and S2).

Table 3. Uni- and multivariate analyses of factors associated with reduction in intra-session MFI of immunodominant DSAs.

	DSA Class I		DSA Class II	
	Univariate p-Value	Multivariate p-Value	Univariate p-Value	Multivariate p-Value
Volume of treated plasma	0.01	0.03	0.07	0.37
Technique of apheresis (IA and PE vs. DFPP)	0.20	0.60 (IA)	0.02 (PE) 0.01 (IA)	<0.01 (PE) <0.01 (IA)
Duration of session	0.89	-	0.10	-
Maximum MFI of DSA	0.39	0.19	<0.01	<0.01

DFPP: double-filtration plasmapheresis; PE: plasmatic exchange; IA: immunoadsorption; DSA: donor-specific antibody; MFI: mean fluorescence intensity.

Inter-session analyses: For class I DSAs, the mean decrease in MFI was 88 ± 50%. In univariate and multivariate analyses, the volume of treated plasma and the IA were associated with a higher inter-session DSA decrease, p = 0.04 and p = 0.03, respectively. For class II DSAs, the mean decrease in MFI was 59 ± 34%. In univariate and multivariate analyses, a higher total volume of treated plasma was significantly associated with a decrease in inter-session MFI (p = 0.02) (Table 4).

Table 4. Uni- and multivariate analyses of factors associated with reduction of inter-session MFI of immunodominant DSAs.

	DSA Class I		DSA Class II	
	Univariate p-Value	Multivariate p-Value	Univariate p-Value	Multivariate p-Value
Volume of treated Plasma	0.24	0.04	0.06	0.02
Technique of apheresis (IA and PE vs. DFPP)	0.86 (PE) 0.11 (IA)	0.83 (PE) 0.03 (IA)	0.22 (PE) 0.76 (IA)	0.18 (PE) 0.38 (IA)
Delay between sessions	0.42	-	0.49	-
Duration of session	0.92	-	0.78	-

DFPP: double-filtration plasmapheresis; PE: plasmatic exchange; IA: immunoadsorption.

The efficacies of the intra-session subtype immunoglobulin reduction are summarized in Table 4. The best reduction rate of IgG was −60.6% (−46; −73) for PE sessions, followed by −60% (−33; −69) for IA, and −40.0% (−30; −50) for DFPP ($p < 0.001$). Figure 2 shows the percentages of IgG reduction according to apheresis techniques. The volume of treated plasma is significantly associated with IgG reduction post apheresis for all techniques, but IA needs a more important volume to remove Ig. The absolute value of IgG at post-session was lower for IA (0.6 ± 0.7 g/L) versus EP (2.1 ± 1 g/L) and DFPP (1.4 ± 1 g/L), $p < 0.001$. The use of the Monet filter was associated with a significantly higher reduction of IgG but also IgM and IgA post session as compared to IA alone (Figure S1).

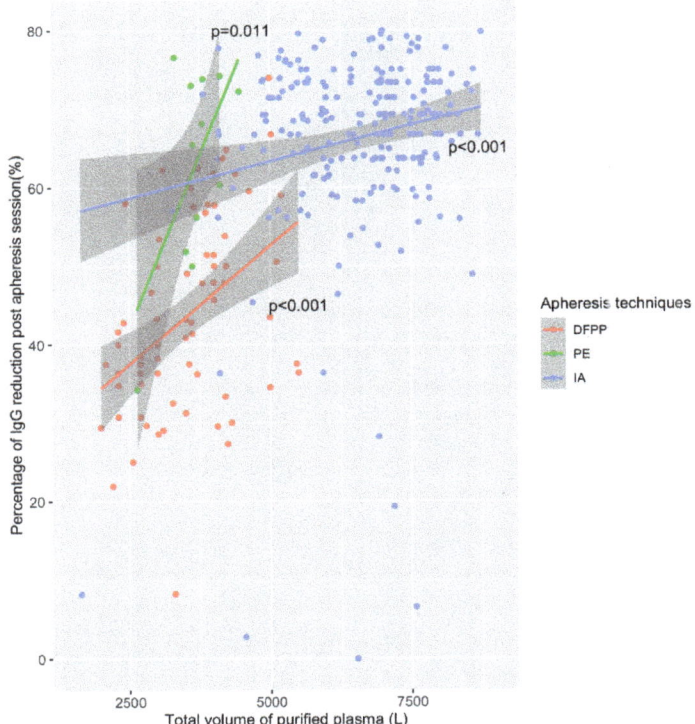

Figure 2. Post session reduction of immunoglobulin-G according to the apheresis technique. DFPP: double-filtration plasmapheresis; PE: plasma exchange; IA: immunoadsorption; IgG: immunoglobulin subtype G. IgG reduction was assessed in all sessions that did not received IV immunoglobulins. The volume of purified plasma is significantly associated with IgG reduction.

3.4. Apheresis Tolerance

Clinical tolerance: serious adverse events occurred in 17 (1.9%) sessions and hemodynamic intolerance occurred in 154 (17.5%) sessions. We assessed the association of serious adverse events with age, trough level of tacrolimus, technique of apheresis, Rituximab, IVIg, Tocilizumab, simultaneous dialysis, vascular access, use of membranous filter, duration of apheresis session, anticoagulation and blood flow rate. DFPP was significantly less well-tolerated compared to IA and PE: serious adverse events occurred in 6.5% of DFPP sessions versus 1.9% and 1.2% for PE and IA, respectively ($p < 0.01$). Trough level of tacrolimus was also associated with serious adverse events ($p = 0.02$). Intrasession hypotension occurred in 39.3% of DFPP sessions versus 20.4% and 14% for PE and IA, respectively ($p < 0.01$). The number of sessions with technical issues that required a nurse's intervention was 88 (10%) and was similar between the three techniques ($p = 0.53$).

Biological tolerance (Table 5): fibrinogen decreased by -46.7% (-23; -60) with a higher loss with DFPP: -1.5% (-55; -69) versus PE -33.3% (-28; -64) and IA -42.9% (-22; -57) ($p < 0.01$). Post-session fibrinogen was lower with DFPP: 0.6 ± 0.4 g/L compared to the other techniques (1.0 ± 0.7 g/L for IA and 1.3 ± 0.7 g/L for PE) ($p < 0.01$). Five (11.1%) patients presented with asymptomatic cytomegalovirus (CMV) DNAemia and 9 (20%) with Epstein—Barr virus (EBV) DNAemia during the desensitization period. Only one patient developed CMV disease with digestive involvement. Red-blood cell transfusion was performed in 82 (9.3%) sessions.

Table 5. Biological parameters according to apheresis techniques.

	DFPP (N = 107)	PE (N = 54)	IA (N = 720)	Total (N = 881)	p-Value
Pre-post IgA evolution (%) Median [IQ]	-55 (-45; -63)	-48 (-1; -71)	-14 (-7; -21)	-17 (-8; -29)	<0.01
Pre-post IgG evolution (%) Median [IQ]	-40 (-31; -50)	-61 (-46; -73)	-60 (-33; -70)	-56 (-33; -69)	<0.01
Pre-post IgM evolution (%) Median [IQ]	-37 (0; -58)	-51 (60; -75)	-17 (0; -54)	-17 (0; -57)	0.10
Pre-post Alb evolution (%) Median [IQ]	1 (14; 2)	10 (14; -3)	9 (14; -1)	9 (15; 0)	0.73
Pre-post fibrinogen evolution (%) Median [IQ]	-61 (-56; -69)	-33 (-29; -64)	-43 (-22; -57)	-47 (-23; -60)	<0.01
Pre-post hemoglobin evolution (%) Median [IQ]	15 (22; -8)	2 (10; -2)	2 (9; -2)	3 (11; -2)	<0.01
Pre-post leukocytes Evolution (%) Median [IQ]	65 (96; 33)	22 (60; 5)	4 (18; 8)	8 (27; 6)	<0.01
Pre-post platelet evolution (%) Median [IQ]	7 (-1; 17)	14 (2; 21)	12 (3; 21)	12 (2; 21)	0.01

DFPP: double-filtration plasmapheresis; PE: plasmatic exchange; IA: immunoadsorption.

4. Discussion

In this cohort, we found that an MFI-stratified apheresis protocol associated with rituximab and a standard immunosuppressive regimen was efficient to desensitize patients in the setting of HLAi KT. Only six patients did not receive a transplant due to failure of desensitization or an intercurrent event. Removal of intra-session class II DSAs was more efficient with IA and PE than with DFPP and when the maximal DSA was lower. The decrease in inter-session class I and II DSAs was associated with the higher volume of treated plasma (in multivariate analyses). IA was also associated with a better class I inter-session decrease.

The very first plasmapheresis technique was performed on dogs in 1914 [10]. In CKD and KT, the main pathologies associated with plasmapheresis are antibody-mediated rejection, focal segmental glomerulosclerosis, and desensitization [11]. Highly sensitized patients without a HLA-compatible donor are difficult to manage. These patients have to wait long periods for a compatible deceased donor, are often on hemodialysis, and have increased morbidity-mortality [12]. Desensitization strategies have significantly improved access to KT from deceased and living donors [5,13].

The goal of desensitization is to obtain a sustained drop in DSA MFI and to allow KT under an acceptable immunological risk. In the 1970s, Cardella et al. considered that PE could remove DSAs involved in acute humoral rejection [14]. In desensitization, plasmapheresis has shown better results compared to IVIg to achieve a negative crossmatch and was associated with a lower rate of antibody-mediated rejection [15]. Anti-HLA antibodies are IgG, with a half-life of 21 days, with a molecular weight about 160,000 Daltons, and a vascular distribution of about 40% [16]. For these reasons, apheresis can remove DSAs from plasma.

To date, there are three different apheresis techniques: PE, DFPP, and IA. PE is a non-selective technique that removes all plasma proteins. In our center, PE has been mostly performed by centrifugation, which allows a decrease in blood flow and reduces the session time [17]. DFPP and IA are more recent techniques that allow selective or semi-selective plasma purification. Selective plasma purification avoids the unnecessary loss of plasma proteins and reduces the need for liquid replacement and increases the efficiency of purification [18].

Böhmig et al., in 2007, showed, in a randomized study, the efficacy of IA to remove antibodies in a setting of acute antibody-mediated rejection post KT [19]. In our study, the most effective apheresis technique was IA. The first use of IA in KT for highly HLA-sensitized cases dates from 1989 [20]. IA has since been used successively as a desensitizing therapy by many teams [21]. The most commonly used IA column in our center has been a Globaffin® column: it uses a synthetic peptide with a high affinity for the constant fraction (Fc) of IgG antibodies of subclasses 1, 2 and 4 [22]. By purifying a high plasmatic volume with IA, Belàk et al. have shown a 87% drop in the initial IgG level and good affinity for IgG 2 and 4 [23]. IA and DFPP allow higher plasma volumes to be treated without excessive loss of plasma [24,25] whereas the main constraint of PE remains the necessary use of a substitute solution.

To the best of our knowledge, only a few studies with very small populations have compared apheresis techniques in the setting of HLAi KT [23,26]. In our study, the percentage IgG reduction was higher with PE, but the absolute value of IgG at post-session was lower with IA. This is partly due to the pore size of DFPP filters, which allows good elimination of IgA and IgM, but low elimination of IgG to avoid loss of albumin with a similar molecular weight [27]. Regarding to HLA antibodies removal and monitoring, the limitation is the measurement itself by Single-Antigen Bead assay. Indeed, high level of HLA antibodies can be missed or underestimated because of IgG detection interference (prozone effect). In order to prevent this, all patients of this study had a dilution test of their serum before the desensitization procedure and none had a prozone effect. Moreover, in our study, the initial MFI of HLA antibody was not similar for IA, PE and DFPP. We may suspect that the reduction of MFI is partially correlated with the amount of antibody which introduce of possible bias in our results.

Apheresis requires both medical and paramedical expertise with a team that is well-trained in the different techniques. Plasmapheresis may be complicated by cardiovascular [28], hemorrhagic [29,30] or allergic [31] complications. In our center, the technique with the most undesirable effects was DFPP. We also found a significant increase in the numbers of leukocytes after DFPP. This may be explained by the bio-incompatibility of the membranes and the frictional forces imposed on blood through these membranes [32]. This activation of the inflammatory system may be partly responsible for the excess risk of hypotension.

Moreover, even if not assessed in this study, we suspect there is improved quality of life for patients that receive a transplant after desensitization compared to those that remain on dialysis.

Finally, desensitization with apheresis was effective at removing HLA antibodies and allowed access to HLAi KT for sensitized patients. IA and EP were more effective to remove IgG and antiHLA antibodies, especially for class II DSAs, and were better tolerated than DFPP.

Supplementary Materials: The following are available online at https://www.mdpi.com/2077-0383/10/6/1316/s1, Figure S1: Percentage of IgM, IgA and IgG reduction post immunoadsorption alone or combined with membrane filtration, Table S1: Mixed model modeling the effect of session type as a fixed and a random effect on DSA class I reduction, Table S2: Mixed model modeling the effect of session type as a fixed and a random effect on DSA class II reduction.

Author Contributions: J.N.: performed the statistical analysis and wrote the paper; A.M.: collected the data and performed the literature search; H.N.B.: manuscript revision; M.D.: collected the data, manuscript revision; D.M.: collected the data, manuscript revision; F.T.: manuscript revision; F.I.: collected the data, manuscript revision; B.B.: analysis and interpretation of data, manuscript revision; G.F.: intellectual content and manuscript revision; R.M.: intellectual content and manuscript revision; B.J.: drafting of the article and manuscript revision; E.C.: manuscript revision P.M.: manuscript revision, verified underlying data and final approval; L.R.: conception design and final approval T.J.: performed statistical analysis, conception, manuscript revision and final approval. All authors have read and agreed to the published version of the manuscript.

Funding: This research received no external funding.

Institutional Review Board Statement: The study was conducted according to the guidelines of the Declaration of Helsinki, and approved by the Institutional Review Board (or Ethics Committee) of CNIL (French National committee for data protection) approval number 1987785v0. N° BRIF: BB-0033-00069.

Informed Consent Statement: Informed consent was obtained from all subjects involved in the study.

Data Availability Statement: The data presented in this study are available on request from the corresponding author.

Conflicts of Interest: The authors declare no conflict of interest.

References

1. Wolfe, R.A.; Ashby, V.B.; Milford, E.L.; Ojo, A.O.; Ettenger, R.E.; Agodoa, L.Y.; Held, P.J.; Port, F.K. Comparison of Mortality in All Patients on Dialysis, Patients on Dialysis Awaiting Transplantation, and Recipients of a First Cadaveric Transplant. *N. Engl. J. Med.* **1999**, *341*, 1725–1730. [CrossRef]
2. Malvezzi, P.; Jouve, T.; Noble, J.; Rostaing, L. Desensitization in the Setting of HLA-Incompatible Kidney Transplant. *Exp. Clin. Transpl.* **2018**, *16*, 367–375.
3. Pruthi, R.; Hilton, R.; Pankhurst, L.; Mamode, N.; Hudson, A.; Roderick, P.; Ravanan, R. UK Renal Registry 16th Annual Report: Chapter 4 Demography of Patients Waitlisted for Renal Transplantation in the UK: National and Centre-Specific Analyses. *Nephron Clin. Pract.* **2013**, *125*, 81–98. [CrossRef]
4. Claas, F.H.J.; Witvliet, M.D.; Duquesnoy, R.J.; Persijn, G.G.; Doxiadis, I.I.N. The Acceptable Mismatch Program as a Fast Tool for Highly Sensitized Patients Awaiting a Cadaveric Kidney Transplantation: Short Waiting Time and Excellent Graft Outcome. *Transplant. J.* **2004**, *78*, 190–193. [CrossRef] [PubMed]
5. Gridelli, B.; Remuzzi, G. Strategies for Making More Organs Available for Transplantation. *N. Engl. J. Med.* **2000**, *343*, 404–410. [CrossRef] [PubMed]
6. Orandi, B.J.; Montgomery, R.A.; Segev, D.L. Kidney Transplants from HLA-Incompatible Live Donors and Survival. *N. Engl. J. Med.* **2016**, *375*, 288–289. [CrossRef] [PubMed]
7. Loupy, A.; Suberbielle-Boissel, C.; Zuber, J.; Anglicheau, D.; Timsit, M.-O.; Martinez, F.; Thervet, E.; Bruneval, P.; Charron, D.; Hill, G.S.; et al. Combined Posttransplant Prophylactic IVIg/Anti-CD 20/Plasmapheresis in Kidney Recipients with Preformed Donor-Specific Antibodies: A Pilot Study. *Transplantation* **2010**, *89*, 1403–1410. [CrossRef]
8. Defendi, F.; Malvezzi, P.; Eskandary, F.; Cesbron, J.-Y.; Rostaing, L.; Böhmig, G.A.; Dumestre-Pérard, C. Effects of Immunoadsorption Combined with Membrane Filtration on Complement Markers-Results of a Randomized, Controlled, Crossover Study. *Transpl. Int.* **2019**, *32*, 876–883. [CrossRef]
9. Shin, B.-H.; Everly, M.J.; Zhang, H.; Choi, J.; Vo, A.; Zhang, X.; Huang, E.; Jordan, S.C.; Toyoda, M. Impact of Tocilizumab (Anti-IL-6R) Treatment on Immunoglobulins and Anti-HLA Antibodies in Kidney Transplant Patients with Chronic Antibody-Mediated Rejection. *Transplantation* **2020**, *104*, 856–863. [CrossRef]
10. Sokolov, A.A.; Solovyev, A.G. Russian Pioneers of Therapeutic Hemapheresis and Extracorporeal Hemocorrection: 100-Year Anniversary of the World's First Successful Plasmapheresis. *Ther. Apher. Dial.* **2014**, *18*, 117–121. [CrossRef]
11. Salvadori, M.; Tsalouchos, A. Therapeutic Apheresis in Kidney Transplantation: An Updated Review. *World J. Transpl.* **2019**, *9*, 103–122. [CrossRef]
12. Sapir-Pichhadze, R.; Tinckam, K.J.; Laupacis, A.; Logan, A.G.; Beyene, J.; Kim, S.J. Immune Sensitization and Mortality in Wait-Listed Kidney Transplant Candidates. *J. Am. Soc. Nephrol.* **2016**, *27*, 570–578. [CrossRef] [PubMed]
13. Sethi, S.; Choi, J.; Toyoda, M.; Vo, A.; Peng, A.; Jordan, S.C. Desensitization: Overcoming the Immunologic Barriers to Transplantation. *J. Immunol. Res.* **2017**, *2017*, 6804678. [CrossRef]
14. Cardella, C.J.; Sutton, D.; Uldall, P.R.; Deveber, G.A. Intensive plasma exchange and renal-transplant rejection. *Lancet* **1977**, *309*, 264. [CrossRef]

15. Stegall, M.D.; Gloor, J.; Winters, J.L.; Moore, S.B.; Degoey, S. A Comparison of Plasmapheresis versus High-Dose IVIG Desensitization in Renal Allograft Recipients with High Levels of Donor Specific Alloantibody. *Am. J. Transpl.* **2006**, *6*, 346–351. [CrossRef]
16. Kaplan, A.A. Toward the Rational Prescription of Therapeutic Plasma Exchange: The Kinetics of Immunoglobulin Removal. *Semin. Dial.* **1992**, *5*, 227–229. [CrossRef]
17. Hafer, C.; Golla, P.; Gericke, M.; Eden, G.; Beutel, G.; Schmidt, J.J.; Schmidt, B.M.W.; De Reys, S.; Kielstein, J.T. Membrane versus Centrifuge-Based Therapeutic Plasma Exchange: A Randomized Prospective Crossover Study. *Int. Urol. Nephrol.* **2016**, *48*, 133–138. [CrossRef]
18. Sanchez, A.P.; Cunard, R.; Ward, D.M. The Selective Therapeutic Apheresis Procedures. *J. Clin. Apher.* **2013**, *28*, 20–29. [CrossRef] [PubMed]
19. Böhmig, G.A.; Wahrmann, M.; Regele, H.; Exner, M.; Robl, B.; Derfler, K.; Soliman, T.; Bauer, P.; Müllner, M.; Druml, W. Immunoadsorption in Severe C4d-Positive Acute Kidney Allograft Rejection: A Randomized Controlled Trial. *Am. J. Transpl.* **2007**, *7*, 117–121. [CrossRef]
20. Palmer, A.; Taube, D.; Welsh, K.; Bewick, M.; Gjorstrup, P.; Thick, M. Removal of Anti-HLA Antibodies by Extracorporeal Immunoadsorption to Enable Renal Transplantation. *Lancet* **1989**, *1*, 10–12. [CrossRef]
21. Rostaing, L.; Congy, N.; Aarnink, A.; Maggioni, S.; Allal, A.; Sallusto, F.; Game, X.; Kamar, N. Efficacy of Immunoadsorption to Reduce Donor-Specific Alloantibodies in Kidney-Transplant Candidates. *Exp. Clin. Transpl.* **2015**, *13* (Suppl. 1), 201–206.
22. Ronspeck, W.; Brinckmann, R.; Egner, R.; Gebauer, F.; Winkler, D.; Jekow, P.; Wallukat, G.; Muller, J.; Kunze, R. Peptide Based Adsorbers for Therapeutic Immunoadsorption. *Ther. Dial.* **2003**, *7*, 91–97. [CrossRef] [PubMed]
23. Belàk, M.; Borberg, H.; Jimenez, C.; Oette, K. Technical and Clinical Experience with Protein a Immunoadsorption Columns. *Transfus. Sci.* **1994**, *15*, 419–422. [CrossRef]
24. Lorenz, M.; Regele, H.; Schillinger, M.; Kletzmayr, J.; Haidbauer, B.; Derfler, K.; Druml, W.; Böhmig, G.A. Peritransplant Immunoadsorption: A Strategy Enabling Transplantation in Highly Sensitized Crossmatch-Positive Cadaveric Kidney Allograft Recipients. *Transplantation* **2005**, *79*, 696–701. [CrossRef] [PubMed]
25. Higgins, R.; Lowe, D.; Hathaway, M.; Lam, F.T.; Kashi, H.; Tan, L.C.; Imray, C.; Fletcher, S.; Chen, K.; Krishnan, N.; et al. Double Filtration Plasmapheresis in Antibody-Incompatible Kidney Transplantation. *Ther. Apher. Dial.* **2010**, *14*, 392–399. [CrossRef] [PubMed]
26. Zhang, Y.; Tang, Z.; Chen, D.; Gong, D.; Ji, D.; Liu, Z. Comparison of Double Filtration Plasmapheresis with Immunoadsorption Therapy in Patients with Anti-Glomerular Basement Membrane Nephritis. *BMC Nephrol.* **2014**, *15*, 128. [CrossRef]
27. Gurland, H.J.; Lysaght, M.J.; Samtleben, W.; Schmidt, B. Comparative Evaluation of Filters Used in Membrane Plasmapheresis. *Nephron* **1984**, *36*, 173–182. [CrossRef]
28. Huestis, D.W. Mortality in Therapeutic Haemapheresis. *Lancet* **1983**, *1*, 1043. [CrossRef]
29. Biesenbach, P.; Eskandary, F.; Ay, C.; Wiegele, M.; Derfler, K.; Schaden, E.; Haslacher, H.; Oberbauer, R.; Böhmig, G.A. Effect of Combined Treatment with Immunoadsorption and Membrane Filtration on Plasma Coagulation—Results of a Randomized Controlled Crossover Study. *J. Clin. Apher.* **2016**, *31*, 29–37. [CrossRef]
30. Keller, A.J.; Chirnside, A.; Urbaniak, S.J. Coagulation Abnormalities Produced by Plasma Exchange on the Cell Separator with Special Reference to Fibrinogen and Platelet Levels. *Br. J. Haematol.* **1979**, *42*, 593–603. [CrossRef]
31. Sutton, D.M.; Nair, R.C.; Rock, G. Complications of Plasma Exchange. *Transfusion* **1989**, *29*, 124–127. [CrossRef] [PubMed]
32. Siami, G.A.; Siami, F.S. Membrane Plasmapheresis in the United States: A Review over the Last 20 Years. *Ther. Apher.* **2001**, *5*, 315–320. [CrossRef] [PubMed]

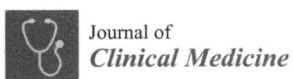

Article

Urinary NGAL Measured after the First Year Post Kidney Transplantation Predicts Changes in Glomerular Filtration over One-Year Follow-Up

Małgorzata Kielar [1], Paulina Dumnicka [2], Agnieszka Gala-Błądzińska [3], Alina Będkowska-Prokop [4], Ewa Ignacak [4], Barbara Maziarz [5], Piotr Ceranowicz [6,*] and Beata Kuśnierz-Cabala [5,*]

1 St. Louis Regional Children's Hospital, Medical Diagnostic Laboratory with a Bacteriology Laboratory, Strzelecka 2 St., 31-503 Kraków, Poland; gkielar@tlen.pl
2 Jagiellonian University Medical College, Faculty of Pharmacy, Department of Medical Diagnostics, 30-688 Kraków, Poland; paulina.dumnicka@uj.edu.pl
3 Medical College of Rzeszów University, Institute of Medical Sciences, Kopisto 2A Avn., 35-310 Rzeszów, Poland; agala.edu@gmail.com
4 Jagiellonian University Medical College, Faculty of Medicine, Department of Nephrology, Jakubowskiego 2 St., 30-688 Kraków, Poland; alina.betkowska-prokop@uj.edu.pl (A.B.-P.); ewa.igncak@uj.edu.pl (E.I.)
5 Jagiellonian University Medical College, Faculty of Medicine, Department of Diagnostics, Kopernika 15A St., 31-501 Kraków, Poland; mbmaziar@cyf-kr.edu.pl
6 Jagiellonian University Medical College, Faculty of Medicine, Department of Physiology, Grzegórzecka 16 St., 31-531 Kraków, Poland
* Correspondence: piotr.ceranowicz@uj.edu.pl (P.C.); mbkusnie@cyf-kr.edu.pl (B.K.-C.); Tel.: +48-12-424-83-65 (B.K.-C.)

Abstract: Currently, serum creatinine and estimated glomerular filtration rate (eGFR) together with albuminuria or proteinuria are laboratory markers used in long-term monitoring of kidney transplant recipients. There is a need for more sensitive markers that could serve as early warning signs of graft dysfunction. Our aim was to assess the urinary concentrations of neutrophil gelatinase-associated lipocalin (NGAL) as a predictor of changes in kidney transplant function after the first year post-transplantation. We prospectively recruited 109 patients with functioning graft at least one year after the transplantation, with no acute conditions over the past three months, during their control visits in kidney transplant ambulatory. Urinary NGAL measured on recruitment was twice higher in patients with at least 10% decrease in eGFR over 1-year follow-up compared to those with stable or improving transplant function. Baseline NGAL significantly predicted the relative and absolute changes in eGFR and the mean eGFR during the follow-up independently of baseline eGFR and albuminuria. Moreover, baseline NGAL significantly predicted urinary tract infections during the follow-up, although the infections were not associated with decreasing eGFR. Additionally, we assessed urinary concentrations of matrix metalloproteinase 9—NGAL complex in a subgroup of 77 patients and found higher levels in patients who developed urinary tract infections during the follow-up but not in those with decreasing eGFR. High urinary NGAL in clinically stable kidney transplant recipients beyond the first year after transplantation may be interpreted as a warning and trigger the search for transient or chronic causes of graft dysfunction, or urinary tract infection.

Keywords: kidney allograft; neutrophil gelatinase-associated lipocalin; matrix metalloproteinase 9-neutrophil gelatinase-associated lipocalin complex; glomerular filtration rate; urinary tract infections

1. Introduction

Renal transplantation is the best therapeutic option for patients with end-stage kidney disease. Both donor—and recipient-related factors are associated with kidney graft function, including metabolic and immunological factors. Acute or chronic rejection, recurrent or de novo nephropathies, side effects of immunosuppressive drugs, comorbidities (including infections), and age-related decline in renal function adversely affect long-term survival of both kidney graft and transplant recipient. According to 2009 Kidney Disease: Improving Global Outcomes (KDIGO) guidelines [1], the monitoring of kidney transplant recipients is based on physical examination, urine volume, the assessment of albuminuria or proteinuria, serum creatinine measurements, glomerular filtration rate (GFR) estimation based on serum creatinine, and the ultrasound imaging. Kidney transplant biopsy and histopathological examination allow precise diagnosis of graft injury. Although protocol-specified biopsies are performed in some centers [2], the biopsy procedure is invasive and is associated with possible adverse events. Therefore, most centers only use graft biopsy in the patients with worsening renal function i.e., suspected acute kidney rejection episodes or a chronic elevation in creatinine and/or the onset of persistent proteinuria (indication or "for cause" biopsies), as recommended by the KDIGO guidelines [1]. This allows the diagnosis of kidney graft injury. However, the indication for graft biopsy based on the clinical assessment, including serum creatinine, eGFR, and albuminuria (proteinuria) may in some cases be controversial.

The studies using protocol biopsies reveal the signs of chronic rejection in a significant proportion of cases without clinical signs of decreasing renal function [3,4]. Still, even subclinical chronic rejection leads to a decrease in graft survival over long-term time periods [4]. There is a need for novel markers that may be used in routine monitoring of patients and would provide earlier warning signal as compared to currently recommended markers used in clinical practice, i.e., serum creatinine, eGFR and albuminuria or proteinuria. Specifically, serum creatinine concentrations, and thus eGFR, may be influenced by extra-renal factors, leading to the intra-individual biological variability that has been estimated for about 5–8% [5–8].

In the last 15 years, neutrophil gelatinase-associated lipocalin (NGAL) became one of the most extensively studied marker of acute kidney injury (AKI) [9,10]. NGAL is a 25 kDa protein that has been originally isolated from the secondary granules of activated neutrophils [11]. It is also produced by hepatocytes, the cells of alimentary and respiratory tracts, the cells of immune system, and, notably, by the epithelial cells of distal renal tubule [12–14]. Both toxic and ischemic kidney injury leads to increased excretion of NGAL in urine which may be noted as soon as two hours from the initial insult [12,14,15]. Three molecular forms of NGAL have been found in urine, namely the NGAL monomer that has been associated with distal tubular cells injury, the NGAL homodimer that has been associated with the presence of neutrophils in urine and urinary tract infections, and the least studied matrix metalloproteinase 9 (MMP 9)-NGAL heterodimer [13,16]. NGAL has been assigned the protective role during acute tubular injury, increasing autophagy in the distal tubular cells, inhibiting apoptosis and inducing regeneration [17–19]. More recently, NGAL has been studied as a marker of chronic kidney disease (CKD), including diabetic kidney disease [20,21], and as a marker of cardiovascular risk [22,23]. In kidney transplantation, NGAL (measured early post-transplant) has been extensively studied as a predictor of delayed graft function [13,24–26]. Also, there are several reports on urinary NGAL as a predictor of acute kidney injury later after transplantation [27,28] and a graft loss after acute kidney injury [29]. However, the diagnostic value of NGAL in kidney transplant patients following the first year after transplantation, in relation to chronic processes leading to a gradual decrease in kidney allograft function, has not been extensively studied [30,31]. Moreover, clinical utility of the published findings is hindered by the use of diverse laboratory methods for urine NGAL measurements, which does not allow directly comparing the measured concentrations and the proposed cut-off values.

Our aim was to assess the concentrations of urinary NGAL with an automated laboratory method in kidney transplant recipients at least one year after transplantation and to study their association with changes in kidney function observed during one-year follow-up. Considering the intra-individual variability of serum creatinine and eGFR that is observed in clinical practice among chronic kidney disease patients, we compared the subgroups of patients with and without at least 10% decrease in eGFR over a 1-year follow-up. Additionally, we performed an exploratory analysis regarding the urinary concentrations of MMP 9-NGAL complex in a subgroup of studied patients.

2. Methods

2.1. Study Design

This was a prospective observational study. Patients were recruited in the ward dedicated to care of kidney transplant recipients, in the Chair and Department of Nephrology, University Hospital, Kraków, Poland between May and July 2019. The inclusion criteria were as follows: age of at least 18 years, at least one year from transplantation, functioning kidney transplant with eGFR at least 15 mL/min/1.73 m^2, and no acute kidney injury fulfilling the definition of KDIGO 2011 [32] or any condition requiring hospital treatment during at least three months before the inclusion into the study. Patients with the signs or symptoms of infection, including urinary tract infection at baseline were excluded from the study.

On recruitment, patients signed an informed consent for the study. They underwent detailed history and physical examination. Urine and venous blood samples were collected for the laboratory tests in the morning of the day of the study visit. The baseline clinical data and the results of routine laboratory tests on enrollment were recorded. The data regarding transplantation procedure (date of transplantation, deceased or living donor, first or second transplant, induction therapy, cold and warm ischemia time, delayed graft function) and the primary cause of kidney disease were based on the available medical records. The data on pretransplant panel reactive antibodies (PRA) and donor/recipient human leukocyte antigens (HLA) mismatches were based on transplantation protocols available for the patients who had undergone transplantation procedure in University Hospital, Kraków, Poland. In September 2020, the follow-up data were collected based on medical records of the patients who remained in control in the kidney transplant recipients' ambulatory, including the clinical course during the follow-up, the serum creatinine concentrations obtained during all control visits, and the results of laboratory tests performed at the last visit of a patient in the kidney transplant recipients' ambulatory.

The study protocol was approved by the Jagiellonian University Bioethical Committee (approval no 1072.6120.46.2019 issued on 28 February 2019).

2.2. Laboratory Tests

The blood and urine samples for laboratory tests were collected in the morning hours after an overnight fast. Routine laboratory test included complete blood count performed in K$_2$EDTA-anticoagulated samples, biochemical and immunochemical tests (serum creatinine, triglycerides, total cholesterol, uric acid, albumin, C-reactive protein, and glucose), and urinalysis. In addition, urine protein, albumin, NGAL and creatinine concentrations were assessed in the samples obtained at the initial study visit. Excess serum and urine samples were aliquoted and frozen in $-80\,^\circ$C within 2 h from samples' collection. Within two months, the thawed samples were centrifuged and the supernatant was analyzed for NGAL and MMP 9-NGAL complex. Urine NGAL was assessed with chemiluminescence microparticle immunoassay (Architect urine NGAL) on Abbott Architect analyzer (Abbott Laboratories, Chicago, IL, USA). The limit of detection for the test was estimated for 0.7 ng/mL by the manufacturer; the intra- and inter-assay precision were $\leq$5.2% and $\leq$6.7%, respectively. The tests were performed in Diagnostic Department of Hospital University, Krakow, Poland, on the day of samples' collection. MMP 9-NGAL complex was assessed in series in duplicate wells per sample using Quantikine ELISA Human MMP-9/NGAL Complex Immunoassay (R&D Systems, McKinley Place, MN, USA). The minimum detectable dose of human MMP 9-NGAL was 0.013 ng/mL. According to the manufacturer of the test, the mean urine concentrations in healthy volunteers was 0.44 ng/mL (ranged from non-detectable to 0.67 ng/mL). The measurements were performed in the Department of Diagnostics, Chair of Clinical Biochemistry, Jagiellonian University Medical College, Krakow, Poland.

2.3. Statistical Analysis

The number of patients and the percentage of the respective group were reported for categories. The contingency tables were analyzed with Pearson's chi-squared test. The mean ± standard deviation (SD) or median with lower and upper quartile (Q1; Q3) were reported for quantitative variables with or without normal distribution, respectively. The variables' distributions were assessed for normality with the Shapiro-Wilk's test. The groups were compared using t-test or Mann-Whitney's test, depending on the variables' distributions. Time-related changes were assessed with the Wilcoxon's matched pairs test as the appropriate variables' distributions differed from normal. Simple correlations were analyzed with the Pearson's correlation coefficient, calculated using log-transformed variables in case of right-skewed distribution. Simple correlations between urinary NGAL, NGAL/creatinine and the number of mismatched HLA were analyzed with the Spearman rank coefficient. Multiple linear regression was used to identify the independent predictors of eGFR changes and eGFR based on mean creatinine during the follow-up period. The regression models included the independent variables that were significantly associated with at least one dependent variable in simple analysis, and were additionally adjusted for time from kidney transplantation (because of the considerable diversity of the time from transplantation in the studied group). Sex-adjusted logistic regression was used to assess the studied laboratory markers as the predictors of urinary tract infections during follow-up. Receiver operating characteristics (ROC) curve analysis was used to assess and compare the diagnostic accuracy of urine NGAL and albumin concentrations (raw and corrected to urine creatinine) for the prediction of at least 10% decrease in eGFR values over the follow-up period. The cut-off values were selected using maximum Youden index. All tests were two-tailed; the results were considered significant at p-value < 0.05. Statistica 12 (StatSoft, Tulsa, OK, USA) and Statistica 13 software (Tibco Software Inc., Tulsa, OK, USA) were used for computation.

3. Results

3.1. Baseline Characteristics of Patients

We recruited 109 adult kidney transplant recipients (43 women and 66 men, aged between 19 and 78 years). The patients were recruited in a single center, the Chair and Department of Nephrology, University Hospital in Kraków, Poland, during the control ambulatory visits. The time from transplantation ranged from 1 year to 22 years, with a median of 7 years. According to 2012 KDIGO guidelines on chronic kidney disease [33], there were 5 (5%) patients in G1T, 29 (27%) in G2T, 22 (20%) in G3aT, 42 (39%) in G3bT, and 11 (10%) in G4T stage as based on baseline eGFR. Forty-nine (45%) patients had normal to mildly increased albuminuria (A1), 39 (36%) moderately increased albuminuria (A2) and 21 (19%) severely increased albuminuria (A3).

The follow-up data were collected during planned control visits over a period of up to 16 months from the enrollment. After a median 12.4-month observation (range 3.2 to 15.4 months; Q1; Q3: 11.2; 13.3 months), 10% or higher decrease in eGFR (i.e., final eGFR ≤90% of initial value) was noted in 30 patients (28%; Table 1). The baseline clinical characteristics of patients with ≥10% decrease in eGFR did not differ significantly from the rest of the group, except for higher maximum panel reactive antibodies' percentage in patients with decreasing eGFR (Table 1).

Table 1. Baseline clinical characteristics of patients according to eGFR changes during follow-up.

Characteristic	eGFR at the End of Follow-Up		p
	≤90% of Initial Value (n = 30)	>90% of Initial Value (n = 79)	
Mean age ± SD, years	54 ± 14	54 ± 13	0.8
Male sex, n (%)	18 (60)	48 (73)	0.9
Median time from transplantation (Q1; Q3), years	8 (5; 14)	7 (3; 13)	0.5
Primary cause of kidney disease glomerular diseases, n (%) tubulointerstitial diseases, n (%) vascular diseases, n (%) cystic/congenital diseases, n (%) unknown, n (%)	 12 (40) 4 (13) 1 (3) 3 (10) 10 (33)	 27 (34) 13 (16) 5 (6) 12 (15) 22 (28)	0.9
First transplant, n (%) Second transplant, n (%)	25 (83) 5 (17)	72 (91) 7 (9)	0.2
Deceased donor, n (%)	30 (100)	78 (99)	1.0
Median number of HLA mismatches (Q1; Q3) *	3 (2; 4)	3 (3; 4)	0.8
Median peak pretransplant PRA (Q1; Q3), % *	10 (0; 30)	0 (0; 3)	0.045
Median last pretransplant PRA (Q1; Q3), % *	0 (0; 10)	0 (0; 0)	0.1
Induction therapy, n (%) no data, n (%)	3 (10) 13 (43)	11 (19) 21 (27)	0.9
Median cold ischemia time (Q1; Q3), min **	1320 (1170; 1566)	1100 (840; 1470)	0.06
Median warm ischemia time (Q1; Q3), min **	35 (29; 50)	32 (27; 40)	0.3
Delayed graft function, n (%) no data, n (%)	11 (37) 10 (33)	21 (27) 19 (24)	0.5
Immunosuppression glucocorticoids, n (%) MMF or MPA, n (%) cyclosporine, n (%) tacrolimus, n (%) mTOR inhibitor, n (%)	 30 (100) 28 (93) 7 (23) 21 (70) 2 (7)	 76 (96) 74 (94) 22 (28) 53 (67) 5 (7)	 0.6 0.9 0.6 0.8 0.9
Diabetes, n (%)	8 (27)	13 (16)	0.2
Hypoglycemic agents oral, n (%) insulin, n (%)	 4 (13) 4 (13)	 9 (11) 5 (6)	 0.8 0.2
Use of RAA blockers, n (%)	11 (37)	35 (44)	0.5
Median daily diuresis (Q1; Q3), mL	2500 (2000; 3000)	2500 (2000; 3000)	0.4
Mean BMI ± SD, kg/m²	25 ± 5	27 ± 5	0.2
Mean systolic pressure ± SD, mmHg	138 ± 15	133 ± 13	0.1
Mean diastolic pressure ± SD, mmHg	84 ± 11	83 ± 10	0.9

* Available in 46 patients (14 with decreasing eGFR and 32 with non-decreasing eGFR) who underwent transplantation procedure in University Hospital, Kraków, Poland; ** Available in 80 patients (19 with decreasing eGFR and 61 with non-decreasing eGFR). BMI, body mass index; eGFR, estimated glomerular filtration rate; MMF, mycophenolate mofetil; MPA, mycophenolic acid; mTOR, mammalian target of rapamycin; PRA, panel reactive antibodies; Q1, first quartile; Q3, third quartile; RAA, renin-angiotensin-aldosterone system; SD, standard deviation.

Urinary albumin and albumin to creatinine ratio (uACR) were significantly higher in patients with ≥10% decrease in eGFR over a follow-up (Table 2). Also, these patients had lower initial eGFR values. Slightly but significantly lower serum albumin and blood hemoglobin concentrations were associated with ≥10% eGFR decrease. Both urinary NGAL concentration and NGAL to creatinine ratio were higher in patients with decreasing eGFR (Table 2).

Table 2. Baseline results of laboratory tests according to eGFR changes during follow-up. Data are shown as mean ± SD or median (Q1; Q3).

Laboratory Test	eGFR at the End of Follow-Up		p
	≤90% of Initial Value (n = 30)	>90% of Initial Value (n = 79)	
Urine albumin, mg/L	165 (20; 731)	21 (8; 67)	0.001
uACR, mg/g	194 (28; 1066)	26 (11; 159)	0.001
Serum creatinine, µmol/L	142 (111; 205)	127 (97; 168)	0.09
eGFR (CKD-EPI$_{Cr}$), mL/min/1.73m^2	38 (31; 54)	49 (38; 70)	0.038
Urine NGAL, µg/L	17.8 (8.0; 30.0)	8.9 (4.0; 21.6)	0.020
Urine NGAL/creatinine, µg/g	25.2 (9.8; 58.5)	13.2 (5.6; 22.7)	0.015
Urine MMP 9-NGAL complex, µg/L *	0.255 (0.141; 0.584)	0.216 (0.13; 0.681)	0.8
Urine MMP 9-NGAL/creatinine, µg/g *	0.35 (0.21; 1.71)	0.39 (0.23; 1.29)	0.9
Hemoglobin, g/dl	12.4 (11.1; 13.4)	13.2 (12.6; 14.5)	0.005
White blood count, ×10^3/µL	7.50 (5.80; 8.38)	7.07 (5.97; 8.51)	0.8
Platelet count, ×10^3/µL	196 ± 53	211 ± 56	0.2
Triglycerides, mmol/L	1.64 (1.28; 2.12)	1.58 (1.21; 2.12)	0.9
Total cholesterol, mmol/L	5.17 (4.20; 5.66)	4.91 (4.21; 5.73)	0.7
Uric acid, mmol/L	378 (342; 431)	379 (334; 431)	0.9
C-reactive protein, mg/L	1.84 (1.00; 4.44)	1.41 (1.00; 2.99)	0.5
Serum albumin, g/L	42 (40; 44)	44 (43; 46)	0.002
Glucose, mmol/L	5.55 (5.16; 6.06)	5.44 (5.07; 6.02)	0.7

* Available in 77 patients (19 with decreasing eGFR and 55 with non-decreasing eGFR). eGFR, estimated glomerular filtration rate; CKD-EPI$_{Cr}$ [33], Chronic Kidney Disease—Epidemiology Collaboration equation based on serum creatinine; NGAL, neutrophil gelatinase-associated lipocalin; MMP 9, matrix metalloproteinase 9; uACR, urinary albumin to creatinine ratio.

3.2. Changes in eGFR over a Follow-Up Period

During the follow-up, we observed both increases and decreases in eGFR values (Figure 1). In the whole studied cohort, this resulted in no difference between initial and final eGFR values ($p = 0.8$; Figure 1A). In patients with final to baseline eGFR ratio ≤90%, the eGFR values decreased by a median of 19% (Q1; Q3: 16; 25%) or by 9 mL/min/1.73 m^2 (Q1; Q3: 6; 14 mL/min/1.73 m^2). On the contrary, we observed a significant increase in eGFR values in the subgroup with final eGFR >90% of baseline eGFR ($p < 0.001$; Figure 1B), resulting in a highly significant difference in final eGFR values between the studied subgroups: median final eGFR was 30 mL/min/1.73 m^2 in patients with final eGFR ≤90% of the baseline values, and 56 mL/min/1.73 m^2 in patients with final eGFR >90% baseline ($p < 0.001$).

Moreover, we analyzed eGFR values calculated based on the arithmetic mean of all serum creatinine measurements performed during the follow-up (excluding the initial eGFR value recorded on enrollment; Figure 1A,B). The median number of visits during the follow-up period was 4 (range 1–7; Q1; Q3: 3; 5) and did not differ significantly between patients with ≥10% decrease in eGFR and the rest of the group ($p = 0.2$). The median eGFR based on mean creatinine during the follow-up period was 48 (Q1; Q3: 37; 68) mL/min/1.73 m^2 and was significantly lower among patients with ≥10% decrease in eGFR as compared to the rest of the group (median 33 and 53 mL/min/1.73 m^2, respectively; $p < 0.001$; Figure 1B).

During the studied period, the attending physicians of kidney transplant ambulatory diagnosed the clinically relevant and sustained decrease in kidney transplant function in nine patients, i.e., 30% of the group with ≥10% decrease in eGFR. It was attributed to chronic rejection in two patients, recurrence of glomerulonephritis in one patient, urological complications with recurrent urinary tract infections in one patient, and due to unknown causes in the remaining five patients (two of them refused to undergo kidney transplant biopsy). Two of these patients progressed to stage G5 CKD and were referred to hemodialysis treatment. Further four patients were diagnosed with urinary tract infection, two with other infections, one with recurrent glomerulonephritis, two with cardiovascular complications, and one with adverse drug reaction that were recognized as resulting in a transient decrease of the transplant function. In the remaining 11 patients, there was no entry in their medical records about the (suspected) cause of eGFR decrease in medical records.

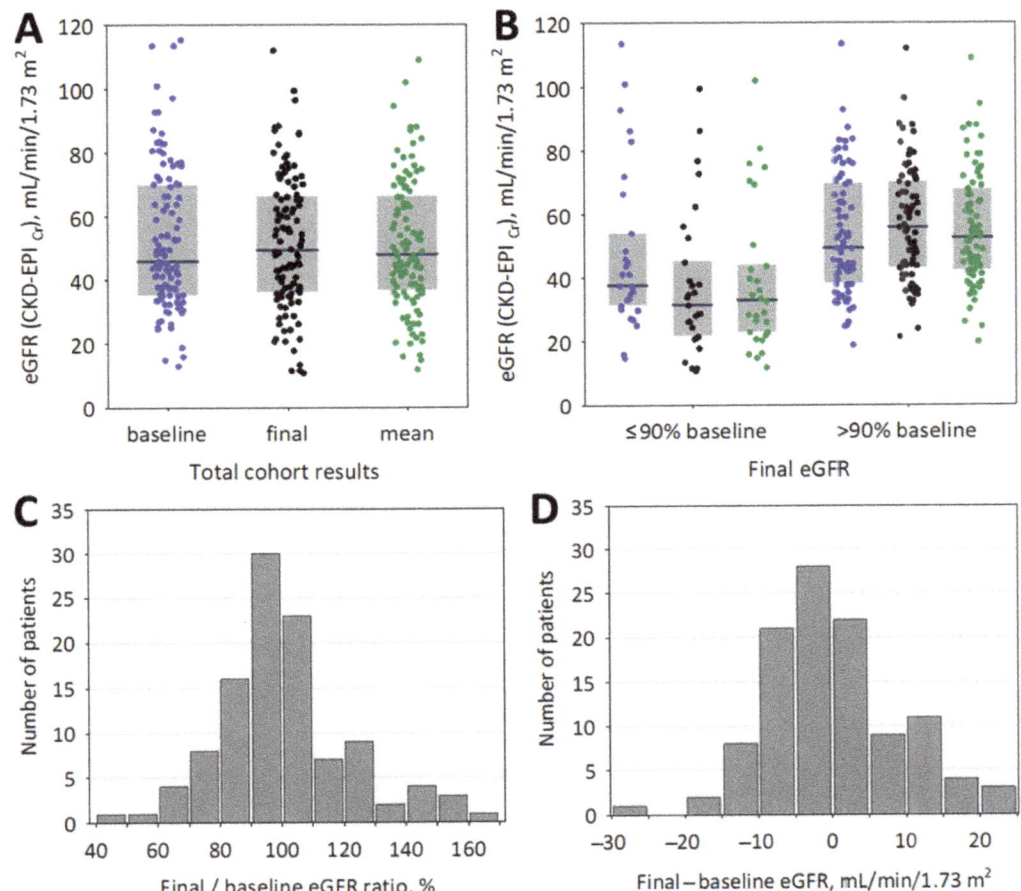

Figure 1. Baseline (blue points), final (black points) eGFR values and eGFR values based on mean creatinine during follow-up ("mean"; green points) in the whole studied cohort of kidney transplant recipients (**A**) and in the subgroups defined by final to baseline eGFR ratio below or above 90% of baseline value (**B**). Data on panels A and B are shown as median (central line), interquartile range (box) and raw data (points). The histograms showing percentage (**C**) and absolute (**D**) changes in eGFR values over the follow-up period in the whole studied group of kidney transplant recipients.

3.3. Associations between Urinary NGAL Concentrations and the Baseline Characteristics of Studied Patients

The baseline urinary concentrations of NGAL (log-transformed: $R = -0.06$; $p = 0.5$) and NGAL to creatinine ratios (log-transformed: $R = -0.09$; $p = 0.4$) did not correlate with the baseline eGFR values either in the total cohort and in the subgroups defined by final to baseline eGFR ratio below or above 90% of the baseline value. Urine NGAL concentration and NGAL to creatinine ratio were significantly correlated with urine albumin and uACR at baseline (R equaled from 0.36 to 0.48 for log-transformed variables; $p \leq 0.001$). Urinary NGAL and NGAL/creatinine were not associated with age ($p > 0.7$), sex ($p > 0.1$), or time from transplantation ($p > 0.5$). Among the patients who had undergone transplantation procedure in our center, there was a marginally significant positive correlation between the urine NGAL concentration and the number of donor/recipient HLA mismatches (Spearman R = 0.31; p = 0.049). Other variables listed in Table 1 showed no associations with urinary NGAL and NGAL/creatinine.

3.4. Associations between Clinical and Laboratory Characteristics and the Changes in eGFR over a Follow-Up Period

Baseline eGFR values, urinary albumin, and albumin to creatinine ratios, urinary NGAL and NGAL to creatinine ratios (but neither MMP 9-NGAL complex concentrations nor MMP 9-NGAl/creatinine ratios), as well as serum uric acid and albumin concentrations were significantly correlated with either the percentage or the absolute changes in eGFR values during the observation (Table 3). Moreover, baseline eGFR, urinary albumin concentration, uACR, urinary NGAL concentration and NGAL/creatinine ratio as well as serum uric acid correlated significantly with eGFR values based on the mean of all serum creatinine results obtained during the follow-up period (Table 3). No significant correlations were observed between the percentage or absolute changes in eGFR and the clinical characteristics, including age, time from transplantation, cold or warm ischemia time, blood pressure values, or daily diuresis (p > 0.1 in all cases). Neither the ratio of follow-up to baseline eGFR (R = 0.15; p = 0.1) nor the absolute difference between the follow-up and the baseline eGFR values (R = 0.14; p = 0.1) correlated with the length of observation. Also, neither the changes in eGFR nor mean follow-up eGFR were associated with sex.

In multiple regression, urine NGAL and serum albumin were identified as the independent predictors of eGFR changes and eGFR values based on mean serum creatinine during the follow-up (Table 3). When uACR and NGAL to creatinine ratio were included in the models instead of uncorrected urine albumin and NGAL concentrations, very similar results were obtained (beta ± SE for NGAL to creatinine ratio: -0.24 ± 0.11; p = 0.025 for final to baseline eGFR ratio as the dependent variable; -0.30 ± 0.10; p = 0.004 for final—baseline eGFR; and -0.12 ± 0.04; p = 0.005 for eGFR based on mean creatinine during the follow-up as the dependent variable, respectively). This results were observed despite the significant correlations of urinary NGAL concentration and NGAL/creatinine ratio with urine albumin and uACR.

ROC curve analysis (Figure 2) showed a weak diagnostic accuracy of baseline urinary NGAL concentration and NGAL/creatinine ratio in the prediction of $\geq$10% decrease in eGFR values during the follow-up. However, the area under the ROC curve (AUC) values for urine NGAL concentration and NGAL/creatinine ratio were not significantly different from the AUC values obtained for urine albumin concentration and uACR (p = 0.7 in all comparisons). The cut-off values selected using maximum Youden index were 9.3 µg/L for urine NGAL concentration (associated with diagnostic sensitivity of 70% and specificity of 54%) and 24.1 µg/g for NGAL/creatinine (sensitivity 53% and specificity 76%), respectively.

We further analyzed the association between the baseline urinary NGAL and the changes in eGFR observed during the study in the subgroups of patients based on the time from transplantation: the correlations were weaker in the patients who were recruited between the end of the first and sixth year post-transplant as compared to those who had longer post-transplant history (Table 4). Moreover, in patients recruited more than six years post-transplantation, we observed significant correlation between urinary NGAL/creatinine (log-transformed) and eGFR at baseline (R = -0.28; p = 0.035).

Table 3. Simple correlations and multiple models showing the associations between studied variables and the changes in eGFR values over the follow-up period (defined either as the follow-up to baseline eGFR ratio or as the difference between follow-up and baseline eGFR) and mean eGFR during the follow-up. The multiple models were adjusted for time from kidney transplantation.

Independent Variable	Dependent Variable											
	Final/Baseline eGFR				Final—Baseline eGFR				eGFR Based on Mean Creatinine during Follow-Up			
	Simple Correlation		Multiple Regression		Simple Correlation		Multiple Regression		Simple Correlation		Multiple Regression	
	R	p	beta ± SE	p	R	p	beta ± SE	p	R	p	beta ± SE	p
Baseline eGFR	−0.09	0.3	−0.04 ± 0.11	0.7	−0.22	0.020	−0.13 ± 0.11	0.2	0.92	<0.001	0.98 ± 0.04	<0.001
log (uAlb)	−0.26	0.006	−0.08 ± 0.12	0.5	−0.16	0.08	−0.01 ± 0.11	0.9	−0.36	<0.001	0.04 ± 0.04	0.4
log (uACR)	−0.24	0.012	not included		−0.14	0.1	not included		−0.36	<0.001	not included	
log (uNGAL)	−0.31	0.001	−0.22 ± 0.10	0.039	−0.32	0.001	−0.28 ± 0.10	0.006	−0.19	0.045	−0.11 ± 0.04	0.008
log (uNGAL/Cr)	−0.31	0.002	not included		−0.29	0.003	not included		−0.22	0.022	not included	
log (uric acid)	0.21	0.028	0.15 ± 0.10	0.2	0.19	0.051	0.08 ± 0.10	0.4	−0.33	0.001	0.10 ± 0.04	0.014
Serum albumin	0.34	<0.001	0.24 ± 0.10	0.018	0.36	<0.001	0.29 ± 0.10	0.004	0.06	0.6	0.11 ± 0.04	0.007

eGFR, estimated glomerular filtration rate; uAlb, urinary albumin; uACR, urine albumin to creatinine ratio; uNGAL, urine neutrophil gelatinase-associated lipocalin; uNGAL/Cr, urine NGAL to creatinine ratio; SE, standard error.

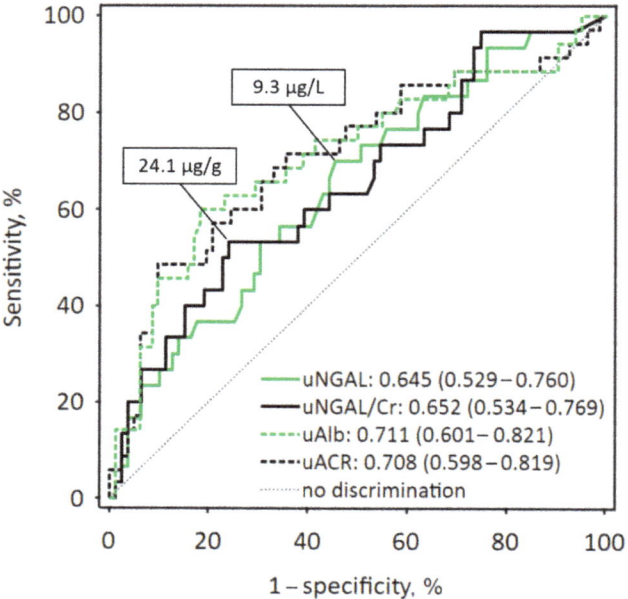

Figure 2. Receiver operating characteristic (ROC) curves for baseline urine NGAL concentration (uNGAL; solid green line) and urine NGAL/creatinine ratio (uNGAL/Cr; solid black line) in the prediction of ≥10% decrease of eGFR during the one-year follow-up. The cut-off values are reported on the graph. For comparison, ROC curves for urine albumin concentration (uAlb) and urine albumin/creatinine ratio are presented using dashed lines. The values of area under the ROC curves (AUC) are shown with 95% confidence intervals in brackets.

Table 4. Correlations between the baseline urine NGAL concentrations (uNGAL) and NGAL to creatinine ratios (uNGAL/Cr) and the changes in eGFR observed during the study as well as the eGFR based on mean serum creatinine during the follow-up.

Variable	Time from Transplantation at the Start of the Study			
	1–6 Years ($n = 49$)		7–22 Years ($n = 60$)	
	uNGAL	uNGAL/Cr	uNGAL	uNGAL/Cr
Final/baseline eGFR	$R = -0.28; p = 0.06$	$R = -0.27; p = 0.07$	$R = -0.34; p = 0.008$	$R = -0.36; p = 0.007$
Final−baseline eGFR	$R = -0.34; p = 0.023$	$R = -0.29; p = 0.05$	$R = -0.31; p = 0.020$	$R = -0.31; p = 0.019$
eGFR based on mean creatinine during follow-up	$R = -0.08; p = 0.6$	$R = -0.06; p = 0.7$	$R = -0.29; p = 0.029$	$R = -0.35; p = 0.007$

3.5. Associations between Urinary NGAL and Persistent or Increasing Proteinuria

We analyzed the laboratory records of studied patients with respect to urine albumin or protein concentrations measured during the one-year follow-up. During the observation, proteinuria persisted or increased in 6 (15%) of 39 patients with A2 albuminuria and 15 (71%) of 21 patients with A3 albuminuria recorded at baseline. In the remaining patients, urine protein concentrations decreased during the observation. The patients with baseline uACR <30 mg/g did not develop increased proteinuria during the study. Among patients with persistent or increasing proteinuria, there were 6 (29%) recipients of second renal transplant, a significantly higher percentage as compared to the rest of the studied group (6 of 88; 7%; $p = 0.004$). Eleven (52%) of the 21 patients were diagnosed with glomerular disease versus 28 (32%) in the rest of the group ($p = 0.08$). Age, time from transplantation, number of donor/recipient HLA mismatches, pretransplant PRA, the use of induction therapy, or transplant ischemia times did not differ between the groups. Persistent proteinuria was associated with higher decline in eGFR during the observation (median final/baseline eGFR 85% versus 101%; $p < 0.001$). The 21 patients with persistent or increased proteinuria were characterized by significantly higher baseline urine NGAL concentrations: median (Q1; Q3) 23.0 (9.25; 45.2) versus 8.75 (3.95; 19.7) µg/L ($p = 0.002$) and NGAL/creatinine ratios: 35.1 (14.7; 84.9) versus 13.1 (5.91; 23.4) µg/g ($p = 0.005$).

3.6. Associations between Urinary NGAL and MMP 9-NGAL Complex and the Incidence of Bacterial Urinary Tract Infections during the Follow-Up Period

During the follow-up, bacterial urinary tract infections were diagnosed in 20 patients: four (14%) in the group that experienced ≥ 10% decrease in eGFR and 16 (20%) in the group with final eGFR >90% of initial value. The incidence of urinary tract infections did not differ significantly between the groups ($p = 0.4$). Also, eGFR values based on the mean serum creatinine during the follow-up did not differ between patients who developed urinary tract infections during the follow-up and those who did not (median 51 and 47 mL/min/1.73 m^2, respectively; $p = 0.9$).

Baseline urine NGAL concentration, NGAL/creatinine ratio, MMP 9-NGAL complex and the complex to creatinine ratio were all significantly associated with bacterial urinary tract infections during the follow-up (Figure 3). The urinary tract infections were more common in women than in men (32% versus 9%, respectively; $p = 0.002$) while they were not associated with diabetes ($p = 0.6$) or immunosuppressive treatment modality ($p > 0.4$). In logistic regression analysis, log-transformed urinary NGAL concentration (odds ratio per unit change 3.46; 95% confidence interval 1.29–9.21; $p = 0.012$) or log-transformed NGAL/creatinine ratio (odds ratio per unit change 3.10; 95% confidence interval 1.20–7.97; $p = 0.018$) predicted urinary tract infections during the follow-up independently of sex. On the contrary, urinary concentration of MMP 9-NGAL complex was significantly associated with sex (median 0.162 in men and 0.552 in women; $p < 0.001$) and did not prove sex-independent predictor of urinary tract infections. Urinary albumin and uACR were not associated with urinary tract infections during the follow-up ($p = 0.3$ for both comparisons).

4. Discussion

In our sample of kidney transplant recipients recruited at least one year after the transplantation, without acute conditions diagnosed before and on enrollment, baseline urinary NGAL measured with the automated laboratory method significantly predicted the changes in eGFR values observed during the following year independently of other predictors, most importantly the baseline eGFR and albuminuria. Although the diagnostic accuracy of urine NGAL in the prediction of eGFR decline was low (the AUC of 0.65 in ROC curve analysis), it was statistically significant and did not differ significantly from the diagnostic accuracy of urine albumin. Higher baseline NGAL was also associated with persistent or increasing proteinuria during one-year observation of the studied patients. Moreover, higher baseline urinary NGAL and MMP 9-NGAL complex were observed in patients who developed urinary tract infections during the follow-up.

Although we recruited "clinically stable" patients, i.e., without any acute conditions (including infections and kidney injury) before and on enrollment, we observed significant changes in eGFR values during the follow-up: the final eGFR values were in the range of 40–170% of the initial values or −30 to +25 mL/min/1.73 m^2. Serum creatinine concentrations (and thus GFR estimate) is dependent of non-renal factors, e.g., water balance, nutritional status, physical exercise, other metabolic factors, or diet [34]. Together with the laboratory imprecision, these factors lead to the variability in serum creatinine and eGFR that must be considered when monitoring the patients with chronic kidney disease. As stated in KDIGO guidelines for the care of kidney transplant recipients [1], because of within-subject variation of serum creatinine, a 25–50% increase of creatinine concentrations over baseline is predictive of the subsequent graft failure and should be considered an indication for graft biopsy (after excluding acute causes such as dehydration or blocked urine output). Considering the well-known inverse hyperbolic association between serum creatinine and GFR, the 50% increase in creatinine may be translated into roughly 25% decrease in GFR [35]. On the other hand, a decrease in GFR of 5 mL/min/1.73 m^2 per year is considered a rapid progression of chronic kidney disease [33]. We believe that a 10% decrease in eGFR over a year should be clinically interpreted as a warning sign, despite the variability observed in clinical practice, and the causes of such a decrease should be sought.

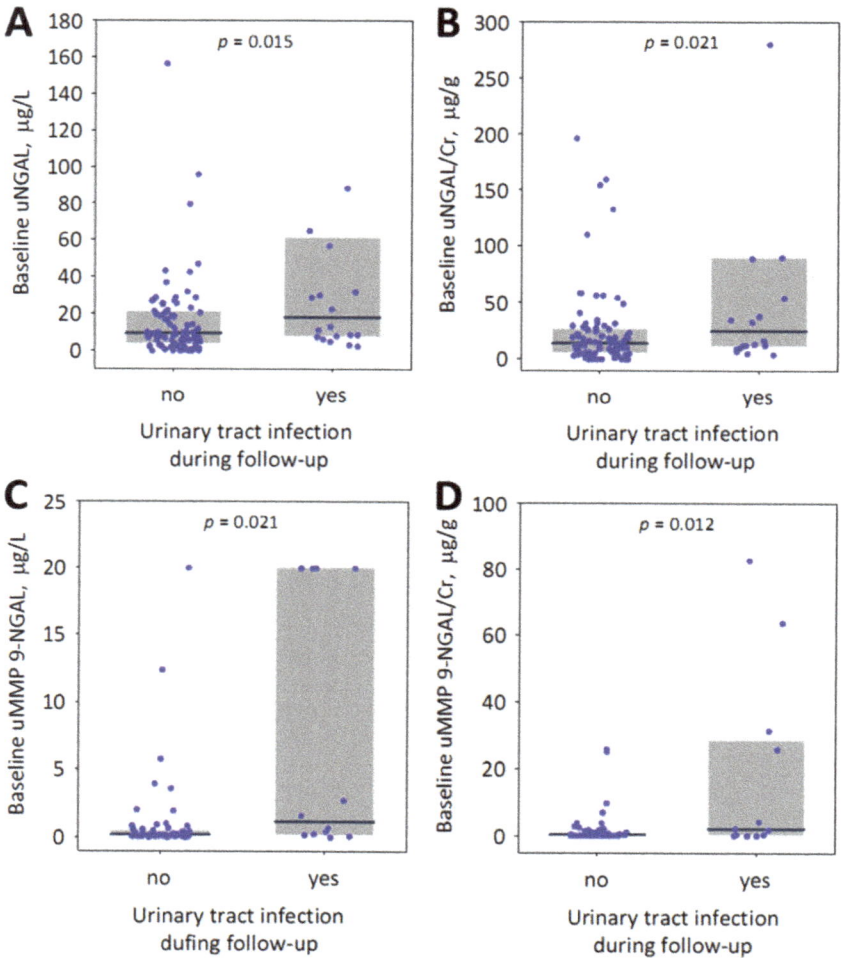

Figure 3. Baseline urine NGAL concentration (uNGAL; (**A**)), urine NGAL to creatinine ratio (uNGAL/Cr; (**B**)), urine MMP 9-NGAL complex concentration (uMMP 9-NGAL; (**C**)) and urine MMP 9-NGAL complex to creatinine ratio (uMMP 9-NGAL/Cr; (**D**)) among studied kidney transplant recipients who did or did not experience bacterial urinary tract infections during the follow-up period. Data are shown as median (central line), interquartile range (box) and raw data (points); p-values are given for the differences between groups. To increase readability of the graphs, we omitted the highest results of urine NGAL (528; 1275; 1401 μg/L; panel (**A**)) and NGAL/creatinine (1251; 1656; 2183 μg/g; panel (**B**)) obtained in three patients who experienced urinary tract infection during follow-up.

According to the recent studies, chronic graft dysfunction is mainly caused by chronic antibody-mediated rejection, interstitial fibrosis, and tubular atrophy (IF/TA) induced by various chronic inflammatory processes, and BK polyoma virus (BKV) nephropathy. In protocol biopsies done in 1000 transplant recipients at 3, 12, 24, 48, and 60 months post-transplant, the signs of chronic rejection were detected in 17% of patients, and IF/TA in 30% [3]. The long-term function of kidney transplant and the risk of graft loss may be predicted based on serum creatinine and proteinuria at one year following kidney transplantation [36]. Moreover, anemia and high systolic blood pressure have been associated with higher risk of graft loss [36]. While overt proteinuria (detectable by urine dipstick) occurring in a kidney transplant recipient is a serious adverse predictor of graft survival, we need a non-invasive biomarker (or markers) that would allow detecting the injury at an earlier stage, before it leads to significant decrease in GFR or overt proteinuria.

Most studies evaluating urinary NGAL in kidney transplant recipients used NGAL concentrations measured early (hours till days) after transplantation procedure. Urinary NGAL measured between 6 and 48 h from the surgery predicted delayed graft function in most studies (although the diagnostic accuracy of serum/plasma NGAL in this context has been better in some studies) [26,37–41]. Consistently, urinary NGAL measured early post-transplant was shown to predict graft function at one year [39,41]. Recently, Maier et al. [42] assessed serum and urine NGAL in 170 kidney transplant recipients during the first week following transplantation and showed the best diagnostic utility of day 2 measurements for the delayed graft function. Both serum and urine NGAL concentrations on day 2 after transplantation predicted delayed graft function independently of serum creatinine and urine output; however, NGAL as an independent variable did not reach statistical significance in the models predicting graft loss or recipient's death at 2 or 5 years post-transplant [42].

We were able to identify only several reports where NGAL has been measured in kidney transplant recipients after the peri-transplantation period. Ramirez-Sandoval et al. [27] measured several tubular biomarkers including urinary NGAL in kidney transplant recipients with acute kidney injury: the median time from transplantation was 3.5 years. The urinary concentrations of NGAL were significantly higher in kidney transplant recipients with AKI as compared to kidney transplant controls with normal eGFR and normal transplant histology. Moreover, urine NGAL/creatinine ratios were higher in patients with immunological rejection as compared to those with prerenal or other causes of acute kidney injury [27]. In a prospective observation of kidney transplant recipients admitted with AKI that occurred after median period of three years from the transplantation, high urinary NGAL (>210 ng/mL) at admission significantly predicted graft loss during subsequent year, independently of baseline eGFR, serum creatinine on admission and time from transplantation [29]. We cannot directly compare our results to that of Ramirez-Sandoval [27,29], as our group did not include patients with clinically detectable acute kidney injury on enrollment. However, their results indicate that urinary NGAL measurements performed years after transplantation may be diagnostically and prognostically useful. In another study, Kaufeld et al. [28] measured urinary NGAL concentration six weeks, three months and six months after kidney transplantation and compared the concentrations between patients with or without acute tubular injury as verified by protocol transplant biopsies done in the same time points. At six weeks, but not at six months, urinary NGAL was higher in patients with tubular injury as compared to those without injury; moreover, women and patients with urinary tract infections on the day of sample collection had higher NGAL concentrations [28]. Kaufeld et al. [28] used enzyme-linked immunosorbent assay for NGAL determination, and, although the total number of patients in the analysis was 140, the measurements in individual time points were available in smaller subgroups (44 patients with tubular injury and 23 patients without tubular injury at six weeks post-transplant; 55 and 16 at six months, respectively). The study design of Kaufeld et al. [28] differed from ours in several aspects (much longer times from transplantation in our patients, automated method of NGAL determination in our study, and no protocol biopsies in our center), thus, the results cannot be directly compared. Most importantly, we were not able to verify the association between morphological changes in kidney and NGAL excretion. However, the association of NGAL with urinary tract infections was shown in both studies. In 2015, Cassidy et al. [30] measured NGAL as one of several urine biomarkers in 34 patients recruited more than one year after kidney transplantation and analyzed the measured concentrations in the context of histologically proven chronic fibrosis and a similar number of kidney transplant recipients with normal renal function. They observed significantly higher urinary NGAL concentrations in patients with chronic allograft nephropathy [30]. Our results remain in line with the findings of Cassidy et al. [30], although the methods of NGAL determination differed (Cassidy et al. used Western-blot and ELISA). Lacquaniti et al. [31] recruited 84 renal transplant recipients one year or more after renal transplantation. They observed higher baseline serum and urine NGAL concentrations (measured by ELISA) in the patients in whom serum creatinine concentrations doubled or who progressed to end-stage kidney failure during five years' observation [31]. Urine NGAL above 71.8 μg/L was predictive of transplant function worsening during the observation (AUC of 0.889) [31]. This cut-off value is higher as compared to our results; however, the "worsening of kidney function" was more severe in the study of Lacquaniti et al. [31]; still, our results are in line with the findings. Finally, Schaub et al. [43] measured urinary concentrations of several renal tubular markers (retinol-binding protein, α1-microglobulin and NGAL) in kidney transplant recipients with median time from transplantation >90 days, who underwent either protocol or indication graft biopsy and were divided into four groups based on the biopsy findings regarding tubular pathology. Patients with clinical tubulitis and other tubular pathology had higher concentrations of measured proteins including NGAL. Moreover, subclinical tubulitis was associated with non-significantly (p = 0.06) higher NGAL as compared to transplant recipients with normal histology [43]. The results of Schaub et al. [43] show that urinary NGAL measured late after the transplantation (median time from transplantation was 158 days in the group with clinical tubulitis and 1163 days in patients with other tubular pathology) is indicative of tubular pathology in kidney transplant recipients.

In non-transplanted chronic kidney disease patients, higher urinary NGAL was associated with a chronic decline in kidney function [21,44]. Moreover, in renal transplant recipients, the presence of tubular proteinuria with increase in urinary concentrations of retinol-binding protein or α1-microglobulin (i.e., low molecular weight proteins that are normally reabsorbed in proximal tubule) after the first year post kidney transplantation has been associated with decline in transplant function during long-term follow-up [45,46], which is in line with our results.

While the NGAL monomer has been associated with tubular injury, and neutrophils seem the main source of NGAL dimer in urine [13,16,47], the complex of MMP 9 (gelatinase B) with NGAL has not been extensively studied in the context of kidney diseases. The 135 kDa complex of MMP 9 (gelatinase B) with NGAL has been originally described and purified from neutrophils isolated from blood and activated with phorbol myristate acetate. Later, the „high molecular weight metalloproteinase", present in urine of patients with cancer, has been characterized as a 125 kDa complex of MMP 9 and NGAL [48]. The MMP 9-NGAL complex has been found in urine of breast cancer patients [49]. According to Yan et al. [48], the complex may be formed in urine from NGAL and MMP 9 that are separately filtered or secreted into urine. Alternatively, the neutrophils present in urine may be a source of the MMP 9-NGAL complex. In our sample of kidney transplant recipients, the latter is consistent with higher concentrations of the MMP 9-NGAL complex among patients who subsequently developed bacterial urinary tract infections as well as in women, more prone to urinary tract infections. Previously, the MMP 9-NGAL complex has been detected in dogs with pyuria and azotemia [50]. Of note, NGAL has been shown to prevent MMP 9 from proteolysis and a complex of MMP 9 with NGAL found in human urine has been shown to exert the gelatinase enzymatic activity [48,49]. This may have pathophysiological implications in kidney disease, as matrix metalloproteinases play a role in IF/TA affecting the transplanted kidney [51,52]. We measured MMP 9-NGAL complex in a subgroup of 77 patients, of whom only 19 had decreasing eGFR, and it is possible that our study was underpowered to find a weak association of the complex urinary concentrations with transplant function.

In our study, in addition to urinary NGAL, serum albumin and uric acid were also associated with the changes in eGFR and mean eGFR during the follow-up. Serum albumin is an indicator and predictor of poor nutritional status in kidney disease, moreover, it is a known negative acute phase protein [53,54]. The association of low serum albumin concentrations with decreasing eGFR and lower mean eGFR in our patients may reflect subclinical inflammatory states or worse nutritional status of the patients with subsequently decreasing kidney function. Of note, NGAL has been associated with low-grade inflammation in kidney disease [55,56]. Serum uric acid has been previously shown to predict adverse outcomes in kidney transplant patients [57].

Our study has several limitations: first, although we included more than 100 patients, the decrease in kidney function was detected in below one third of them, resulting in limited number of such patients. Furthermore, the data on donor/recipient HLA mismatches and PRA were available in a subgroup of patients, and we were not able to report the data on donor-specific antibodies, as these started to be measured in Poland only recently. The causes of decline in transplant function were not verified in histopathological examination because the protocol biopsies are not practiced in our center, and because there were patients who did not agree to indication biopsy. A longer follow-up time would allow studying the association of baseline NGAL with subsequent graft loss, a more robust end-point as compared to the one chosen in our study. In our group only two patients started dialysis treatment due to the end-stage graft failure. However, it was our aim to seek for the predictors of less severe decline in transplant function.

The strength of our study is that we measured urinary NGAL with a robust automated method that may be used in routine clinical practice (and indeed it is available in many centers). Although several studies show the diagnostic utility of urine NGAL for the prediction of adverse outcomes in kidney transplant recipients, the lack of standardization between the assays hinders the use of NGAL in clinical practice. We believe that the automated methods should be used in the studies if we want to translate the studies' results into practice.

In summary, our study indicates that the urinary NGAL and NGAL to creatinine ratio predicts changes in kidney graft function over subsequent year in kidney transplant recipients with long-term functioning graft. The association between urinary NGAL concentration and the follow-up graft function is moderate but independent of baseline eGFR and albuminuria. To which extent this prognostic utility of NGAL may be associated with the prediction of urinary tract infections, remains to be elucidated. Based on our observation, we may hypothesize that a high urinary NGAL measured as an additional marker in a clinically stable kidney transplant recipient should be interpreted as a warning sign, leading to detailed evaluation of a patient in search of either transient or chronic causes of graft dysfunction, or urinary tract infection. Low urinary NGAL is associated with a low risk of kidney graft dysfunction over a subsequent year. However, this clinical hypothesis must be verified in larger studies, at best involving the detailed characterization of graft state with the use of protocol biopsies.

Author Contributions: Conceptualization: M.K., P.D., and B.K.-C.; methodology: B.K.-C., and B.M.; validation: M.K., P.D., P.C., A.G.-B., B.K.-C.; formal analysis: P.D. and B.K.-C.; investigations: M.K., B.K.-C., and B.M.; resources: A.B.-P., E.I., A.G.-B.; data curation: M.K , B.K.-C., A.B.-P., and E.I.; writing-original draft preparation: M.K., P.D., and B.K.-C.; writing—review and editing: P.D., M.K., P.C., and B.K.-C., supervision: P.D., and B.K.-C.; project administration: P.C., and B.K.-C., funding acquisition: P.C., B.K.-C. All authors have read and agreed to the published version of the manuscript.

Funding: The study has been financed from the Jagiellonian University Medical College grant No. N42/DBS/000171.

Institutional Review Board Statement: The study was conducted according to the guidelines of the Declaration of Helsinki, and approved by the Jagiellonian University Bioethical Committee (approval no 1072.6120.46.2019 issued on 28 February 2019).

Informed Consent Statement: Informed consent was obtained from all subjects involved in the study.

Data Availability Statement: The data are available from the corresponding author upon reasonable request.

Acknowledgments: The authors thank Marek Kuźniewski for his support and inspiring.

Conflicts of Interest: The authors declare no conflict of interest.

References

1. Kidney Disease: Improving Global Outcomes (KDIGO) Transplant Work Group KDIGO Clinical Practice Guideline for the Care of Kidney Transplant Recipients. *Am. J. Transplant.* **2009**, *9*, S1–S155. [CrossRef] [PubMed]
2. Sakai, K.; Oguchi, H.; Muramatsu, M.; Shishido, S. Protocol graft biopsy in kidney transplantation. *Nephrology* **2018**, *23*, 38–44. [CrossRef] [PubMed]
3. Van Loon, E.; Senev, A.; Lerut, E.; Coemans, M.; Callemeyn, J.; Van Keer, J.M.; Daniëls, L.; Kuypers, D.; Sprangers, B.; Emonds, M.-P.; et al. Assessing the Complex Causes of Kidney Allograft Loss. *Transplantation* **2020**, *104*, 2557–2566. [CrossRef] [PubMed]
4. Cosio, F.G.; El Ters, M.; Cornell, L.D.; Schinstock, C.A.; Stegall, M.D. Changing kidney allograft histology early posttransplant: Prognostic implications of 1-year protocol biopsies. *Am. J. Transplant.* **2016**, *16*, 194–203. [CrossRef] [PubMed]
5. Reinhard, M.; Erlandsen, E.J.; Randers, E. Biological variation of cystatin C and creatinine. *Scand. J. Clin. Lab. Investig.* **2009**, *69*, 831–836. [CrossRef] [PubMed]
6. Bandaranayake, N.; Ankrah-Tetteh, T.; Wijeratne, S.; Swaminathan, R. Intra-individual variation in creatinine and cystatin C. *Clin. Chem. Lab. Med.* **2007**, *45*. [CrossRef] [PubMed]
7. Carobene, A.; Graziani, M.S.; Cascio, C.L.; Tretti, L.; Cremonese, E.; Yabarek, T.; Gambaro, G.; Ceriotti, F. Age dependence of within-subject biological variation of nine common clinical chemistry analytes. *Clin. Chem. Lab. Med.* **2012**, *50*, 841–844. [CrossRef] [PubMed]
8. Carobene, A.; Marino, I.; Coskun, A.; Serteser, M.; Unsal, I.; Guerra, E.; Bartlett, W.A.; Sandberg, S.; Aarsand, A.K.; Sverredotter Sylte, M.; et al. The EuBIVAS project: Within- and between-subject biological variation data for serum creatinine using enzymatic and alkaline picrate methods and implications for monitoring. *Clin. Chem.* **2017**, *63*, 1527–1536. [CrossRef]
9. Hall, P.S.; Mitchell, E.D.; Smith, A.F.; Cairns, D.A.; Messenger, M.; Hutchinson, M.; Wright, J.; Vinall-Collier, K.; Corps, C.; Hamilton, P.; et al. The future for diagnostic tests of acute kidney injury in critical care: Evidence synthesis, care pathway analysis and research prioritisation. *Health Technol. Assess. (Rockv).* **2018**, *22*, 1–274. [CrossRef]
10. Kashani, K.; Cheungpasitporn, W.; Ronco, C. Biomarkers of acute kidney injury: The pathway from discovery to clinical adoption. *Clin. Chem. Lab. Med.* **2017**, *55*, 1074–1089. [CrossRef]
11. Kjeldsen, L.; Johnsen, A.H.; Sengelov, H.; Borregaard, N. Isolation and primary structure of NGAL, a novel protein associated with human neutrophil gelatinase. *J. Biol. Chem.* **1993**, *268*, 10425–10432. [PubMed]
12. Devarajan, P. Neutrophil gelatinase-associated lipocalin (NGAL): A new marker of kidney disease. *Scand. J. Clin. Lab. Investig.* **2008**, *68*, 89–94. [CrossRef]
13. Ramirez-Sandoval, J.C.; Herrington, W.; Morales-Buenrostro, L.E. Neutrophil gelatinase-associated lipocalin in kidney transplantation: A review. *Transplant. Rev.* **2015**, *29*, 139–144. [CrossRef] [PubMed]
14. Mishra, J.; Qing, M.A.; Prada, A.; Mitsnefes, M.; Zahedi, K.; Yang, J.; Barasch, J.; Devarajan, P. Identification of neutrophil gelatinase-associated lipocalin as a novel early urinary biomarker for ischemic renal injury. *J. Am. Soc. Nephrol.* **2003**, *14*, 2534–2543. [CrossRef] [PubMed]
15. Cai, L.; Rubin, J.; Han, W.; Venge, P.; Xu, S. The Origin of Multiple Molecular Forms in Urine of HNL/NGAL. *Clin. J. Am. Soc. Nephrol.* **2010**, *5*, 2229–2235. [CrossRef]
16. Lippi, G.; Aloe, R. Neutrophil gelatinase associated lipocalin (NGAL): Analytical issues. *LigandAssay* **2013**, *14*, 332–336.
17. Li, J.; Chen, Y.; Deng, F.; Zhao, S. Protective effect and mechanisms of exogenous neutrophil gelatinase-associated lipocalin on lipopolysaccharide-induced injury of renal tubular epithelial cell. *Biochem. Biophys. Res. Commun.* **2019**, *515*, 104–111. [CrossRef]
18. Mori, K.; Lee, H.T.; Rapoport, D.; Drexler, I.R.; Foster, K.; Yang, J.; Schmidt-Ott, K.M.; Chen, X.; Li, J.Y.; Weiss, S.; et al. Endocytic delivery of lipocalin-siderophore-iron complex rescues the kidney from ischemia-reperfusion injury. *J. Clin. Investig.* **2005**, *115*, 610–621. [CrossRef]
19. Kashiwagi, E.; Tonomura, Y.; Kondo, C.; Masuno, K.; Fujisawa, K.; Tsuchiya, N.; Matsushima, S.; Torii, M.; Takasu, N.; Izawa, T.; et al. Involvement of neutrophil gelatinase-associated lipocalin and osteopontin in renal tubular regeneration and interstitial fibrosis after cisplatin-induced renal failure. *Exp. Toxicol. Pathol.* **2014**, *66*, 301–311. [CrossRef]
20. Bhavsar, N.A.; Köttgen, A.; Coresh, J.; Astor, B.C. Neutrophil Gelatinase-Associated Lipocalin (NGAL) and Kidney Injury Molecule 1 (KIM-1) as Predictors of Incident CKD Stage 3: The Atherosclerosis Risk in Communities (ARIC) Study. *Am. J. Kidney Dis.* **2012**, *60*, 233–240. [CrossRef]

21. Gala-Błądzińska, A.; Dumnicka, P.; Kuśnierz-Cabala, B.; Rybak, K.; Drozdz, R.; Zyłka, A.; Kuźniewski, M. Urinary Neutrophil Gelatinase-Associated Lipocalin Is Complementary to Albuminuria in Diagnosis of Early-Stage Diabetic Kidney Disease in Type 2 Diabetes. *BioMed Res. Int.* **2017**, *2017*, 4691389. [CrossRef] [PubMed]
22. Gala-Błądzińska, A.; Romanek, J.; Mazur, D.; Stepek, T.; Braun, P.; Szafarz, P.; Chlebuś, M.; Przybylski, A. Reduced Albuminuria and Potassemia Indicate Early Renal Repair Processes after Resynchronization Therapy in Cardiorenal Syndrome Type 2. *Cardiol. Res. Pract.* **2020**, *2020*, 2727108. [CrossRef] [PubMed]
23. Bolignano, D.; Coppolino, G.; Lacquaniti, A.; Buemi, M. From kidney to cardiovascular diseases: NGAL as a biomarker beyond the confines of nephrology. *Eur. J. Clin. Investig.* **2010**, *40*, 273–276. [CrossRef] [PubMed]
24. Li, Y.M.; Li, Y.; Yan, L.; Wang, H.; Wu, X.J.; Tang, J.T.; Wang, L.L.; Shi, Y.Y. Comparison of urine and blood NGAL for early prediction of delayed graft function in adult kidney transplant recipients: A meta-analysis of observational studies. *BMC Nephrol.* **2019**, *20*, 1–10. [CrossRef]
25. Hollmen, M.E.; Kyllönen, L.E.; Inkinen, K.A.; Lalla, M.L.T.; Merenmies, J.; Salmela, K.T. Deceased donor neutrophil gelatinase-associated lipocalin and delayed graft function after kidney transplantation: A prospective study. *Crit. Care* **2011**, *15*, R121. [CrossRef]
26. Cappuccilli, M.; Capelli, I.; Comai, G.; Cianciolo, G.; La Manna, G. Neutrophil Gelatinase-Associated Lipocalin as a Biomarker of Allograft Function After Renal Transplantation: Evaluation of the Current Status and Future Insights. *Artif. Organs* **2018**, *42*, 8–14. [CrossRef]
27. Ramirez-Sandoval, J.C.; Barrera-Chimal, J.; Simancas, P.E.; Correa-Rotter, R.; Bobadilla, N.A.; Morales-Buenrostro, L.E. Tubular urinary biomarkers do not identify aetiology of acute kidney injury in kidney transplant recipients. *Nephrology* **2014**, *19*, 352–358. [CrossRef]
28. Kaufeld, J.K.; Gwinner, W.; Scheffner, I.; Haller, H.G.; Schiffer, M. Urinary NGAL Ratio Is Not a Sensitive Biomarker for Monitoring Acute Tubular Injury in Kidney Transplant Patients: NGAL and ATI in Renal Transplant Patients. *J. Transplant.* **2012**, *2012*, 1–8. [CrossRef]
29. Ramírez-Sandoval, J.C.; Barrera-Chimal, J.; Simancas, P.E.; Rojas-Montaño, A.; Correa-Rotter, R.; Bobadilla, N.A.; Morales-Buenrostro, L.E. Urinary neutrophil gelatinase-associated lipocalin predicts graft loss after acute kidney injury in kidney transplant. *Biomarkers* **2014**, *19*, 63–69. [CrossRef]
30. Cassidy, H.; Slyne, J.; O'Kelly, P.; Traynor, C.; Conlon, P.J.; Johnston, O.; Slattery, C.; Ryan, M.P.; McMorrow, T. Urinary biomarkers of chronic allograft nephropathy. *Proteom. Clin. Appl.* **2015**, *9*, 574–585. [CrossRef]
31. Lacquaniti, A.; Caccamo, C.; Salis, P.; Chirico, V.; Buemi, A.; Cernaro, V.; Noto, A.; Pettinato, G.; Santoro, D.; Bertani, T.; et al. Delayed graft function and chronic allograft nephropathy: Diagnostic and prognostic role of neutrophil gelatinase-associated lipocalin. *Biomarkers* **2016**, *21*, 371–378. [CrossRef] [PubMed]
32. Kellum, J.A.; Lameire, N.; Aspelin, P.; Barsoum, R.S.; Burdmann, E.A.; Goldstein, S.L.; Herzog, C.A.; Joannidis, M.; Kribben, A.; Levey, A.S.; et al. Kidney disease: Improving global outcomes (KDIGO) acute kidney injury work group. KDIGO clinical practice guideline for acute kidney injury. *Kidney Int. Suppl.* **2012**, *2*, 1–138. [CrossRef]
33. Kidney Disease: Improving Global Outcomes (KDIGO) KDIGO 2012 Clinical Practice Guideline for the Evaluation and Management of Chronic Kidney Disease. *Kidney Int. Suppl.* **2013**, *3*, 1–150.
34. Wyss, M.; Kaddurah-Daouk, R. Creatine and creatinine metabolism. *Physiol. Rev.* **2000**, *80*, 1107–1213. [CrossRef]
35. Stevens, L.A.; Coresh, J.; Greene, T.; Levey, A.S. Assessing kidney function—Measured and estimated glomerular filtration rate. *N. Engl. J. Med.* **2006**, *354*, 2473–2483. [CrossRef]
36. Denisov, V.; Zakharov, V.; Ksenofontova, A.; Onishchenko, E.; Golubova, T.; Kichatyi, S.; Zakharova, O. Clinical Course and Outcomes of Late Kidney Allograft Dysfunction. *J. Transplant.* **2016**, *2016*, 1–6. [CrossRef]
37. Cui, L.-Y.; Zhu, X.; Yang, S.; Zhou, J.-S.; Zhang, H.-X.; Liu, L.; Zhang, J. Prognostic Value of Levels of Urine Neutrophil Gelatinase-associated Lipocalin and Interleukin-18 in Patients With Delayed Graft Function After Kidney Transplantation. *Transplant. Proc.* **2015**, *47*, 2846–2851. [CrossRef]
38. Hollmen, M.E.; Kyllönen, L.E.; Inkinen, K.A.; Lalla, M.L.T.; Salmela, K.T. Urine neutrophil gelatinase-associated lipocalin is a marker of graft recovery after kidney transplantation. *Kidney Int.* **2011**, *79*, 89–98. [CrossRef]
39. Fonseca, I.; Oliveira, J.C.; Almeida, M.; Cruz, M.; Malho, A.; Martins, L.S.; Dias, L.; Pedroso, S.; Santos, J.; Lobato, L.; et al. Neutrophil Gelatinase-Associated Lipocalin in Kidney Transplantation Is an Early Marker of Graft Dysfunction and Is Associated with One-Year Renal Function. *J. Transplant.* **2013**, *2013*, 1–12. [CrossRef]
40. Parikh, C.R.; Jani, A.; Mishra, J.; Ma, Q.; Kelly, C.; Barasch, J.; Edelstein, C.L.; Devarajan, P. Urine NGAL and IL-18 are predictive biomarkers for delayed graft function following kidney transplantation. *Am. J. Transplant.* **2006**, *6*, 1639–1645. [CrossRef]
41. Choi, H.M.; Park, K.T.; Lee, J.W.; Cho, E.; Jo, S.K.; Cho, W.Y.; Kim, H.K. Urine neutrophil gelatinase-associated lipocalin predicts graft outcome up to 1 year after kidney transplantation. *Transplant. Proc.* **2013**, *45*, 122–128. [CrossRef] [PubMed]
42. Maier, H.T.; Ashraf, M.I.; Denecke, C.; Weiss, S.; Augustin, F.; Messner, F.; Vallant, N.; Böcklein, M.; Margreiter, C.; Göbel, G.; et al. Prediction of delayed graft function and long-term graft survival by serum and urinary neutrophil gelatinase–associated lipocalin during the early postoperative phase after kidney transplantation. *PLoS ONE* **2018**, *13*, e0189932. [CrossRef] [PubMed]
43. Schaub, S.; Mayr, M.; Hönger, G.; Bestland, J.; Steiger, J.; Regeniter, A.; Mihatsch, M.J.; Wilkins, J.A.; Rush, D.; Nickerson, P. Detection of subclinical tubular injury after renal transplantation: Comparison of urine protein analysis with allograft histopathology. *Transplantation* **2007**, *84*, 104–112. [CrossRef] [PubMed]

44. Zyłka, A.; Gala-Błądzińska, A.; Dumnicka, P.; Ceranowicz, P.; Kuźniewski, M.; Gil, K.; Olszanecki, R.; Kuśnierz-Cabala, B.; Żyłka, A.; Gala-Błądzińska, A.; et al. Is Urinary NGAL Determination Useful for Monitoring Kidney Function and Assessment of Cardiovascular Disease? A 12-Month Observation of Patients with Type 2 Diabetes. *Dis. Markers* **2016**, *2016*, 1–8. [CrossRef] [PubMed]
45. Câmara, N.O.S.; Silva, M.S.; Nishida, S.; Pereira, A.B.; Pacheco-Silva, A. Proximal tubular dysfunction is associated with chronic allograft nephropathy and decreased long-term renal-graft survival. *Transplantation* **2004**, *78*, 269–275. [CrossRef] [PubMed]
46. Teppo, A.M.; Honkanen, E.; Finne, P.; Törnroth, T.; Grönhagen-Riska, C. Increased urinary excretion of α1-microglobulin at 6 months after transplantation is associated with urinary excretion of transforming growth factor-β1 and indicates poor long-term renal outcome. *Transplantation* **2004**, *78*, 719–724. [CrossRef] [PubMed]
47. Wu, P.H.; Hsu, W.L.; Tsai, P.S.J.; Wu, V.C.; Tsai, H.J.; Lee, Y.J. Identification of urine neutrophil gelatinase-associated lipocalin molecular forms and their association with different urinary diseases in cats. *BMC Vet. Res.* **2019**, *15*, 1–10. [CrossRef]
48. Yan, L.; Borregaard, N.; Kjeldsen, L.; Moses, M.A. The high molecular weight urinary matrix metalloproteinase (MMP) activity is a complex of gelatinase B/MMP-9 and neutrophil gelatinase-associated lipocalin (NGAL): Modulation of MMP-9 activity by NGAL. *J. Biol. Chem.* **2001**, *276*, 37258–37265. [CrossRef]
49. Fernández, C.A.; Yan, L.; Louis, G.; Yang, J.; Kutok, J.L.; Moses, M.A. The matrix metalloproteinase-9/neutrophil gelatinase-associated lipocalin complex plays a role in breast tumor growth and is present in the urine of breast cancer patients. *Clin. Cancer Res.* **2005**, *11*, 5390–5395. [CrossRef]
50. Hsu, W.L.; Chiou, H.C.; Tung, K.C.; Belot, G.; Virilli, A.; Wong, M.L.; Lin, F.Y.; Lee, Y.J. The different molecular forms of urine neutrophil gelatinase-associated lipocalin present in dogs with urinary diseases. *BMC Vet. Res.* **2014**, *10*, 1–8. [CrossRef]
51. Hirt-Minkowski, P.; Marti, H.-P.; Hönger, G.; Grandgirard, D.; Leib, S.L.; Amico, P.; Schaub, S. Correlation of serum and urinary matrix metalloproteases/tissue inhibitors of metalloproteases with subclinical allograft fibrosis in renal transplantation. *Transpl. Immunol.* **2014**, *30*, 1–6. [CrossRef] [PubMed]
52. Mazanowska, O.; Kamińska, D.; Krajewska, M.; Żabińska, M.; Kopeć, W.; Boratyńska, M.; Chudoba, P.; Patrzalek, D.; Klinger, M. Imbalance of Metallaproteinase/Tissue Inhibitors of Metalloproteinase System in Renal Transplant Recipients With Chronic Allograft Injury. *Transplant. Proc.* **2011**, *43*, 3000–3003. [CrossRef] [PubMed]
53. Maraj, M.; Kuśnierz-Cabala, B.; Dumnicka, P.; Gala-Błądzińska, A.; Gawlik, K.; Pawlica-Gosiewska, D.; Ząbek-Adamska, A.; Mazur-Laskowska, M.; Ceranowicz, P.; Kuźniewski, M. Malnutrition, inflammation, atherosclerosis syndrome (MIA)and diet recommendations among end-stage renal disease patients treated with maintenance hemodialysis. *Nutrients* **2018**, *10*, 69. [CrossRef] [PubMed]
54. Gama-Axelsson, T.; Heimbürger, O.; Stenvinkel, P.; Bárány, P.; Lindholm, B.; Qureshi, A.R. Serum albumin as predictor of nutritional status in patients with ESRD. *Clin. J. Am. Soc. Nephrol.* **2012**, *7*, 1446–1453. [CrossRef]
55. Choi, J.W.; Fujii, T.; Fujii, N. Significance of Neutrophil Gelatinase-Associated Lipocalin Level-to-Serum Creatinine Ratio for Assessing Severity of Inflammation in Patients with Renal Dysfunction. *BioMed Res. Int.* **2015**, *2015*. [CrossRef]
56. Chakraborty, S.; Kaur, S.; Guha, S.; Batra, S.K. The multifaceted roles of neutrophil gelatinase associated lipocalin (NGAL) in inflammation and cancer. *Biochim. Biophys. Acta Rev. Cancer* **2012**, *1826*, 129–169. [CrossRef] [PubMed]
57. Kim, D.G.; Choi, H.Y.; Kim, H.Y.; Lee, E.J.; Huh, K.H.; Kim, M.S.; Nam, C.M.; Kim, B.S.; Kim, Y.S. Association between post-transplant serum uric acid levels and kidney transplantation outcomes. *PLoS ONE* **2018**, *13*, e0209156. [CrossRef]

A Review of Current and Emerging Trends in Donor Graft-Quality Assessment Techniques

Natalia Warmuzińska, Kamil Łuczykowski and Barbara Bojko *

Department of Pharmacodynamics and Molecular Pharmacology, Faculty of Pharmacy, Collegium Medicum in Bydgoszcz, Nicolaus Copernicus University in Torun, 85-089 Bydgoszcz, Poland; n.warmuzinska@cm.umk.pl (N.W.); k.luczykowski@cm.umk.pl (K.Ł.)
* Correspondence: bbojko@cm.umk.pl

Abstract: The number of patients placed on kidney transplant waiting lists is rapidly increasing, resulting in a growing gap between organ demand and the availability of kidneys for transplantation. This organ shortage has forced medical professionals to utilize marginal kidneys from expanded criteria donors (ECD) to broaden the donor pool and shorten wait times for patients with end-stage renal disease. However, recipients of ECD kidney grafts tend to have worse outcomes compared to those receiving organs from standard criteria donors (SCD), specifically increased risks of delayed graft function (DGF) and primary nonfunction incidence. Thus, representative methods for graft-quality assessment are strongly needed, especially for ECDs. Currently, graft-quality evaluation is limited to interpreting the donor's recent laboratory tests, clinical risk scores, the visual evaluation of the organ, and, in some cases, a biopsy and perfusion parameters. The last few years have seen the emergence of many new technologies designed to examine organ function, including new imaging techniques, transcriptomics, genomics, proteomics, metabolomics, lipidomics, and new solutions in organ perfusion, which has enabled a deeper understanding of the complex mechanisms associated with ischemia-reperfusion injury (IRI), inflammatory process, and graft rejection. This review summarizes and assesses the strengths and weaknesses of current conventional diagnostic methods and a wide range of new potential strategies (from the last five years) with respect to donor graft-quality assessment, the identification of IRI, perfusion control, and the prediction of DGF.

Keywords: kidney transplantation; graft quality assessment; biomarkers; machine perfusion; IRI; DGF

1. Introduction

Kidney transplantation (KTx) is a life-saving treatment for patients with end-stage renal dysfunction that is characterized by higher survival rates and greater quality of patient life compared to dialysis treatment [1]. Unfortunately, the number of patients placed on kidney transplant waiting lists is rapidly increasing, resulting in a growing gap between organ demand and the availability of kidneys for transplantation. Standard criteria donors (SCD) are preferred for kidney transplants because organs from these individuals typically result in more favourable outcomes compared to other donor types [2]. However, the shortage of available kidneys has forced medical professionals to utilize marginal kidneys from expanded criteria donors (ECD) to broaden the donor pool and shorten wait times for patients with end-stage renal disease. Nonetheless, it is well known that donor organ quality affects long-term outcomes for renal transplant recipients, and ECD kidney grafts have been shown to have worse outcomes compared to SCD grafts, including an increased risk of delayed graft function (DGF) and primary nonfunction incidence (PNF) [2,3]. Thus, representative methods of assessing graft-quality are urgently needed, especially for ECDs. Currently, the surgeon decides whether to accept or decline a kidney based on their interpretation of the donor's recent laboratory tests and a visual evaluation of the organ, with a biopsy being employed in some cases for direct tissue analysis [4,5].

Notably, the rapid emergence of techniques such as imaging, omics, and organ perfusion has provided surgeons with a wide range of new potential tools and biomarkers that could be used to evaluate graft quality.

In this paper, we review and evaluate the limits and advantages of current conventional diagnostic methods and a range of new potential tools (from the last five years) with respect to donor graft-quality assessment, the identification of ischemia-reperfusion injury (IRI), perfusion control, and the prediction of DGF (Figure 1).

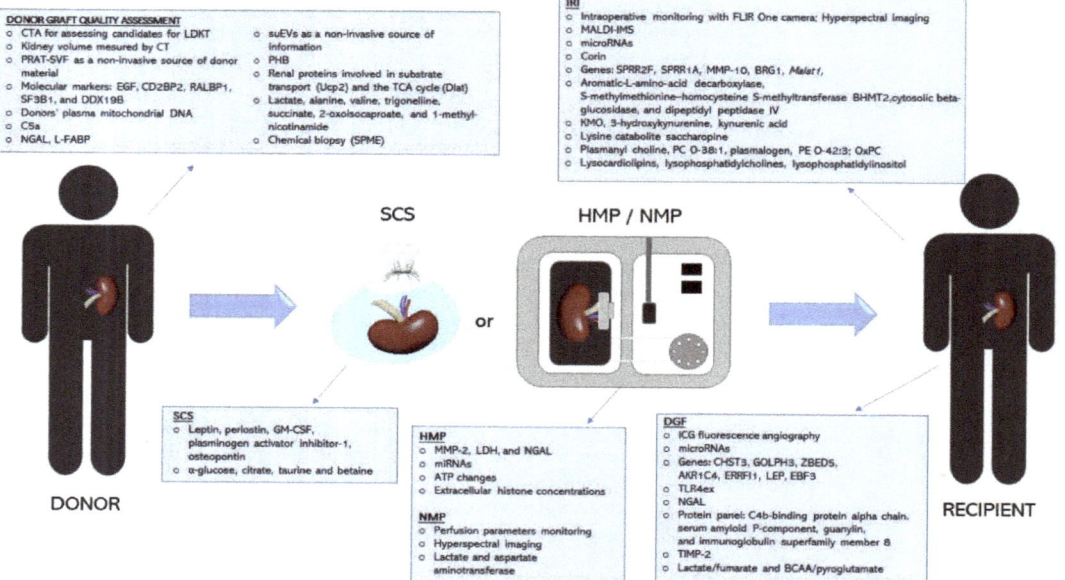

Figure 1. Emerging techniques and biomarkers in graft quality assessment, the identification of ischemia-reperfusion injury, perfusion control, and the prediction of DGF.

2. Current Conventional Diagnostic Methods

2.1. Visual Assessment

A visual evaluation of the kidney by the transplant team is a critical step in determining whether it will be accepted for transplantation or rejected. Macroscopic examination is useful for identifying kidney tumors, anatomical changes, damage, fibrosis, and scars that indicate the quality of the graft. However, this method is subjective and depends on the transplant team's level of experience [4]. Recent findings showed that surgeons were able to reliably predict the occurrence of postperfusion syndrome through visual assessments of liver graft quality, thus emphasizing the importance of visual appraisals by the surgical team [6]. However, no prior studies have evaluated intra-observer variability and the predictive value of visual kidney assessment. Thus, there is a need for new standardized diagnostic solutions for graft-quality assessment.

2.2. Clinical Risk Scores

Clinical information and laboratory results for a potential donor are crucial for an initial assessment of organ quality. Consequently, several scoring systems have been created to comprehensively analyse the risk of long-term graft failure or DGF [7–10]. At present, the Kidney Donor Risk Index (KDRI) and the Kidney Donor Profile Index (KDPI) are recognized as the most effective systems for scoring kidney graft quality. The KDRI was created by Rao et al., to quantify the risk of graft failure from deceased donors (DDs) based on donor and transplant variables, such as age, serum creatinine (CR), diabetes, HCV status, and cause of death [10]. The KDPI is a percentile measure based on the KDRI that was designed to assess how long a kidney from a DD is expected to function relative to all kidneys recovered in the U.S. during the previous year. The KDPI score is calculated based on ten variably weighted donor parameters that relevantly affect organ quality, with an emphasis on nephron mass. Lower KDPI scores are linked with longer estimated organ function, while higher KDPI scores are associated with a shorter estimated organ lifespan [11,12]. The KDRI and KDPI are regarded as reliable predictors of graft outcomes, and they are expected to increase the prevalence of marginal kidney grafting and reduce the unnecessary discard rate [11,13]. However, these indexes are not intended to be used as the only metric for determining donor suitability; rather, they should be utilized as a part of a comprehensive assessment along with other factors, including pre-implant biopsy histopathology and hypothermic machine perfusion (HMP) parameters [11,14]. Because age is the most influential factor in calculating the KDRI and KDPI scores, it is unclear whether the scores for these indexes can be applied to elderly and pediatric DDs. Recent studies suggest that the KDPI does not precisely predict pediatric kidney graft survival, while the KDRI has been found to be more reliable for elderly DDs. Overall, more research is needed to assess how reliably KDPI and KDRI scores predict postoperative renal function for grafts using kidneys from pediatric and elderly donors [13,15].

2.3. Biopsy

Pretransplant biopsy is currently one of the most widely used diagnostic methods and is recognized as the gold standard for confirming allograft injury. However, the frequency with which biopsies are performed varies between medical facilities and countries. In the United States, up to 85% of higher-risk kidneys are biopsied, whereas pretransplant biopsies are rarely conducted in European medical facilities. Histological evaluation is usually applied selectively, predominantly in ECD and donor after cardiac death (DCD) kidneys, and can help surgeons decide whether a kidney should be selected for transplantation or rejected [4,5,16].

In contrast to most laboratory data, histopathological assessments of biopsies do not yield a single value; rather, they produce comprehensive diagnoses that consider all available information. Although glomerulosclerosis, vascular disease, and interstitial fibrosis are the most frequently reported kidney parameters associated with worse graft outcomes [4,16], there is no consensus on the relative importance of each factor and which threshold values should be used to define the acceptable limit values. A further difficulty is the low reproducibility of kidney biopsy evaluations between on-call pathologists and renal pathologists described in many prior studies. The clear need to improve reproducibility and to objectivize the procedure and reporting of results prompted the development of several new composite histopathological scoring systems, including the Remuzzi score, the Maryland Aggregate Pathology Index, Banff criteria, and the Chronic Allograft Damage Index. Nevertheless, even with all these scoring systems, there are still doubts relating to the sampling, processing, and evaluation of biopsies [4,5,16].

In daily practice, it may be necessary to obtain quick results. In such circumstances, frozen section (FS) evaluation is often used for decision making. Producing paraffin sections (PS) is time consuming, which can cause histological evaluations to require up to 3 h to complete, even with the use of high-speed processing methods [5,17,18]. However, reports of reproducibility and prognostic value are based on paraffin-embedded tissue [18]. Recent studies have shown discrepancies in the results obtained with the use of FS and PS, but these variances had no significant impact on the outcomes for the transplanted organs [18]. Observed changes could be subtler in frozen sections than in paraffin sections, which may be a limitation, particularly in the hands of inexperienced pathologists [17,19]. On the other hand, it is also critical to consider logistics when choosing an optimal biopsy technique. For instance, FS is able to provide a diagnosis in less than 30 min, whereas PS requires at least 3 h. In selecting the proper technique, it is important to strike a balance between the benefits and risks associated with increased cold ischemia [4,18].

A lack of uniformity with respect to procedural standards has resulted in the use of a variety of biopsy techniques. The majority of medical facilities seem to prefer wedge biopsy (WB) over needle biopsy (NB) because NB carries a greater risk of injuring larger blood vessels, potentially resulting in uncontrolled bleeding after reperfusion. However, most recent reports comparing WB and NB have found that NB provides a much better evaluation of vascular lesions and has a higher overall correlation with the state of the whole kidney [5,16,17].

Ultimately, the most crucial factor is how the histopathological results correlate with long-term graft survival. Many studies have attempted to address the predictive value of renal biopsy with respect to graft outcomes, but the results of these studies have been predominantly inconclusive [20–23]. For instance, Traynor et al., conducted a retrospective study that examined kidney transplants over a 10-year period to determine whether pretransplant histology is able to predict graft outcomes at 5 years, and whether donor histology adds incremental data to the current clinical parameters. While the results of these reports suggest that that histological assessment adds little additional prognostic information aside from clinical parameters [20], Yap et al., found that the histological evaluation of ECD kidneys was associated with improved long-term graft survival. Their results suggest that pretransplant biopsy assessment can enable ECD kidneys to be used as a safe and viable option during persistent shortages of kidney donors [21]. The divergence between recent studies highlights the need for a prospective controlled trial to evaluate the predictive value of pretransplant biopsies. Until a standardized and comprehensive evaluation protocol has been developed, biopsy findings remain only one component of a donor organ assessment and should not be taken as the sole determinant in deciding whether to discard or transplant donor kidneys [19,24,25].

2.4. Perfusion Control

Static cold storage (SCS) and HMP are the main techniques of kidney graft preservation [26]. HMP has become a frequently and widely used procedure in kidney transplantation over the past few years [26–28]. Indeed, several reports have shown that the HMP reconditioning effect results in better postoperative outcomes with respect to reducing DGF and better long-term graft survival after transplantation [29–31]. An important benefit of HMP is that it enables the monitoring of perfusion parameters that could predict post-transplant organ viability. In particular, flow rate and renal resistance (RR) have been among the most frequently used perfusion parameters in predicting post-transplant function [27,32–34]. Previous studies have produced findings suggesting that real-time RR detection provides good predictive value. As Bissolati et al., showed, the RR trend during HMP can be used to predict post-transplantation outcomes, especially in relation to kidneys procured from ECD [28]. Patel et al., conducted a retrospective study that included 190 kidneys in order to evaluate the prognostic utility of HMP in DD transplantation. Their findings showed that resistances at two hours and beyond predicted DGF, while initial resistance to machine perfusion predicted one-year graft survival post-transplantation [35]. On the other hand, some studies found no association between hemodynamic parameters during HMP and the development of DGF [27]. Thus, due to these inconclusive results, the perfusion parameters cannot be regarded as stand-alone criteria. However, the undoubted advantage of perfusion parameters is that they are easy to obtain in a non-invasive manner. As such, Jochmans et al., and Zheng et al., have suggested that HMP parameters should be included as part of a comprehensive graft assessment [14,32]. DGF has a complex pathogenesis and cannot be predicted with precision using the HMP parameters as a stand-alone assessment tool. However, RR represents an additional source of information that can help clinicians in their decision-making process. Attaining more accurate predictions of graft outcomes will require integrating the perfusion parameters into multifactorial graft quality scoring systems. A combination of the donor's clinical data, kidney pre-implant histopathology, and HMP parameters may provide a more effective prediction of DGF than any of the measures alone [14,32].

2.5. Microbiological Analysis of Preservation Fluid

Organ transplant recipients are prone to infectious complications, and despite many advances, post-operative infections remain associated with significant morbidity and mortality [36–38]. Early post-transplant infections among kidney transplant recipients may be transmitted via the donor, or the donated organ may be contaminated during the transplantation procedure [36,38]. Moreover, pathogens can be transmitted via preservation solution, which is required to maintain kidney viability, but due to its biochemical characteristics, it can also keep microorganisms alive and serve as an infection vector [36,38,39]. For that reason, some transplant centres collect preservation fluid for microbiological analysis in addition to standard screening for donor infections. However, there are no widely accepted recommendations for managing positive preservation fluid cultures [36,38]. Moreover, it remains unanswered whether intra-operative preservation fluid routine screening should be performed because the clinical impact of this practice is still not well established. Some studies have evaluated the risk factors associated with culture-positive preservation fluid and determined the benefit of routine screening of preservation solutions for the management of kidney transplant recipients [36–38,40]. Corbel et al., demonstrated that 24% of DD preservation fluid cultures were positive, and these contaminations were mainly a consequence of procurement procedures [37]. Reticker et al. [36] and Oriol et al. [38] showed that the prevalence of culture-positive preservation fluid was up to 60%; however, the vast majority of microbial growth was consistent with skin flora or low-virulence pathogens. In addition, Oriol et al., indicated that pre-emptive antibiotic therapy for recipients with high-risk culture-positive preservation fluid might improve the outcomes and help to avoid preservation-fluid-related infections [38]. Moreover, Stern et al., reported that fungal contamination of preservation fluid was infrequent, although yeast contamination of preservation solutions was associated with high mortality [40]. In parallel, Reticker et al., suggested that antibiotic therapy for recipients with preservation solutions contaminated by low virulence pathogens may not be necessary, reducing antibiotic overuse [36]. In conclusion, routine screening of preservation solutions could improve graft outcomes and pre-emptive antibiotic therapy and be helpful to avoid preservation-fluid-related infections. However, future studies are needed to establish guidelines for preservation fluid microbiological analysis and handling culture-positive preservation fluid.

3. Emerging Techniques

3.1. Imaging

Diagnostic imaging methods are mainly used to evaluate kidneys from living donors (LD) prior to acceptance for transplantation, as well as for assessing post-renal transplant complications. In the case of living donor surgeries, non-invasive preoperative evaluation of the quality of the graft organ is especially critical, which allows surgeons to assess certain vital features, such as size, the presence/absence of focal cystic or solid lesions, and the condition of vascular structures, to establish whether it is appropriate for transplantation. While most of these features can be visualized via Doppler ultrasound, computed tomography angiography (CTA) is usually necessary for a more accurate assessment of the vascular anatomy [41–43]. However, given the critical role of careful evaluation and suitable preparation when dealing with living donor transplantation, it will be imperative to continue to conduct new research aimed at improving transplantation outcomes.

Sarier et al., conducted a retrospective study wherein they compared pretransplant CTA images to intraoperative findings to evaluate renal artery variations in a large sample of LD. They found that laparoscopic donor nephrectomy enabled the detection of the same number of renal arteries as CTA in 97.9% of the analysed kidneys, but less than CTA in the remaining 2.1%. Notably, a greater number of renal arteries were not detected in any of the studied kidneys via nephrectomy compared to CTA. These results indicate that CTA is more accurate than intraoperative findings, and is an effective method for evaluating candidate donors for living donor kidney transplantation (LDKT), as well as for identifying renovascular variations [42].

Al-Adra et al., employed computed tomography (CT) scans to assess the influence of donor kidney volume on recipient estimated glomerular filtration rate (eGFR) in a large cohort of patients undergoing LDKT. The resultant statistical models showed a significant correlation between donor kidney volume and recipient eGFR at 1, 3, and 6 months ($p < 0.001$). These findings indicate that donor kidney volume is a strong independent predictor of recipient eGFR in LDKT and may therefore be a valuable addition to predictive models of eGFR after transplantation. Further research could examine whether addition of donor kidney volume in matching algorithms can improve recipient outcomes [43].

Although the ability to monitor graft status intraoperatively is limited at present, several novel solutions have been proposed over the past few years to evaluate graft quality during transplantation and predict DGF.

In 2019, Fernandez et al., proposed a novel approach that utilized infrared imaging to monitor the reperfusion phase during kidney transplantation in real-time. To this end, they used a long-wave infrared camera (FLIR One) with a visual resolution of 1440×1080 pixels and a thermal resolution of 160×120 to study the grafts in 10 pediatric patients undergoing kidney transplantation. During the study, images were acquired at several key time points. The authors observed a correlation between changes in intraoperative graft temperature and decreases in postoperative creatinine levels in all of the analysed subjects. Given these results, Fernandez et al., concluded that infrared thermal imaging could be a promising option for non-invasive graft perfusion monitoring. However, additional work is required to confirm Fernandez et al.'s results because they were somewhat limited due to the relatively small number of patients included and the short follow-up period [44].

In another study, Sucher et al., employed Hyperspectral Imaging (HSI) as a noncontact, non-invasive, and non-ionizing method of acquiring quantitative information relating to kidney viability and performance during transplantation. Specifically, they used HSI to study seventeen consecutive deceased donor kidney transplants prior to transplantation, while stored on ice, and again at 15 and 45 min after reperfusion. After computation time of less than 8 s, the analysis software was able to provide an RGB image and 4 false color images representing the physiological parameters of the recorded tissue area, namely, tissue oxygenation, perfusion, organ hemoglobin, and tissue water index. The obtained results revealed that allograft oxygenation and microperfusion were significantly lower in patients with DGF. Future applications might also utilize HSI during donor surgery to assess kidney quality prior to cold perfusion and procurement. However, HSI can only be used intraoperatively and requires a direct view of the kidney because the maximum penetration depth for microcirculation measurements is currently 4–6 millimetres, making transcutaneous applications impossible. Thus, this technique's main limitations are its inability to provide continuous or intermittent transcutaneous follow-up measurements, as well as its small sample size. Thus, further studies are required to confirmed these results [45].

In the recent article, Gerken et al., documented a prospective diagnostic study that they had conducted in two German transplantation centres wherein allograft microperfusion was assessed intraoperatively via near-infrared fluorescence angiography with indocyanine green (ICG). While previous studies have shown that ICG fluorescence angiography can be applied safely during kidney transplantation, none have provided a quantitative assessment of the use of fluorescence video. To fill this gap, Gerken et al., evaluated the benefits of coupling quantitative intraoperative fluorescence angiography with ICG to predict postoperative graft function and the occurrence of DGF. Their findings indicated that the impairment of intraoperative microperfusion in the allograft cortex is a risk factor for the occurrence of DGF, and that ICG Ingress is an independent predictor of DGF. Further studies are warranted to analyse the effect of applying early therapeutic approaches to prevent DGF in kidney transplant recipients, thus improving long-term graft success [46].

The use of imaging techniques to diagnose post-renal transplant complications has been discussed extensively in recent reviews [47–49]; therefore, the present work will only examine a few of the most recent studies in this field. Promising results have been reported with respect to combining positron emission tomography (PET) with CT or magnetic resonance imaging (MRI) using the glucose analogue radiotracer, 2-deoxy-2-fluoro-D-glucose (FDG), to detect acute kidney allograft rejection, for diagnostic applications, for the functional assessment of grafts, and for therapeutic monitoring [50,51]. In another study, the utility of arterial spin labeling (ASL) magnetic resonance imaging was evaluated for its ability to identify kidney allografts with underlying pathologies. ASL uses endogenous water as a tracer, and it has previously been used in applications relating to the brain. Moreover, there have been reports demonstrating that ASL can be used to categorize stages of chronic kidney disease [52]. Wang et al., demonstrated that ASL might be a non-invasive tool for differentiating kidneys with subclinical pathology from those with stable graft function. However, more research should be performed to verify these findings [53].

3.2. Omics

The last few years has seen the emergence of many new technologies that examine organ function on a molecular level, which has enabled the discovery of numerous potential biomarkers of renal injury. High-throughput omics technologies allow researchers to obtain a large amount of data about specific types of molecules, providing a holistic picture that captures the complex and dynamic interactions within a biological system. These innovative methods, including transcriptomics, genomics, proteomics, metabolomics, and lipidomics, provide a deeper understanding of the complex mechanisms associated with IRI, inflammatory processes, and graft rejection [5,54]. This section surveys some promising methods and techniques that could be successfully translated to clinical settings in the foreseeable future (Table 1).

3.2.1. Transcriptomics/Genomics

Several studies have examined how graft quality and donor category impact graft and patient survival. Giraud et al., proposed an open-ended approach based on microarray technology to understand IRI occurring in DCD kidneys in a preclinical porcine model that had been subjected to warm ischemia (WI) followed by cold ischemia. Giraud et al.'s findings indicated that hundreds of cortex and corticomedullary junction genes were significantly regulated after WI or after WI followed by cold storage compared to healthy kidneys. In addition, they also analysed the kinetics of the most differentially expressed genes. They hypothesized that these genes played a key role in IRI and could be divided into eight categories: mitochondria and redox state regulation; inflammation and apoptosis; and protein folding and proteasome; cell cycle, cellular differentiation and proliferation; nucleus genes and transcriptional regulation; transporters; metabolism regulation; mitogen-activated protein kinase and GTPase (guanosine triphosphate, GTP) activity [55].

Boissier et al., performed a comparative study of cellular components, transcriptomics, and the vasculogenic profiles obtained from 22 optimal donors and 31 deceased ECDs. They hypothesized that as an easily accessible source of donor-derived material, perirenal adipose tissue (PRAT) can be used to assess the quantitative and functional features that characterize donor cells. In addition, adipose tissue can be enzymatically processed to obtain stromal vascular fraction (SVF), which is a heterogeneous cellular mixture free of adipocytes. In their study, Bossier et al., performed a transcriptomic analysis in order to differentiate the PRAT-SVF molecular transcript in ECD and other donors. The upregulated genes demonstrated a strong association with the inflammatory response, cytokine secretion, and circulatory system development, while the downregulated genes were associated with regulating metabolic processes and circulatory system development. Importantly, Bossier et al.'s findings provide new evidence that PRAT-SVF serves as a non-invasive source of donor material that can be highly valuable in the assessment of inflammatory features affecting the quality and function of the graft [56].

The midterm outcomes of kidney transplant recipients with early borderline changes between ECD, SCD, and LD were compared in a retrospective observational study. In the ECD group, microarray analysis showed a higher expression of 244 transcripts than the SCD group, and 437 more than the LD group. Compared to both the SCD and LD groups, gene annotation analysis of transcripts with elevated expression in ECD group revealed enhancement in the inflammatory response, the response to wounding, the defence response, and the ECM-receptor interaction pathway. ECD-related transcripts were likely increased by already occurred vascular changes compared to SCD group, and, similarly in SCD group, by longer ischemia compared with LD group. Therefore, chronic vascular changes and cold ischemia time enhance inflammation and thus contribute to poor outcomes for these grafts [57].

Another novel organ-evaluation tool was proposed in a retrospective open-cohort study that examined donors' plasma mitochondrial DNA (mtDNA), which can be easily and non-invasively assayed in the pre-transplant period, and may be a promising predictive biomarker for allograft function [58]. The mtDNA levels in the plasma of DCD were determined via real-time polymerase chain reaction (RT-PCR) and then statistically analysed in relation to the recipient's mtDNA levels and DGF. The linear prediction model, which included plasma mtDNA, donor serum creatinine, and warm ischemia time (WIT), showed high predictive value for reduced graft function. Moreover, the findings indicated that plasma mtDNA might be a novel non-invasive predictor of DGF and allograft function at six months after transplantation, in addition to correlating to allograft survival. Furthermore, mtDNA may serve as a surrogate predictive marker for PNF [58].

The vast majority of studies aiming to identify novel biomarkers involved in IRI have used murine or rat models. A growing body of evidence indicates that the aberrant expression of microRNAs (miRNA/miR) is closely associated with IRI pathogenesis [59–64]. MiRNAs are small, noncoding RNAs that mediate mRNA cleavage, translational repression, or mRNA destabilization [59]. For instance, Chen et al.'s findings suggest that miR-16 may serve as a potential biomarker of IRI-induced acute kidney injury (AKI) [59], while Zhu et al., found that miR-142-5p and miR-181a might be responsible for modulating renal IRI development [63]. On the other hand, some studies have pointed that miR-17-92, miR-139-5p, and miR-27a may play a protective role in IRI [61,62,64]. For example, Song et al., suggest that the overexpression of miR-17-92 could partly reverse the side-effects of IRI on the proximal tubules in vivo [61]. Furthermore, Wang et al., have reported that the overexpression of miR-27a results in the downregulation of toll-like receptor 4 (TLR4), which in turn inhibits inflammation, cell adhesion, and cell death in IRI [62].

Other murine-model-based studies have explored new candidate genes associated with renal IRI. In one such study, Su et al., found that IRI caused the upregulation of SPRR2F, SPRR1A, MMP-10, and long noncoding RNA (lncRNA) *Malat1* in kidney tissues. These genes are involved in keratinocyte differentiation, regeneration, and the repair of kidney tissues; extracellular matrix degradation and remodeling; inflammation; and cell proliferation in renal IRI [64]. In a separate study, Liu et al., investigated the role of BRG1 in IRI-induced AKI with a focus on its role in regulating IL-33 expression in endothelial cells. Their findings revealed that endothelial BRG1 deficiency reduces renal inflammation following ischemia-reperfusion in mice with a simultaneous reduction in IL-33 levels [65].

Comparisons of IRI in murine-based models and clinical studies have yielded valuable results [66,67]. For instance, Cippà et al., employed RNA-sequencing-mediated transcriptional profiling and machine learning computational approaches to analyse the molecular responses associated with IRI, which emphasized early markers of kidney disease progression and outlined transcriptional programs involved in the transition to chronic injury [66]. Other studies have demonstrated that Corin is downregulated in renal IRI and may be associated with DGF after kidney transplantation. Researchers have also screened differentially expressed genes in a murine model of IRI, with findings identifying Corin as one of the most relevant downregulated genes among 2218 differentially expressed genes. Moreover, 11 recipients with complications due to DGF and 16 without DGF were recruited for an ELISA to determine their plasma Corin concentrations. The findings of this study showed downregulation of plasma Corin concentrations in transplant recipients with DGF complications, indicating that Corin could be a potential biomarker of DGF [67]. DGF may result from early ischemic injury and potentially contribute to poor long-term survival following kidney transplantation [68,69]. For this reason, much research has been devoted to devising reliable methods for predicting the extent of IRI, and hence, DGF.

Hence, as with the IRI, miRNA was evaluated as a biomarker of DGF. In one study, Khalid et al., quantified microRNAs in urine samples from kidney transplant patients to determine whether this approach can be used to predict who will develop DGF following kidney transplantation. To this end, they used unbiased profiling to identify microRNAs that are predictive of DGF following kidney transplantation (i.e., miR-9, -10a, -21, -29a, -221, and -429), and afterward confirmed their findings by measuring specific microRNAs via RT-PCR. The biomarker panel was then assessed using an independent cohort at a separate transplant centre, with urine samples being collected at varying times during the first week after transplantation. When considered individually, all miRs in the panel showed a trend towards an increase or relevant increase in patients with DGF [68].

Wang et al., used high-throughput sequencing to investigate the miRNA expression profiling of exosomes in the peripheral blood of kidney recipients with and without DGF, and explain the regulation of miRNAs in the DGF pathogenesis [69]. Exosomes are cell-derived membrane vesicles present in numerous bodily fluids that play a crucial role in processes such as the regulation of cellular activity, intercellular communication, and waste management [69,70]. Wang et al., identified 52 known and 5 conserved exosomal miRNAs specifically expressed in transplant recipients with DGF. Additionally, their findings showed that transplant recipients with DGF also exhibited the upregulation of three co-expressed miRNAs: hsa-miR-33a-5p R-1, hsa-miR-98-5p, and hsa-miR-151a-5p. Moreover, hsa-miR-151a-5p was positively correlated with the kidney recipients' serum CR, blood urea nitrogen (BUN), and uric acid (UA) levels in the first week post-transplantation [69].

MicroRNA expression in kidney transplant recipients with DGF has also been assessed in another recently published study [71]. In this work, the researchers employed RT-PCR to analyse the expression of miRNA-146-5p in peripheral blood and renal tissue obtained from kidney transplant recipients who had undergone a surveillance graft biopsy during the DGF period. In the renal tissue, the expression of miR-146a-5p was significantly increased among the DGF patients compared to the stable and acute rejection (AR) patients. Similarly, microRNA 146a-5p had heightened expression in the peripheral blood samples from the DGF group compared to those of the acute rejection and stable groups; however, these differences were not statistically significant ($p = 0.083$) [71].

Overall, all these reports indicate that miRNAs are emerging as essential biomarkers in the molecular diagnosis of DGF. The above-discussed findings identify biomarkers that could contribute to the development of tools for predicting DGF and, as such, represent an important area of focus for future research.

Zmonarski et al., applied PCR to nonstimulated peripheral blood mononuclear cells (PBMCs) to examine the averaged mRNA toll-like receptor 4 expression (TLR4ex). The sample for this study consisted of 143 kidney transplant patients, 46 of whom had a history of DGF, and a control group of 38 healthy volunteers. The patients with a history of DGF were divided into two subgroups based on the median TLRex: low-TLR4 expression and high-TLR expression. Zmonarski et al.'s findings showed that patients with DGF had a much lower TLR4ex and worse parameters of kidney function. In addition, while a comparison of the DGF patients with low and high TLR4ex revealed no initial differences in kidney transplant function, differences were observed in the post-follow-up period. Furthermore, regression analysis showed that TLR4ex was related to recipient age, tacrolimus concentration, and uremic milieu. Consequently, the authors concluded that the low TLR4 expression in patients with DGF may be associated with poor graft-capacity prognosis, and that analysis of changes in TLR4ex may be valuable for assessing immunosuppression efficacy [72].

Another study aiming to identify potential biomarkers of DGF and AKI was recently conducted by Bi et al. [73]. In this study, the authors obtained two mRNA expression profiles from the National Center of Biotechnology Information Gene Expression Omnibus repository, including 20 DGF and 68 immediate graft function (IGF) samples. Differentially expressed genes (DEGs) in the DGF and IGF groups were identified, and pathway analysis of these DEGs was conducted using the Gene Ontology and Kyoto Encyclopedia of Genes and Genomes. Next, a protein–protein interaction analysis extracted hub genes. The essential genes were then searched in the literature and cross-validated based on the training dataset. In total, 330 DEGs were identified in the DGF and IGF samples, including 179 upregulated and 151 downregulated genes. Of these, OLIG3, EBF3, and ETV1 were transcription factor genes, while LEP, EIF4A3, WDR3, MC4R, PPP2CB, DDX21, and GPT served as hub genes in the PPI network. In addition, the findings suggested that EBF3 may be associated with the development of AKI following renal transplantation because it was significantly upregulated in the validation dataset (GSE139061), which is consistent with the initial gene differential expression analysis. Moreover, the authors found that LEP had a good diagnostic value for AKI (AUC = 0.740). Overall, these findings provided more profound insights into the diagnosis of AKI following kidney transplantation [73].

Elsewhere, McGuinness et al., combined epigenetic and transcriptomic data sets to determine a molecular signature for loss of resilience and impaired graft function. Notably, at a translational level, this study also provided a platform for developing a universal IRI signature and the ability to link it to post-transplant outcomes. Furthermore, McGuinness et al.'s findings relate DNA methylation status to reperfusion injury and DGF outcome. In this study, 24 paired pre- and post-perfusion renal biopsies defined as either meeting the extreme DGF phenotype or exhibiting IGF were selected for analysis. The findings of this analysis showed that the molecular signature contained 42 specific transcripts, related through IFNγ signaling, which, in allografts displaying clinically impaired function (DGF), exhibited a major change in transcriptional amplitude and increased expression of noncoding RNAs and pseudogenes, which is consistent with increased allostatic load. This phenomenon was attended by an increase in DNA methylation within the promoter and intragenic regions of the DGF panel in pre-perfusion allografts with IGF. Overall, McGuinness et al.'s findings suggest that kidneys exhibiting DGF suffer from an impaired ability to restore physiological homeostasis in response to stress that is commensurate to their biological age and associated allostatic load. This outcome is reflected in changes in the epigenome and transcriptome, as well as in the dysregulation of RNA metabolism [3].

3.2.2. Proteomics

Proteomics approaches have also been used to identify donor biomarkers that may predict graft dysfunction in order to alleviate organ shortages and address the lack of representative methods for assessing graft quality. To date, several studies have focused on identifying novel proteomic biomarkers of graft quality in donor urine [74–77]. Koo et al.'s study aimed to investigate the viability of using the levels of neutrophil gelatinase-associated lipocalin (NGAL), kidney injury molecule-1 (KIM-1), and L-type fatty acid binding protein (L-FABP) in donor urine samples to predict reduced graft function (RGF). In addition, Koo et al., also created a prediction model of early graft dysfunction based on these donor biomarkers. This model, which includes donor urinary NGAL, L-FABP, and serum CR, has been shown to provide better predictive value for RGF than donor serum CR alone. Based on this model, a nomogram for a scoring method to predict RGF was created to help guide the allocation of DD and maximize organ utilization [74]. On the other hand, another large prospective study has shown that donor injury biomarkers such as microalbumin, NGAL, KIM-1, IL-18, and L-FABP have limited utility in predicting outcomes among kidney transplant recipients [75]. This study evaluated the associations between injury biomarkers in the urine of DD and donor AKI, recipient DGF, and recipient six-month eGFR. Each of the tested biomarkers was strongly associated with donor AKI in the adjusted analyses. However, although the levels of all five donor biomarkers were higher in recipients with DGF than in those without DGF, the fully adjusted analyses revealed an association between higher donor urinary NGAL concentrations and a modest increase in the relative risk of recipient DGF. Moreover, the results of this study indicated that donor urinary biomarkers add minimal value in predicting recipient allograft function at six months post-transplantation [75]. In both studies, the tested biomarkers were strongly associated with donor AKI, while NGAL concentration was associated with DGF. A potential explanation for the different conclusions of these studies may be that Koo et al., used RGF as an outcome in their study, while Reese et al., used DGF due to different donor characteristics. Furthermore, it is worth emphasizing that, while these proteins are upregulated and secreted in urine in response to tubular injury, they were reported to have low specificity for tubular epithelial cell injury and were observed to increase in patients with urinary tract infections and sepsis [78,79].

In another study, the potential utility of C3a and C5a in DD urine samples as biomarkers for early post-transplant outcomes was investigated [76]. The results of this large, prospective, observational cohort study indicated a three-fold increase in C5a concentrations in urine samples from donors with stage 2 and 3 AKI compared to donors without AKI. In addition, donor C5a was positively correlated with the occurrence of DGF in recipients. In adjusted analyses, C5a remained independently correlated with recipient DGF only for donors without AKI. Moreover, the authors observed a tendency to indicate better 12-month organ functioning from donors with the lowest urinary C5a [76].

Monocyte chemoattractant protein-1 (MCP-1) has also been proposed as a potential biomarker of donor kidney quality. For example, Mansour et al., evaluated the association between graft outcomes and levels of MCP-1 in urine from DD at the time of organ procurement. In particular, they measured MCP-1 concentration to determine its correlation to donor AKI, recipient DGF, six-month estimated eGFR, and graft failure. Unfortunately, Mansour et al.'s results suggested that urinary MCP-1 has minimal clinical utility. Although median urinary MCP-1 concentrations were elevated in donors with AKI compared to those without AKI, higher MCP-1 levels were independently associated with a higher six-month eGFR in those without DGF. However, MCP-1 was not independently associated with DGF, and no independent associations between MCP-1 and graft failure were observed over a median follow-up of ~two years [77].

Recently, Braun et al., demonstrated the potential of using small urinary extracellular vesicles (suEVs) as a non-invasive source of data regarding early molecular processes in transplant biology. Their unbiased proteomic analysis revealed temporal patterns in the signature of suEV proteins, as well as cellular processes involved in both early response and longer-term graft adaptation. In addition, a subsequent correlative analysis identified potential prognostic markers of future graft function, such as phosphoenol pyruvate carboxykinase (PCK2). However, while Braun et al.'s study showed the potential of suEVs as biomarkers, the small number of patients in their sample did not allow for a conclusive statement on the predictive value of suEV PCK2. Therefore, the potential use of this biomarker will depend on larger trials in the future [80].

Studies focusing on the use of kidney tissue as a sample matrix to evaluate donor organ quality have also been performed. Using a rabbit model of brain death (BD), Li et al., employed two-dimensional gel electrophoresis and Matrix Assisted Laser Desorption/Ionization Time-of-Flight Mass Spectrometry (MALDI-TOF-MS)-based comparative proteomic analysis to profile the differentially-expressed proteins between BD and renal tissue collected from a control group. The authors were able to acquire five downregulated proteins and five upregulated proteins, which were then classified according to their function, including their association with proliferation and differentiation, signal transduction, protein modification, electron transport chain, and oxidation-reduction. Moreover, immunohistochemical analysis indicated that the expression of prohibitin (PHB) gradually elevated in a time-dependent manner. These data showed alterations in the levels of certain proteins in the organs from the BD group, even in the case of non-obvious functional and morphological changes. Given their results, Li et al., suggested that PHB may be an innovative biomarker for the primary assessment of the quality of kidneys from BD donors [81].

Conversely, van Erp et al., used a multi-omics approach and a rat model to investigate organ-specific responses in the kidneys and liver during BD. The application of proteomics analysis enabled them to quantify 50 proteins involved in oxidative phosphorylation, tricarboxylic acid (TCA) cycle, fatty acid oxidation (FAO), substrate transport, and several antioxidant enzymes in isolated hepatic and renal mitochondria. The most relevant changes were observed in the reduced peptide levels in the kidneys, which were related to complex I (Ndufs1), the TCA cycle (Aco2, Fh, and Suclg2), FAO (Hadhb), and the connection between FAO and the electron transport chain (Etfdh). The expression of two renal proteins, which were associated with substrate transport (Ucp2) and the TCA cycle (Dlat), was significantly increased in samples from the BD group compared to the sham-operated group. Interestingly, van Erp et al.'s findings showed that BD pathophysiology affects systemic metabolic processes, alongside organ-explicit metabolic changes, manifest in the kidneys by metabolic shutdown and suffering from oxidative stress, and a shift to anaerobic energy production, while kidney perfusion decreases. Ultimately, van Erp et al., concluded that an organ-specific strategy focusing on metabolic changes and graft perfusion should be part of novel procedures for assessing graft quality in organs from brain-dead donor, and may be the key to improving transplantation outcomes [82].

The vast majority of studies focusing on IRI have used animal models. In one proteo-metabolomics study using rat models, coagulation, complement pathways, and fatty acid (FA) signaling were observed following the elevation of proteins belonging to acute phase response due to IRI. Moreover, after 4 h of reperfusion, analysis of metabolic changes showed an increase in glycolysis, lipids, and FAs, while mitochondrial function and adenosine triphosphate (ATP) production were impaired after 24 h [83]. The authors of another study that used a porcine model of IRI found that integrative proteome analysis can provide a panel of potential—and predominantly renal—biomarkers at many levels, as changes occurring in the tissue are reflected in serum and urine protein profiles. This conclusion was based on the use of urine, serum, and renal cortex samples. In the renal cortex proteome, the authors observed an elevation in the synthesis of proteins in the ischemic kidney (vs. the contralateral kidney), which was highlighted by transcription factors and epithelial adherens junction proteins. Intersecting the set of proteins up- or downregulated in the ischemic tissue with both serum and urine proteomes, authors identified six proteins in the serum that may provide a set of targets of kidney injury. In addition, four urinary proteins with predominantly renal gene expression were also identified: aromatic-L-amino-acid decarboxylase (AADC), S-methylmethionine–homocysteine S-methyltransferase BHMT2 (BHMT2), cytosolic beta-glucosidase (GBA3), and dipeptidyl peptidase IV (DPPIV) [84]. Recent research by Moser et al., has examined kidney preservation injury and the nephroprotective activity of doxycycline (Doxy). In this work, rat kidneys were cold perfused with and without Doxy for 22 h, followed by the extraction of proteins from the renal tissue. Subsequent analysis showed a significant difference in eight enzymes involved in cellular and mitochondrial metabolism. Interestingly, the levels of N(G),N(G)-dimethylarginine dimethylaminohydrolase and phosphoglycerate kinase 1 decreased during cold perfusion on its own but increased during cold perfusion with Doxy [85]. The influence of perfusion type on graft quality has also been evaluated by Weissenbacher et al., who applied proteomics analysis to determine the differences between normothermically perfused (normothermic machine perfusion, NMP) human kidneys with urine recirculation (URC) and urine replacement (UR). Their findings revealed that damage-associated patterns in the kidney tissue decreased after 6 h of NMP with URC, suggesting decreased inflammation. Furthermore, they also observed that vasoconstriction in the kidneys was also attenuated with URC, as indicated by a reduction in angiotensinogen levels. The kidneys became metabolically active during NMP, which could be improved and prolonged by applying URC. The application of URC also enhanced mitochondrial succinate dehydrogenase enzyme levels and carbonic anhydrase, which contributed to pH stabilization. Key enzymes involved in glucose metabolism increased after 12 and 24 h of NMP with URC, including mitochondrial malate dehydrogenase and glutamic-oxaloacetic transaminase, predominantly in DCD tissue. The authors concluded that NMP with URC can prolong organ preservation and revitalize metabolism to possibly better mitigate IRI in discarded kidneys [86].

Ischemic injury may result in DGF, which is associated with a more complicated post-operative course, including a higher risk of AR [87]. Therefore, the early evaluation of kidney function following transplantation is essential for predicting graft outcomes [88]. Several studies have applied proteomic analysis to recipient urine samples in an attempt to identify protein biomarkers of DGF [87–89]. For instance, Lacquaniti et al., evaluated the usefulness of NGAL levels both for the early detection of DGF and as a long-term predictor of graft outcome. Their findings revealed that serum and urine samples from DGF patients contained high levels of NGAL beginning the first day after transplantation. Moreover, in patients who had received a kidney from a living related donor with excellent allograft function, NGAL concentrations lowered quickly during the first 24 h post-transplant period, reflecting a more pronounced reversible short-term injury. Importantly, NGAL levels in urine provided a better diagnostic profile than serum NGAL. Hence, urinary biomarkers on day 1 post-transplant may not only be useful in predicting who will need dialysis within one week, but they may also allow clinicians to discriminate between more subtle allograft recovery patterns [88]. However, as mentioned above, NGAL is characterized by low specificity; hence, its clinical application is limited due to inconclusive results [78,79]. Williams et al., used a Targeted Urine Proteome Assay (TUPA) to identify biomarkers of DGF following kidney transplantation. After employing data quality consideration and rigorous statistical analysis, they identified a panel of the top 4 protein biomarkers, including the C4b-binding protein alpha chain, serum amyloid P-component, guanylin, and immunoglobulin superfamily member 8, which had an AUC of 0.891, a specificity of 82.6%, and a sensitivity of 77.4% [87]. Similarly, urinary tissue inhibitor of metalloproteinases-2 (TIMP-2) and insulin-like growth factor binding protein-7 (IGFBP7) have been evaluated as biomarkers for DGF [89]. The findings of these studies indicated that TIMP-2 was able to adequately identify patients with DGF and prolonged DGF (AUC 0.89 and 0.77, respectively), whereas IGFBP7 was not. Moreover, correcting TIMP-2 for urine osmolality improved predictability (AUC 0.91 for DGF, AUC 0.80 for prolonged DGF), and 24-h urinary CR excretion and TIMP-2/mOsm were found to be significant predictors of DGF, with an AUC of 0.90. Hence, the obtained results indicated that TIMP-2 might be a promising, non-invasive indicator for predicting the occurrence and duration of DGF in individual patients [89].

3.2.3. Metabolomics and Lipidomics

In the absence of good quantitative biomarkers correlating to pre-transplantation organ quality, van Erp et al., examined metabolic alterations during BD using hyperpolarized magnetic resonance (MR) spectroscopy and ex vivo graft glucose metabolism during normothermic isolated perfused kidney (IPK) machine perfusion [90]. To this end, they employed hyperpolarized ^{13}C-labeled pyruvate MR spectroscopy to quantify pyruvate metabolism in the kidneys and liver at three time points during BD in a rat model. Following BD, glucose oxidation was measured using tritium-labeled glucose ($_D$-6-3H-glucose) during IPK reperfusion. In addition, enriched ^{13}C-pyruvate was injected repetitively to evaluate the metabolic profile at T = 0, T = 2, and T = 4 h via the relative conversion of pyruvate into lactate, alanine, and bicarbonate. The rats showed significantly higher lactate levels immediately following the induction of BD, with alanine production decreasing in the kidneys 4 h post-BD. However, it should be emphasized that this study's results did not assess whether these metabolic alterations can be associated with graft quality, or if they are suitable predictors of transplant outcome [90].

Another study using a rodent model of IRI examined the potential of using Hyperpolarized ^{13}C-labeled pyruvate to evaluate the metabolic profile directly in the kidneys [91]. The in vivo responses observed at 24 h and 7 d following ischemic injury demonstrated a similar trend towards a general decrease in the overall metabolism in the ischemic kidney and a compensatory increase in anaerobic metabolism, which is evidenced by elevated lactate production, compared to aerobic metabolism. In addition, a correlation was found between the intra-renal metabolic profile 24 h after reperfusion and 7 d after injury induction, as well as a correlation with the plasma CR. As a result, the authors suggest that using hyperpolarized ^{13}C-labeled pyruvate to identify the balance between anaerobic and aerobic metabolism has great future potential as a prognostic biomarker [91].

Increased lactate levels due to IRI were also observed in another study [92]. However, analysis of urine samples via nuclear magnetic resonance (NMR) spectroscopy showed higher levels of valine and alanine and decreased levels of metabolites such as trigonelline, succinate, 2-oxoisocaproate, and 1-methyl-nicotinamide following IRI, which was likely due to altered kidney function or metabolism [92].

A novel and minimally invasive metabolomic and lipidomic diagnostic protocol based on solid-phase microextraction (SPME) has been proposed to address the lack of representative methods of assessing graft quality [93,94]. The small size of the SPME probe allows the performance of chemical biopsy, which enables metabolites to be extracted directly from the kidney without any tissue collection. Furthermore, SPME's minimally invasive nature permits multiple analyses over time. For instance, ischemia-induced alterations in the metabolic profile of the kidneys and oxidative stress as a function of cold storage were observed in one study that used an animal model, with the most pronounced alterations being observed in the levels of essential amino acids and purine nucleosides [93]. However, more work is required to discriminate a set of characteristic compounds that could serve as biomarkers of graft quality and indicators of possible development of organ dysfunction.

In response to reports that the pharmacological inhibition of kynurenine 3-monooxygenase (KMO), and, separately, the transcriptional blockage of the Kmo gene, reduces 3-hydroxykynurenine formation and protects against secondary AKI, Zheng et al., investigated whether mice lacking functional KMO (Kmo^{null} mice) are protected from AKI experimentally induced by the direct induction of renal IRI [95]. KMO plays a crucial role in kynurenine metabolism. Kynurenine metabolites are generated by tryptophan catabolism and are involved in the regulation of various biological processes, including host-microbiome signaling, immune cell response, and neuronal excitability. The kynurenine pathway diverges into two distinct branches, which are regulated by kynurenine aminotransferases (KATs) and KMO, respectively. KMO is the only route of 3-hydroxykynurenine production that is known to be injurious to cells and tissue. Kynurenine may also be metabolized into kynurenic acid by KATs and to anthranilic acid by kynureninase [95]. Following the experimental induction of AKI via renal IRI, Zheng et al., observed that the Kmo^{null} mice had kept renal function, decreased renal tubular cell injury, and fewer infiltrating neutrophils than the wild-type control mice. Given these results, they suggested that KMO is a critical regulator of renal IRI. Moreover, higher levels of kynurenine and kynurenic acid were observed in the Kmo^{null} IRI mice compared to the Kmo^{null} sham-operated mice. This result may indicate that these metabolites help to protect against AKI after renal IRI, particularly because kynurenic acid has been demonstrated to have protective properties in other inflammatory situations due to its activity at glutamate receptors [95].

A 12.5-fold increase in the lysine catabolite saccharopine in IRI kidneys was observed in a recent study examining the differences between renal allograft acute cellular rejection (ACR) and IRI. The findings of this work indicated that the accumulation of saccharopine causes mitochondrial toxicity and may contribute to IRI pathophysiology. Moreover, similar to other reports, increased levels of itaconate and kynurenine were also observed in ACR kidneys. However, the detected changes in metabolites seemed to be unique for IRI and ACR, respectively, indicating that these two conditions have distinct tissue metabolomic signatures [96].

Several reports have also demonstrated that IRI can alter the lipidome. For example, Rao et al., evaluated lipid changes in an IRI mouse model using sequential window acquisition of all theoretical spectra-mass spectrometry (SWATH-MS) lipidomics. Their findings indicated that four lipids increased significantly at 6 h after IRI: plasmanyl choline, phosphatidylcholine (PC) O-38:1 (O-18:0, 20:1), plasmalogen, and phosphatidylethanolamine (PE) O-42:3 (O-20:1, 22:2). As anticipated, statistically significant changes were observed in many more lipids at 24 h after IRI. Interestingly, elevated levels of PC O-38:1 persisted at 24 h post-IRI, while renal levels of PE O-42:3 decreased alongside all ether PEs detected by SWATH-MS at this later time point. Overall, the authors found that coupling SWATH-MS lipidomics with MALDI-IMS (Imaging Mass Spectrometry, IMS) for lipid localization provided a better understanding of the role played by lipids in the pathobiology of acute kidney injury [97].

Researchers have also tested whether oxidized phosphatidylcholine (OxPC) molecules are generated following renal IRI. Solati et al., identified fifty-five distinct OxPC molecules in rat kidneys following IRI, including various fragmented (aldehyde and carboxylic-acid-containing species) and nonfragmented products. Among these, 1-stearoyl-2-linoleoyl-phosphatidylcholine (SLPC-OH) and 1-palmitoyl-2-azelaoyl-sn-glycero-3-phosphocholine (PAzPC) were the most abundant after 6 h and 24 h IRI, respectively. The total number of fragmented aldehyde OxPC molecules was significantly elevated in the 6 h and 24 h IRI groups compared to the sham-operated group, while an increase in the level of fragmented carboxylic acid was observed in the 24 h group compared to the sham and 6 h groups. In addition, fragmented OxPC levels were found to be significantly correlated with CR levels [98].

In their recent paper, van Smaalen et al., introduced and employed an interesting new approach based on IMS to rapidly and accurately evaluate acute ischemia in kidney tissue from a porcine model. First, ischemic tissue damage was systematically evaluated by two pathologists; this was followed by the application of MALDI-IMS to study the spatial distributions and compositions of lipids in the same tissues. Whereas the histopathological analysis revealed no significant difference between the tested groups, the MALDI-IMS analysis provided detailed discrimination of severe and mild ischemia based on the differential expression of characteristic lipid-degradation products throughout the tissue. In particular, elevated levels of lysolipids, including lysocardiolipins, lysophosphatidylcholines, and lysophosphatidylinositol, were present after severe ischemia. This data shows IMS's potential for use in differentiating and identifying early ischemic injury molecular patterns, and as a future tool that can be deployed in kidney assessment [99].

Because ischemia and reperfusion are inevitable consequences of kidney transplantation, and because DGF is a manifestation of IRI, Wijermars et al., used kidney transplantation as a clinical model of IRI to evaluate the role of the hypoxanthine-xanthine oxidase (XO) axis in human IRI. The sample group for this study consisted of patients undergoing renal allograft transplantation (n = 40), who were classified into three groups based on the duration of ischemia: short, intermediate, and prolonged. The results of the analysis confirmed the progressive accumulation of hypoxanthine during ischemia. However, differences in arteriovenous concentrations of UA and an in situ enzymography of XO did not indicate relevant XO activity in IRI kidney grafts. Moreover, renal malondialdehyde and isoprostane levels and allantoin formation were assessed during the reperfusion period to determine whether a putative association exists between hypoxanthine accumulation and renal oxidative stress. The absence of the release of these markers indicated the lack of an association between ischemic hypoxanthine accumulation and post-reperfusion oxidative stress. Based on these results, the authors suggest that the hypoxanthine-xanthine oxidase axis is not involved in the initial phase of clinical IRI [100]. In their clinical study, Kostidis et al., employed NMR spectroscopy to analyse the urinary metabolome of DCD transplant recipients at multiple time points in an attempt to identify markers that predict the prolonged duration of functional DGF [79]. To this end, urine samples were collected at 10, 42, 180, and 360 days post-transplantation. Their analysis revealed that samples collected on day 10 had a different profile than samples obtained at the other time points. At day 10, D-glucose, 2-aminobutyrate, valine, p-hydroxyhippurate, fumarate, 2-ethylacrylate, leucine, and lactate were significantly elevated in patients with DGF compared to those without DGF, while asparagine, DMG, 3-hydroxyisobutyrate, 3-hydroxyisovalerate, 2-hydroxy-isobutyrate, and histidine were significantly reduced in the DGF group. Urine samples from patients with prolonged DGF (≥21 days) showed increased levels of lactate and lower levels of pyroglutamate compared to participants with limited DGF (<21 days). Moreover, the ratios of all metabolites were analysed via logistic regression analysis in an attempt to further distinguish prolonged DGF from limited DGF. The results of this analysis showed that the combination of lactate/fumarate and branched chain amino acids (BCAA)/pyroglutamate provided the best outcome, predicting prolonged DGF with an AUC of 0.85. Given these results, the authors concluded that it is possible to identify kidney transplant recipients with DGF based on their altered urinary metabolome, and that it may also be possible to use these two ratios to predict prolonged DGF [79].

In another study, Lindeman et al., examined possible metabolic origins of clinical IRI by integrating data from 18 pre- and post-reperfusion tissue biopsies with 36 sequential arteriovenous blood samplings from grafts in three groups of subjects, including LD and DD grafts with and without DGF. The integration of metabolomics data enabled Lindeman et al., to determine a discriminatory profile that can be used to identify future DGF. This profile was characterized by impaired recovery of the high-energy phosphate-buffer, phosphocreatine, in DGF grafts post-reperfusion, as well as by persistent post-reperfusion ATP/GTP catabolism and significant ongoing tissue damage. The impaired recovery of high-energy phosphate occurred despite the activation of glycolysis, fatty acid oxidation, glutaminolysis, autophagia and was found to be related to a defect at the level of the oxoglutarate dehydrogenase complex in the Krebs cycle. Hence, Lindeman et al.'s findings suggest that DGF is preceded by a post-reperfusion metabolic collapse, leading to an inability to sustain the organ's energy requirements. Thus, efforts aimed at preventing DGF should aim to preserve or restore metabolic competence [101].

3.3. New Solutions in Perfusion Control

Organ-preservation technologies have been garnering significant interest for graft quality assessment, advanced organ monitoring, and treating transplanted kidneys during machine perfusion. As mentioned above, SCS and HMP are two of the more common methods of hypothermic preservation applied in clinical settings at present. In SCS, the kidney is submerged in a cold preservation fluid and placed on ice in an icebox; in HMP, a device pumps cold preservation fluid through the renal vasculature, which has been revealed to improve post-transplant outcomes [102]. NMP is another dynamic preservation strategy that involves the circulation of a perfusion solution through the kidney. The NMP conditions are designed to nearly replicate physiological conditions, which makes a real-life assessment of the graft possible prior to transplantation [103,104]. NMP has been recently translated into clinical practice, but this application is still at an experimental stage. However, early clinical results are promising [103,105]. Because preservation/perfusion solutions serve as a non-invasive source for the analysis of biomarkers, numerous studies have employed it for the purposes of graft quality assessment. In this section of this paper, we summarize the latest findings and studies that have used preservation/perfusion fluid and perfusion control in kidney transplantation (Table 1).

Coskun et al., used proteomic techniques to analyse the protein profiles of preservation fluid used in SCS kidneys. Their findings revealed significant correlations between protein levels and donor age (23 proteins), cold ischemia time (5 proteins), recipients' serum BUN (12 proteins), and CR levels (7 proteins). The identified proteins belonged to groups related to the structural constituent of the cytoskeleton, serine-type endopeptidase inhibitor activity, peptidase inhibitor activity, cellular component organization or biogenesis, and cellular component morphogenesis, among others [106]. In another proteomic study of preservation fluid, five potential biomarkers (leptin, periostin, granulocyte-macrophage colony-stimulating factor (GM-CSF), plasminogen activator inhibitor-1, and osteopontin) were identified in a discovery panel for differentiating kidneys with immediate function from those with DGF. Further analysis yielded a prediction model based on leptin and GM-CSF. Receiver-operating characteristic analysis revealed an AUC of 0.87, and the addition of recipient BMI significantly increased the model's predictive power, resulting in an AUC of 0.89 [107]. The metabolomic study compared the level of metabolites in perfusate samples collected prior to transplantation, during static cold storage, and between the allografts exhibiting DGF and IGF, while an integrated NMR-based analysis revealed a significant elevation in α-glucose and citrate levels, and significant decreases in taurine and betaine levels in the perfusate of DGF allografts [108].

In the last few years, several studies have documented the benefits of HMP over SCS, including improved short-term outcomes and reduced risk of DGF [109–111]. However, reports suggesting that HMP improves long-term graft function are inconclusive [102,111]. Some research groups have compared HMP with SCS to evaluate HMP's potential to improve kidney-graft outcomes [109,112] and to better understand the long-term benefits associated with its use [111,113]. At the same time, other groups have investigated how the use of oxygenated HMP impacts post-transplant outcomes, and how it can be used to further optimize kidney preservation, thereby expanding the number of organs available for transplant [102,114]. Furthermore, perfusion solution has been used in the search for useful biomarkers of graft quality and potential therapeutic targets. The analysis of perfusates from donor after brain death (DBD), DCD, and LD kidneys showed that DCD kidneys contained the highest levels of matrix metalloproteinase-2 (MMP-2), lactate dehydrogenase (LDH), and NGAL, followed by DBD and LD kidneys, respectively, suggesting a greater amount of injury in the DCD kidneys. Moreover, the DCD kidney perfusate contained significantly higher levels of protein compared to the DBD and LD perfusates, with quantitative analysis of the protein spots revealing significant differences between the groups in relation to seven spots: peroxiredoxin-2, FABP, A1AT, heavy chain of immunoglobulin, serum albumin, fragment of collagen 1, and protein deglycase (DJ-1) [115]. In another proteomic study, perfusate analysis of DBD kidneys preserved via HMP was performed to identify differences between the proteomic profiles of kidneys with good (GO) and suboptimal outcomes (SO) one-year post-transplantation. Analysis of samples collected 15 min after the start of HMP (T1) and before the termination of HMP (T2) indicated that the 100 most abundant proteins demonstrated discrimination between grafts, with a GO and SO at T1. Increased proteins were involved in classical complement cascades at both T1 and T2, while a decreased abundance of lipid metabolism at T1 and cytoskeletal proteins at T2 in GO (vs. SO) was also observed. Perfusate analysis at T1 revealed a predictive value of 91% for ATP-citrate synthase and fatty acid-binding protein 5, and analysis at T2 showed a predictive value of 86% for immunoglobulin heavy variable 2–26 and desmoplakin. In summary, HMP perfusate profiles for DBD kidneys can distinguish between outcomes one-year post-transplantation, providing a potential non-invasive method of assessing donor organ quality [2].

MicroRNAs in kidney machine perfusion solutions have also been considered as new biomarkers for graft function. For instance, Gómez dos Santos et al., conducted a prospective cohort study to investigate graft dysfunction in kidney transplantation from ECD. To this end, they employed a mean expression value approach, which confirmed the significance of a subset of the miRNAs previously identified with the development of delayed graft function, namely, miR-486-5p, miR-144-3p, miR-142-5p, and miR-144-5p. These results confirmed that perfusion fluid can be a valuable pre-transplantation source of organ-viability biomarkers [116].

In another study, Tejchman et al., assessed oxidative stress markers from the hypothermic preservation of transplanted kidneys. In particular, they sought to analyse the activity of enzymes and levels of non-enzymatic compounds involved in antioxidant defense mechanisms. These compounds, which included glutathione (GSH), glutathione peroxidase (GPX), catalase (CAT), superoxide dismutase (SOD), glutathione reductase (GR), glutathione transferase (GST), thiobarbituric acid reactive substances (TBARS), malondialdehyde (MDA), were measured in preservation solutions before the transplantation of human kidneys grafted from DBD. The study group was divided into two groups based on the method of kidney storage, with Group 1 consisting of HMP kidneys (n = 26) and Group 2 consisting of SCS kidneys (n = 40). There were aggregations of significant correlations between kidney function parameters after KTx and oxidative stress markers, namely: diuresis and CAT; Na^+ and CAT; K^+ and GPX; and urea and GR. Moreover, there were aggregations of correlations between recipient blood count and oxidative stress markers, including CAT and monocyte count; SOD and white blood cell count; and SOD and monocyte count. However, there was an issue of unequivocal interpretation because none of the observed aggregations constituted conditions that supported the authors' hypothesis that kidney function after KTx can be predicted based on oxidative stress markers measured during preservation. Moreover, it would be hard to conclude that the blood count alterations observed in the repeated measurements after KTx were unrelated to factors other than oxidative stress or acidosis. As the authors suggest, many other factors may modify blood count, including operative stress, bleeding, immunosuppression, and microaggregation [117].

Longchamp et al., presented an interesting and non-invasive method of assessing graft quality during perfusion based on the use of ^{31}P pMRI spectroscopy to detect high-energy phosphate metabolites, such as ATP. Thus, pMRI can be used to predict the energy state of a kidney and its viability before transplantation. In addition, Longchamp et al., also performed gadolinium perfusion sequences, which allowed them to observe the internal distribution of the flow between the cortex and the medulla. pMRI showed that warm ischemia caused a reduction in ATP levels, but not its precursor, adenosine monophosphate (AMP). Moreover, they found that ATP levels and cortical and medullary gadolinium elimination were inversely correlated with the severity of kidney histological injury. Thus, the measured parameters may be considered as biomarkers of kidney injury after warm ischemia, and Longchamp et al.'s method provides an innovative non-invasive approach to assessing kidney viability prior to transplantation [118].

Other researchers have examined whether a correlation exists between the level of extracellular histones in machine perfusates and the viability of DD kidneys. Extracellular histone levels were significantly elevated in the perfusates of kidneys with post-transplant graft dysfunction, and they were considered an independent risk factor for DGF and one-year graft failure, but not for PNF. One-year graft survival was 12% higher in the low-histone-concentration group ($p = 0.008$) compared to the higher-histone-concentration group. Hence, the quantitation of extracellular histones might contribute to the evaluation of post-transplant graft function and survival [119].

NMP is an emerging approach for donor organ preservation and functional improvements in kidney transplantation. However, methods for evaluating organs via NMP have yet to be developed, and the development of novel graft quality assessment solutions has only recently come into focus.

Kaths et al., used a porcine model to investigate whether NMP is suitable for graft quality assessment prior to transplantation. They found that intra-renal resistance was lowest in the HBD group and highest in the severely injured DCD group (60 min of warm ischemia), and that the initiation of NMP was correlated with post-operative renal function. Markers of acid-base homeostasis (pH, HCO_3^-, base excess) correlated with post-transplantation renal function. Furthermore, concentrations of lactate and aspartate aminotransferase were lowest in perfusate from non-injured grafts (vs. DCD kidneys) and were correlated with post-transplantation kidney function. Kaths et al., found that perfusion characteristics and clinically available perfusate biomarkers during NMP were correlated with post-transplantation kidney graft injury and function. However, further research is needed to identify perfusion parameter thresholds for DGF and PNF [120].

HSI combined with NMP was introduced as a novel approach for monitoring physiological kidney parameters. The experimental results of an HSI-based oxygen-saturation calculation indicated that HSI is useful for monitoring oxygen saturation distribution and identifying areas with a reduced oxygen supply prior to transplantation. Moreover, camera-based measurements are easy to integrate with a perfusion setup and allow the fast and non-invasive measurement of tissue characteristics [121]. Subsequent research has explored how to improve algorithms for determining kidney oxygen saturation [122]. Unfortunately, the application of HSI is limited by the propagating light's low penetration depth, which makes it impossible to detect deeper tissue injuries. However, based on the fact that most metabolic activity occurs in the kidney cortex, the combined use of HSI and NMP offers a promising and easy-to-use method for assessing the status of the organ and for chemical imaging [121,122].

Hyperpolarized MRI and spectroscopy (MRS) using pyruvate and other ^{13}C-labeled molecules offers a novel approach to monitoring the state of ex vivo perfused kidneys. In one study, the state of a porcine kidney was quantified using acquired anatomical, functional, and metabolic data. The findings showed an apparent reduction in pyruvate turnover during renal metabolism compared with the typical in vivo levels observed in pigs, while perfusion and blood gas parameters were found to be in the normal ex vivo range. Mariager et al.'s findings demonstrate the applicability of these techniques for monitoring ex vivo graft metabolism and function in a large animal model that resembles human renal physiology [123].

In another study, researchers sought to investigate the link between the urinary biomarkers, endothelin-1 (ET-1), NGAL, and KIM-1, and NMP parameters in order to improve kidney assessment prior to transplantation. Fifty-six kidneys from DD were used in this work, with each kidney being subjected to 1 h of NMP, followed by assessment based on macroscopic examination, renal blood flow, and urine output. The levels of ET-1 and NGAL measured in the urine samples after 1 h of NMP were significantly associated with perfusion parameters during NMP. These biomarkers and NMP perfusion parameters were also significantly associated with terminal graft function in the donor. However, KIM-1 was not correlated with the perfusion parameters or the donor's renal function. Larger studies are required to determine the usefulness of using these biomarkers with NMP to predict transplant outcomes. Despite this limitation, this study undoubtedly demonstrates that measuring urinary biomarkers during NMP provides additional information about graft quality [124].

Table 1. Emerging trends in donor graft quality assessment techniques.

Application	Category	Model	Type of Sample	Main Conclusions	Author
Evaluation of gene expression profile of kidney submitted to ischemic injury	Donor graft quality	Pig	Tissue	• ischemia leads to the full reprogramming of the transcriptome of major pathways such those related to oxidative stress responses, cell reprogramming, cell-cycle, inflammation and cell metabolism	Giraud et al. [55]
Investigation of the features of perirenal adipose tissue as an indicator of the detrimental impact of the ECD microenvironment on a renal transplant	Donor graft quality	Human	Perirenal adipose tissue	• ↑ genes associated with the inflammatory response, cytokine secretion, and circulatory system development • ↓ genes associated with regulating metabolic processes and regulating the circulatory system development	Boissier et al. [56]
Evaluation of donor category influence on borderline changes in kidney allografts by molecular fingerprints	Donor graft quality	Human	Tissue	• early borderline changes in ECD kidneys were characterized by the most increased regulation of inflammation, extracellular matrix remodeling, and AKI transcripts compared to SCD and LD groups	Hruba et al. [57]

Table 1. Cont.

Application	Category	Model	Type of Sample	Main Conclusions	Author
Exploration of the association between plasma mtDNA levels and post-transplant renal allograft function	Donor graft quality	Human	Plasma	• plasma mtDNA may be a non-invasive predictor of DGF and allograft function at 6 months after transplantation, and it also correlates with allograft survival • mtDNA may serve as a surrogate predictive marker for PNF	Han et al. [58]
Searching for urinary miRs that can be a biomarker for AKI	IRI	• Mouse • Human	• Urine; Tissue • Urine; Serum	• urinary miR-16 may serve as a valuable indicator for AKI patients	Chen et al. [59]
Determination of the role of miR-17-92 in IRI-induced AKI	IRI	Mouse	Tissue	• overexpression of miR-17-92 may antagonize the side-effects of IRI on the proximal tubules in vivo	Song et al. [61]
Investigation of the expression of renal miRNAs following renal IRI	IRI	Rat	Tissue	• ↑ miR-27a downregulated the expression of TLR 4, which resulted in inhibition of inflammation, cell adhesion and cell death in IRI	Wang et al. [62]
Identification of candidate genes involved in renal IRI	IRI	Mouse	Tissue	• IRI induces changes in the expression of SPRR2F, SPRR1A, MMP-10, Malat1, and miR-139-5p in the kidney, suggesting the utility of this panel as a biomarker of the renal IRI	Su et al. [64]
Examination of a link between activation of IL-33 transcription by BRG1 in endothelial cells and renal IRI	IRI	Mouse	Tissue	• endothelial BRG1 deficiency alleviates renal inflammation following IRI in mice with a concomitant reduction in IL-33 levels	Liu et al. [65]
Screening for differentially expressed genes in renal IR-injured mice using a high-throughput assay	IRI; DGF	• Mouse • Human	• Tissue, Serum • Plasma	• plasma Corin was downregulated in kidney transplantation recipients complicated with DGF • Corin might be a potential biomarker that is associated with DGF of kidney transplantation	Hu et al. [67]
Unbiased urinary microRNA profiling to identify DGF predictors after kidney transplantation.	DGF	Human	Urine	• combined measurement of six microRNAs (miR-9, miR-10a, miR-21, miR-29a, miR-221, miR-429) had predictive value for DGF following KT	Khalid et al. [68]
High-throughput sequencing to expression profiling of exosomal miRNAs obtained from the peripheral blood of patients with DGF	DGF	Human	Plasma	• ↑ hsa-miR-33a-5p R-1, hsa-miR-98-5p, hsa-miR-151a-5p in kidney recipients with DGF	Wang et al. [69]
Examination of miR-146a-5p expression in kidney transplant recipients with DGF	DGF	Human	Tissue; Whole blood	• miR-146a-5p expression has a unique pattern in the renal tissue and perhaps in a blood sample in the presence of DGF	Milhoransa et al. [71]
Evaluation of PBMC TLR4 expression of renal graft recipients with DGF	DGF	Human	Tissue; Whole blood	• low TLR4 expression in patients with DGF may be related to a poor prognosis for graft capability • analysis of TLR4 expression change may be a valuable parameter for the evaluation of immunosuppression effectiveness	Zmonarski et al. [72]

Table 1. *Cont.*

Application	Category	Model	Type of Sample	Main Conclusions	Author
Profiling of molecular changes associated with decreased resilience and impaired function of human renal allografts	DGF	Human	Tissue	• identified 42 transcripts associated with IFNγ signaling, which in allografts with DGF exhibited a greater magnitude of change in transcriptional amplitude and higher expression of noncoding RNAs and pseudogenes identified	McGuinness et al. [3]
Searching for urinary biomarkers that predict reduced graft function after DD kidney transplantation	RGF	Human	Urine	• utility of donor urinary NGAL, KIM-1, L-FABP levels in predicting RGF • the model including donor urinary NGAL, L-FABP, and serum CR showed a better predictive value for RGF than donor serum CR alone	Koo et al. [74]
Evaluation of associations between DD urine injury biomarkers and kidney transplant outcomes	DGF	Human	Urine	• higher urinary NGAL and L-FABP levels correlated with slightly decreased 6-month eGFR only among patients without DGF • donor urine injury biomarkers correlate with donor AKI but have poor predictive value for outcomes in kidney transplant recipients	Reese et al. [75]
Assessment of C3a and C5a in urine samples as biomarkers for post-transplant outcomes	DGF	Human	Urine	• urinary C5a was associate with the degree of donor AKI • in the absence of clinical donor AKI, donor urinary C5a concentrations associate with recipient DGF	Schröppel et al. [76]
Assessment of urinary and perfusate concentrations of MCP-1 from kidneys on HMP as an organ function indicator	AKI; DGF	Human	Urine; Perfusate	• higher concentrations of uMCP-1 are independently associated with donor AKI • donor uMCP-1 concentrations were modestly associated with higher recipient six-month eGFR in those without DGF • donor uMCP-1 has low clinical utility due to the lack of correlation with graft failure	Mansour et al. [77]
Evaluation of the proteome of suEVs and its changes throughout LD transplantation	Donor graft quality	Human	Urine; Tissue	• the abundance of PCK2 in the suEV proteome 24 h after transplantation may have a predictive value for overall kidney function one year after transplantation	Braun et al. [80]
Proteomic study of differentially expressed proteins in BD rabbits kidneys	Donor graft quality	Rabbit	Tissue; Serum	• the results indicated alterations in levels of several proteins in the kidneys of those with BD, even if the primary function and the structural changes were not obvious • PHB may be a novel biomarker for primary quality evaluation of kidneys from DBD	Li et al. [81]
Investigation of the influence of BD on systemic and specifically hepatic and renal metabolism in a rodent BD model	Donor graft quality	Rat	Plasma; Urine; Tissue	• the kidneys undergo metabolic arrest and oxidative stress, turning to anaerobic energy generation as renal perfusion diminishes	Van Erp et al. [82]

Table 1. Cont.

Application	Category	Model	Type of Sample	Main Conclusions	Author
Unbiased integrative proteo-metabolomic study in combination with mitochondrial function analysis of kidneys exposed to IRI to investigate its effects at the molecular level	IRI	Rat	Tissue	• proteins belonging to the acute phase response, coagulation and complement pathways, and FA signaling were elevated after IRI • metabolic changes showed increased glycolysis, lipids, and FAs after 4 h reperfusion • mitochondrial function and ATP production were impaired after 24 h	Huang et al. [83]
Integrative proteome analysis of potential and predominantly renal injury biomarkers considering changes occurring in the tissue and echo in serum and urine protein profiles	IRI	Pig	Serum; Urine; Tissue	• four urinary proteins with primarily renal gene expression were changed in response to managed kidney IRI and may be biomarkers of kidney dysfunction: aromatic-L-amino-acid decarboxylase (AADC), S-methylmethionine–homocysteine S-methyltransferase BHMT2 (BHMT2), cytosolic beta-glucosidase (GBA3), and dipeptidyl peptidase IV (DPPIV)	Malagrino et al. [84]
Evaluation of the changes in the proteome of kidney subjected to ischemia during machine cold perfusion with doxycycline	IRI	Rat	Tissue; Perfusate	• analysis showed a significant difference in 8 enzymes, all involved in cellular and mitochondrial metabolism • N(G),N(G)-dimethylarginine dimethylaminohydrolase and phosphoglycerate kinase 1 were decreased by cold perfusion, and perfusion with Doxy led to an increase in their levels	Moser et al. [85]
Proteomics analysis determinating the molecular differences between NMP human kidneys with URC and UR	IRI	Human	Tissue	• NMP with URC permits prolonged preservation and revitalizes metabolism to possibly better cope with IRI in discarded kidneys	Weissenbacher et al. [86]
TUPA to identify protein biomarkers of delayed recovery following KTx	DGF	Human	Urine	• C4b-binding protein alpha chain, serum amyloid P-component, Guanylin, and Immunoglobulin Super-Family Member 8 were identified that together distinguished DGF with a sensitivity of 77.4%, specificity of 82.6%	Williams et al. [87]
Assessment of the diagnostic and prognostic role of NGAL in DGF and chronic allograft nephropathy	DGF	Human	Serum; Urine	• high levels of NGAL characterized DGF patients since the first day after transplantation in urine and serum • urine NGAL presented a better diagnostic profile than serum NGAL	Lacquaniti et al. [88]
Investigation of changes of urinary TIMP-2 and IGFBP7 in the first days after KTx and their diagnostic utility for predicting DGF outcomes	DGF	Human	Urine	• urinary TIMP-2, but not IGFBP7, is a potential biomarker to predict the occurrence and duration of DGF in DCD kidney transplant recipients	Bank et al. [89]

Table 1. Cont.

Application	Category	Model	Type of Sample	Main Conclusions	Author
Investigation of organ-specific metabolic profiles of the liver and kidney during BD and afterwards during NMP of the kidney	Donor graft quality	Rat	Tissue; Plasma; Urine	• immediately following BD induction, BD animals demonstrated significantly increased lactate levels, and after 4 h of BD, alanine production decreased in the kidney • during IPK perfusion, renal glucose oxidation was decreased following BD vs sham animals	van Erp et al. [90]
Investigation of the acute and prolonged metabolic consequences associated with IRI, and elucidation whether the early injury mediated metabolic reprogramming can predict the outcome of the injury	IRI	Rat	Tissue; Plasma	• significant correlation between the intra-renal metabolic profile 24 h after reperfusion and 7 d after injury induction • identifying the balance between the anaerobic and aerobic metabolism with the use of hyperpolarized ^{13}C-labeled pyruvate has a great potential to be used in the future as a prognostic biomarker	Nielsen et al. [91]
NMR identification of metabolic alterations to the kidney following IRI	IRI	Mouse	Urine; Serum; Tissue	• higher levels of valine and alanine and decreased metabolites such as trigonelline, succinate, 2-oxoisocaproate, and 1-methyl-nicotinamide were found in urine following IRI due to altered kidney function or metabolism	Chihanga et al. [92]
Monitoring of the effect of oxidative stress and ischemia on the condition of kidneys using SPME-LC-HRMS platform	Organ ischemia	Rabbit	Tissue	• pronounced alterations in metabolic profile in kidneys induced by ischemia and oxidative stress as a cold storage function were reflected in levels of essential amino acids and purine nucleosides	Stryjak et al. [93]
Assessment of the role of kynurenine 3-monooxygenase as an essential regulator of renal IRI	IRI	Mouse	Plasma; Urine; Tissue	• KMO is highly expressed in the kidney and exerts major metabolic control over the biologically active kynurenine metabolites 3-hydroxykynurenine, kynurenic acid, and downstream metabolites • mice lacking functional KMO kept renal function, decreased renal tubular cell injury, and fewer infiltrating neutrophils compared with control mice	Zheng et al. [95]
Unbiased tissue metabolomic profiling of IRI and ACR in murine models to identify novel biomarkers and to provide a better understanding of the pathophysiology	IRI; ACR	Mouse	Tissue	• the lysine catabolite saccharopine 12.5-fold was increased in IRI kidneys and caused mitochondrial toxicity • itaconate and kynurenine increased levels were found in ACR kidneys	Beier et al. [96]

Table 1. Cont.

Application	Category	Model	Type of Sample	Main Conclusions	Author
Detection of early lipid changes in AKI using SWATH lipidomics coupled with MALDI tissue imaging	IRI	Mouse	Tissue	• increase in plasmanyl choline, phosphatidylcholine (PC) O-38:1 (O-18:0, 20:1), plasmalogen, and phosphatidylethanolamine (PE) O-42:3 (O-20:1, 22:2) concentrations at 6 h after IRI • PC O-38:1 elevations were maintained at 24 h post-IR, while renal PE O-42:3 levels reduced, as were all ether PEs detected by SWATH-MS at this later time point	Rao et al. [97]
Determination of the individual OxPC molecules generated during renal IRI	IRI	Rat	Tissue	• SLPC-OH and PAzPC were the most abundant OxPC species after 6 h and 24 h IRI, respectively • total fragmented aldehyde OxPC were significantly elevated in IRI groups than sham groups • fragmented carboxylic acid elevated in 24 h group compared with other groups	Solati et al. [98]
Rapid identification of IRI in renal tissue by Mass-Spectrometry Imaging	IRI	Pig	Tissue	• MALDI-IMS provided of detailed discrimination of severe and mild ischemia by differential expression of characteristic lipid-degradation products throughout the tissue • lysolipids, including lysocardiolipins, lysophosphatidylcholines, and lysophosphatidylinositol were elevated after severe ischemia	Van Smaalen et al. [99]
Evaluation of the involvement of the hypoxanthine-XO axis in the IRI that occurs during kidney transplantation	IRI	Human	Plasma; Tissue	• arteriovenous concentration differences of UA and in situ enzymography of XO did not indicate significant XO activity in IRI kidney grafts • absent release of malondialdehyde, isoprostane and allantoin is not consistent with an association between ischemic hypoxanthine accumulation and postreperfusion oxidative stress	Wijermars et al. [100]
Prediction of prolonged duration of DGF in DCD kidney transplant recipients by urinary metabolites profiling	DGF	Human	Urine	• the metabolites associated with prolonged DGF are handled by proximal tubular epithelial cells and reflect tubular (dys)function • lactate/fumarate and BCAAs/pyroglutamate ratios were useful to predict prolonged duration of DGF	Kostidis et al. [79]
Explorative metabolic assessment based on an integrated, time-resolved strategy involving sequential evaluation of AV differences over reperfused grafts and parallel profiling of graft biopsies	DGF	Human	Tissue; Plasma	• DGF is preceded by a post-reperfusion metabolic collapse, leading to an inability to sustain the organ's energy requirements	Lindeman et al. [101]

Table 1. Cont.

Application	Category	Model	Type of Sample	Main Conclusions	Author
Analysis of the proteins and peptides that are passed from the kidneys to the preservation fluid during organ preservation	Perfusion control	Human	Preservation fluid	• the relevant correlations between the levels of proteins and donors' age (23 proteins), cold ischemia time (5), recipients' serum BUN (12), and CR (7) levels were observed • identified proteins belonged to groups related to the structural constituent of the cytoskeleton, serine-type endopeptidase inhibitor activity, peptidase inhibitor activity, cellular component organization or biogenesis, and cellular component morphogenesis	Coskun et al. [106]
Searching for proteins accumulating in preservation solutions during SCS as biomarkers to predict posttransplantation graft function	Perfusion control	Human	Preservation fluid	• five potential biomarkers (leptin, periostin, GM-CSF, plasminogen activator inhibitor-1, and osteopontin) were identified in a discovery panel, differentiating kidneys with IGF versus DGF • prediction model based on leptin and GM-CSF and recipient BMI showed an AUC of 0.89	van Balkom et al. [107]
Analysis of perfusates during SCS to obtain the metabolite profiles of DGF and IGF allografts	Perfusion control	Human	Preservation fluid	• significant elevation in α-glucose and citrate levels and significant decreases in taurine and betaine levels in the perfusate of DGF allografts	Wang et al. [108]
Proteomic study of perfusate from HMP of transplant kidneys	Perfusion control	Human	Perfusate	• the highest levels of MMP-2, LDH, and NGAL were seen for the DCD kidneys, followed by the DBD kidneys and then LD • total protein in the perfusate from DCD was significantly increased than that in the perfusate from other donors	Moser et al. [115]
Proteomic perfusate analysis of DBD kidneys preserved using HMP to identify the differences between proteomic profiles of kidneys with a good and suboptimal outcome	Perfusion control	Human	Perfusate	• DBD kidney HMP perfusate profiles can distinguish between outcome one year after transplantation • increased proteins involved in classical complement cascades and a decreased levels of lipid metabolism at T1 and cytoskeletal proteins at T2 in GO versus SO were observed	van Leeuwen et al. [2]
Evaluation of miRNAs in kidney machine perfusion fluid as novel biomarkers for graft function	Perfusion control	Human	Perfusate	• confirmation of the significance of a subset of the miRNAs previously identified for DGF development and composed of miRNAs miR-486-5p, miR-144-3p, miR-142-5p, and miR-144-5p	Gómez-Dos-Santos et al. [116]
Influence of method of kidney storage on oxidative stress and post-transplant kidney function parameters	Perfusion control	Human	Perfusate; Whole blood	• correlations between kidney function parameters after KTx and oxidative stress markers: diuresis or Na^+ and CAT, K^+ and GPX, urea and GR were found	Tejchman et al. [117]

Table 1. Cont.

Application	Category	Model	Type of Sample	Main Conclusions	Author
Ex vivo evaluation of kidney graft viability during perfusion using ^{31}P MRI spectroscopy	Perfusion control	Pig	n.a.	• warm ischemia induced significant histological damages, delayed cortical and medullary Gadolinium elimination (perfusion), and decreased ATP levels, but not AMP • ATP levels and kidney perfusion are both inversely linked to the degree of kidney histological damage	Longchamp et al. [118]
Assessment of an association between the presence of extracellular histones in machine perfusates and deceased donor kidney viability	Perfusion control	Human	Perfusate	• extracellular histone concentrations were significantly higher in perfusates of kidneys with posttransplant graft dysfunction and were an independent risk factor for DGF and one-year graft failure, but not for primary nonfunction	van Smaalen et al. [119]
Organ quality assessment during NMP	Perfusion control	Pig	Perfusate; Whole blood; Urine	• intra-renal resistance was lowest in the HBD group and highest in the severely injured DCD group and at the initiation of NMP correlated with postoperative renal function • markers of acid-base homeostasis, lactate and aspartate aminotransferase perfusate concentrations were correlated with post-transplantation renal function	Kaths et al. [120]
Hyperpolarized MRI and spectroscopy using pyruvate and other 13C-labeled molecules as a novel tool for monitoring the state of ex vivo perfused kidneys	Perfusion control	Pig	n.a.	• renal metabolism displayed an apparent reduction in pyruvate turnover compared with pigs' usual in vivo levels • perfusion and blood gas parameters were in the normal ex vivo range	Mariager et al. [123]
Examination of the relationship between urinary biomarkers and NMP parameters in a series of human kidneys	Perfusion control	Human	Urine; Serum	• urinary ET-1 and NGAL assessed after 1 h of NMP were significantly associated with perfusion parameters during NMP and terminal renal function in the donor • KIM-1 was not linked with perfusion parameters or donor's renal function	Hosgood et al. [124]

↑—increase of expression; ↓—decrease of expression; n.a—not applicable.

4. Conclusions

New diagnostic solutions for accurately assessing renal graft quality are needed to improve the process for selecting suitable donors, more efficiently managing complications, and prolonging graft survival. Rapid advances in imaging, omics technology, and perfusion methods have led to the development of a wide range of new tools and biomarkers that could be applied to evaluate graft quality. Unfortunately, most of the methods mentioned in the review are based on animal models or require sophisticated technology with a long turn-around time to obtain the results, which significantly limits their potential for clinical use in the form of rapid commercial tests at present. However, non-invasive solutions, including imaging and the measurement of biomarkers in urine, blood, and perfusion fluid, appear to be promising with respect to their ability to be translated to a clinical setting. These studies include mtDNA and miRNAs determination based on commercially available kits for the isolation of genetic material in combination with the RT-PCR technique widely used in laboratory practice. A similar clinical potential is demonstrated by the determination of biomarkers such as NGAL, KIM-1, L-FABP and C5a in urine by ELISA, also routinely used in diagnostics. Nevertheless, the translation of biomarkers from the discovery stage to clinical practice is still challenging due to the complex and multifactorial type of injuries, the absence of standard guidelines for method validation, and adequate prospective and retrospective cohort studies. Larger, multi-centre validation studies are needed before new solutions can be widely implemented in clinics. Moreover, it will be imperative for future research to explore new technologies and integrate molecular measurements from large data sets reported in different experiments.

Author Contributions: Writing—original draft preparation, N.W.; designing writing—review and editing, N.W., K.Ł., B.B.; funding acquisition, B.B. All authors have read and agreed to the published version of the manuscript.

Funding: This study was funded by National Science Centre, grant Opus number 2017/27/B/NZ5/01013.

Data Availability Statement: No new data were created or analyzed in this study. Data sharing is not applicable to this article.

Conflicts of Interest: The authors declare no conflict of interest.

Abbreviations

ACR	acute cellular rejection
AKI	acute kidney injury
AMP	adenosine monophosphate
AR	acute rejection
ASL	arterial spin labelling
ATP	adenosine triphosphate
AUC	area under the curve
BCAA	branched chain amino acids
BD	brain death
BMI	body mass index
BUN	blood urea nitrogen
CAT	catalase
CR	creatinine
CTA	computed tomography
CTA	computed tomography angiography
DBD	donor after brain death
DCD	donor after cardiac death
DD	deceased donors
DEG	Differentially expressed genes
DGF	delayed graft function
DJ-1	protein deglycase
Doxy	doxycycline
ECD	expanded criteria donors
eGFR	estimated glomerular filtration rate
ET-1	endothelin-1
FA	fatty acid
FABP	fatty acid-binding protein
FAO	fatty acid oxidation
FC	fold change
FS	frozen section
GM-CSF	Granulocyte-macrophage colony-stimulating factor
GO	good outcome
GPX	glutathione peroxidase
GR	glutathione reductase

GSH	glutathione
GST	glutathione transferase
GTP	guanosine triphosphate
HMP	Hypothermic machine perfusion
HSI	Hyperspectral Imaging
ICG	indocyanine green
IGF	immediate graft function
IGFBP7	insulin-like growth factor binding protein-7
IL-18	Interleukin-18
IPK	normothermic isolated perfused kidney
IRI	ischemia-reperfusion injury
KATs	kynurenine aminotransferases
KDPI	Kidney Donor Profile Index
KDRI	Kidney Donor Risk Index
KIM-1	kidney injury molecule-1
KMO	kynurenine 3-monooxygenase
KTx	Kidney transplantation
LD	living donor
LDH	lactate dehydrogenase
LDKT	living donor kidney transplantation
L-FABP	L-type fatty acid binding protein
lncRNA	long noncoding RNA
MALDI-IMS	Matrix Assisted Laser Desorption/Ionization-Imaging Mass Spectrometry
MALDI-TOF-MS	Matrix Assisted Laser Desorption/Ionization Time-of-Flight Mass Spectrometry
MCP-1	Monocyte chemoattractant protein-1
MDA	malondialdehyde
miRNA/miR	microRNA
MMP-2	matrix metalloproteinase-2
MR	magnetic resonance
MRI	magnetic resonance imaging
MRS	magnetic resonance spectroscopy
MS	mass spectrometry
MSI	mass spectrometry imaging
mtDNA	mitochondrial DNA
NB	needle biopsy
NGAL	neutrophil gelatinase-associated lipocalin
NMP	normothermic machine perfusion
NMR	nuclear magnetic resonance
OxPC	oxidized phosphatidylcholine
PBMC	peripheral blood mononuclear cells
PC	phosphatidylcholine
PCK2	phosphoenol pyruvate carboxykinase
PE	phosphatidylethanolamine
PET	positron emission tomography
PHB	prohibitin
pMRI	^{31}P magnetic resonance imaging
PNF	primary nonfunction
PRAT	perirenal adipose tissue
PS	paraffin sections
RGB	Red Green Blue (colour model)
RGF	reduced graft function
RR	renal resistance
RT-PCR	real-time polymerase chain reaction
SCD	standard criteria donors
SCS	Static cold storage
SO	suboptimal outcome
SOD	superoxide dismutase
SPME	solid-phase microextraction
suEVs	small urinary extracellular vesicles

SVF	stromal vascular fraction
SWATH-MS	sequential window acquisition of all theoretical spectra-mass spectrometry
TBARS	thiobarbituric acid reactive substances
TCA	tricarboxylic acid
TIMP-2	tissue inhibitor of metalloproteinases-2
TLR4	Toll-like receptor 4
TUPA	Targeted Urine Proteome Assay
UA	uric acid
UR	urine replacement
URC	urine recirculation
WB	wedge biopsy
WI	warm ischemia
WIT	warm ischemia time
XO	hypoxanthine-xanthine oxidase

References

1. Swanson, K.J.; Aziz, F.; Garg, N.; Mohamed, M.; Mandelbrot, D.; Djamali, A.; Parajuli, S. Role of novel biomarkers in kidney transplantation. *World J. Transplant.* **2020**, *10*, 230–255. [CrossRef]
2. Van Leeuwen, L.L.; Spraakman, N.A.; Brat, A.; Huang, H.; Thorne, A.M.; Bonham, S.; van Balkom, B.W.M.; Ploeg, R.J.; Kessler, B.M.; Leuvenink, H.G.D. Proteomic analysis of machine perfusion solution from brain dead donor kidneys reveals that elevated complement, cytoskeleton and lipid metabolism proteins are associated with 1-year outcome. *Transpl. Int.* **2021**, *34*, 1618–1629. [CrossRef]
3. McGuinness, D.; Mohammed, S.; Monaghan, L.; Wilson, P.A.; Kingsmore, D.B.; Shapter, O.; Stevenson, K.S.; Coley, S.M.; Devey, L.; Kirkpatrick, R.B.; et al. A molecular signature for delayed graft function. *Aging Cell* **2018**, *17*, e12825. [CrossRef]
4. Dare, A.J.; Pettigrew, G.J.; Saeb-parsy, K. Preoperative Assessment of the Deceased-Donor Kidney: From Macroscopic Appearance to Molecular Biomarkers. *Transplantation* **2014**, *97*, 797–807. [CrossRef]
5. Moeckli, B.; Sun, P.; Lazeyras, F.; Morel, P.; Moll, S.; Pascual, M.; Bühler, L.H. Evaluation of donor kidneys prior to transplantation: An update of current and emerging methods. *Transpl. Int.* **2019**, *32*, 459–469. [CrossRef] [PubMed]
6. Kork, F.; Rimek, A.; Andert, A.; Becker, N.J.; Heidenhain, C.; Neumann, U.P.; Kroy, D.; Roehl, A.B.; Rossaint, R.; Hein, M. Visual quality assessment of the liver graft by the transplanting surgeon predicts postreperfusion syndrome after liver transplantation: A retrospective cohort study. *BMC Anesthesiol.* **2018**, *18*, 29. [CrossRef] [PubMed]
7. Nyberg, S.L.; Matas, A.J.; Kremers, W.K.; Thostenson, J.D.; Larson, T.S.; Prieto, M.; Ishitani, M.B.; Sterioff, S.; Stegall, M.D. Improved scoring system to assess adult donors for cadaver renal transplantation. *Am. J. Transplant.* **2003**, *3*, 715–721. [CrossRef] [PubMed]
8. Schold, J.D.; Kaplan, B.; Baliga, R.S.; Meier-Kriesche, H.-U. The broad spectrum of quality in deceased donor kidneys. *Am. J. Transplant.* **2005**, *5*, 757–765. [CrossRef] [PubMed]
9. Watson, C.J.E.; Johnson, R.J.; Birch, R.; Collett, D.; Bradley, J.A. A simplified donor risk index for predicting outcome after deceased donor kidney transplantation. *Transplantation* **2012**, *93*, 314–318. [CrossRef] [PubMed]
10. Rao, P.S.; Schaubel, D.E.; Guidinger, M.K.; Andreoni, K.A.; Wolfe, R.A.; Merion, R.M.; Port, F.K.; Sung, R.S. A comprehensive risk quantification score for deceased donor kidneys: The kidney donor risk index. *Transplantation* **2009**, *88*, 231–236. [CrossRef]
11. U.S. Department of Health and Human Services. Organ Procurement and Transplantation Network: KDPI Calculator. Available online: https://optn.transplant.hrsa.gov/resources/guidance/kidney-donor-profile-index-kdpi-guide-for-clinicians (accessed on 9 November 2021).
12. Dahmen, M.; Becker, F.; Pavenstädt, H.; Suwelack, B.; Schütte-Nütgen, K.; Reuter, S. Validation of the Kidney Donor Profile Index (KDPI) to assess a deceased donor's kidneys' outcome in a European cohort. *Sci. Rep.* **2019**, *9*, 11234. [CrossRef]
13. Jun, H.; Yoon, H.E.; Lee, K.W.; Lee, D.R.; Yang, J.; Ahn, C.; Han, S.Y. Kidney Donor Risk Index Score Is More Reliable Than Kidney Donor Profile Index in Kidney Transplantation From Elderly Deceased Donors. *Transplant. Proc.* **2020**, *52*, 1744–1748. [CrossRef]
14. Zheng, J.; Hu, X.; Ding, X.; Li, Y.; Ding, C.; Tian, P.; Xiang, H.; Feng, X.; Pan, X.; Yan, H.; et al. Comprehensive assessment of deceased donor kidneys with clinical characteristics, pre-implant biopsy histopathology and hypothermic mechanical perfusion parameters is highly predictive of delayed graft function. *Ren. Fail.* **2020**, *42*, 369–376. [CrossRef] [PubMed]
15. Parker, W.F.; Thistlethwaite, J.R., Jr.; Ross, L.F. Kidney Donor Profile Index (KDPI) Does Not Accurately Predict the Graft Survival of Pediatric Deceased Donor Kidneys. *Transplantation* **2016**, *100*, 2471–2478. [CrossRef]
16. Hopfer, H.; Kemény, E. Assessment of donor biopsies. *Curr. Opin. Organ. Transplant.* **2013**, *18*, 306–312. [CrossRef] [PubMed]
17. Naesens, M. Zero-time renal transplant biopsies: A comprehensive review. *Transplantation* **2016**, *100*, 1425–1439. [CrossRef] [PubMed]
18. Sagasta, A.; Sánchez-Escuredo, A.; Oppenheimer, F.; Paredes, D.; Musquera, M.; Campistol, J.M.; Solé, M. Pre-implantation analysis of kidney biopsies from expanded criteria donors: Testing the accuracy of frozen section technique and the adequacy of their assessment by on-call pathologists. *Transpl. Int.* **2016**, *29*, 234–240. [CrossRef] [PubMed]

19. Cooper, M.; Formica, R.; Friedewald, J.; Hirose, R.; O'Connor, K.; Mohan, S.; Schold, J.; Axelrod, D.; Pastan, S. Report of National Kidney Foundation Consensus Conference to Decrease Kidney Discards. *Clin. Transplant.* **2019**, *33*, e13419. [CrossRef]
20. Traynor, C.; Saeed, A.; O'Ceallaigh, E.; Elbadri, A.; O'Kelly, P.; de Freitas, D.G.; Dorman, A.M.; Conlon, P.J.; O'Seaghdha, C.M. Pre-transplant histology does not improve prediction of 5-year kidney allograft outcomes above and beyond clinical parameters. *Ren. Fail.* **2017**, *39*, 671–677. [CrossRef]
21. Yap, Y.T.; Ho, Q.Y.; Kee, T.; Ng, C.Y.; Chionh, C.Y. Impact of pre-transplant biopsy on 5-year outcomes of expanded criteria donor kidney transplantation. *Nephrology* **2021**, *26*, 70–77. [CrossRef]
22. De Vusser, K.; Lerut, E.; Kuypers, D.; Vanrenterghem, Y.; Jochmans, I.; Monbaliu, D.; Pirenne, J.; Naesens, M. The predictive value of kidney allograft baseline biopsies for long-term graft survival. *J. Am. Soc. Nephrol.* **2013**, *24*, 1913–1923. [CrossRef]
23. Phillips, B.L.; Kassimatis, T.; Atalar, K.; Wilkinson, H.; Kessaris, N.; Simmonds, N.; Hilton, R.; Horsfield, C.; Callaghan, C.J. Chronic histological changes in deceased donor kidneys at implantation do not predict graft survival: A single-centre retrospective analysis. *Transpl. Int.* **2019**, *32*, 523–534. [CrossRef]
24. Liapis, H.; Gaut, J.P.; Klein, C.; Bagnasco, S.; Kraus, E.; Farris III, A.B.; Honsova, E.; Perkowska-Ptasinska, A.; David, D.; Goldberg, J.; et al. Banff Histopathological Consensus Criteria for Preimplantation Kidney Biopsies. *Am. J. Transplant.* **2017**, *17*, 140–150. [CrossRef]
25. Hall, I.E.; Parikh, C.R.; Schröppel, B.; Weng, F.L.; Jia, Y.; Thiessen-Philbrook, H.; Reese, P.P.; Doshi, M.D. Procurement biopsy findings versus kidney donor risk index for predicting renal allograft survival. *Transplant. Direct* **2018**, *4*, e373. [CrossRef] [PubMed]
26. Peng, P.; Ding, Z.; He, Y.; Zhang, J.; Wang, X.; Yang, Z. Hypothermic Machine Perfusion Versus Static Cold Storage in Deceased Donor Kidney Transplantation: A Systematic Review and Meta-Analysis of Randomized Controlled Trials. *Artif. Organs* **2019**, *43*, 478–489. [CrossRef] [PubMed]
27. Peris, A.; Fulceri, G.E.; Lazzeri, C.; Bonizzoli, M.; Li Marzi, V.; Serni, S.; Cirami, L.; Migliaccio, M.L. Delayed graft function and perfusion parameters of kidneys from uncontrolled donors after circulatory death. *Perfusion* **2021**, *36*, 299–304. [CrossRef]
28. Bissolati, M.; Gazzetta, P.G.; Caldara, R.; Guarneri, G.; Adamenko, O.; Giannone, F.; Mazza, M.; Maggi, G.; Tomanin, D.; Rosati, R.; et al. Renal Resistance Trend During Hypothermic Machine Perfusion Is More Predictive of Postoperative Outcome Than Biopsy Score: Preliminary Experience in 35 Consecutive Kidney Transplantations. *Artif. Organs* **2018**, *42*, 714–722. [CrossRef] [PubMed]
29. Moers, C.; Smits, J.M.; Maathuis, M.-H.J.; Treckmann, J.; van Gelder, F.; Napieralski, B.P.; van Kasterop-Kutz, M.; van der Heide, J.J.H.; Squifflet, J.-P.; van Heurn, E.; et al. Machine Perfusion or Cold Storage in Deceased-Donor Kidney Transplantation. *N. Engl. J. Med.* **2009**, *360*, 7–19. [CrossRef] [PubMed]
30. Lindell, S.L.; Muir, H.; Brassil, J.; Mangino, M.J. Hypothermic Machine Perfusion Preservation of the DCD Kidney: Machine Effects. *J. Transplant.* **2013**, *2013*, 802618. [CrossRef]
31. De Deken, J.; Kocabayoglu, P.; Moers, C. Hypothermic machine perfusion in kidney transplantation. *Curr. Opin. Organ. Transplant.* **2016**, *21*, 294–300. [CrossRef]
32. Jochmans, I.; Moers, C.; Smits, J.M.; Leuvenink, H.G.D.; Treckmann, J.; Paul, A.; Rahmel, A.; Squifflet, J.P.; van Heurn, E.; Monbaliu, D.; et al. The prognostic value of renal resistance during hypothermic machine perfusion of deceased donor kidneys. *Am. J. Transplant.* **2011**, *11*, 2214–2220. [CrossRef]
33. Mozes, M.F.; Skolek, R.B.; Korf, B.C. Use of perfusion parameters in predicting outcomes of machine-preserved kidneys. *Transplant. Proc.* **2005**, *37*, 350–351. [CrossRef]
34. Bunegin, L.; Tolstykh, G.P.; Gelineau, J.F.; Cosimi, A.B.; Anderson, L.M. Oxygen consumption during oxygenated hypothermic perfusion as a measure of donor organ viability. *ASAIO J.* **2013**, *59*, 427–432. [CrossRef] [PubMed]
35. Patel, S.K.; Pankewycz, O.G.; Nader, N.D.; Zachariah, M.; Kohli, R.; Laftavi, M.R. Prognostic utility of hypothermic machine perfusion in deceased donor renal transplantation. *Transplant. Proc.* **2012**, *44*, 2207–2212. [CrossRef] [PubMed]
36. Reticker, A.; Lichvar, A.; Walsh, M.; Gross, A.E.; Patel, S. The Significance and Impact of Screening Preservation Fluid Cultures in Renal Transplant Recipients. *Prog. Transplant.* **2021**, *31*, 40–46. [CrossRef] [PubMed]
37. Corbel, A.; Ladrière, M.; Le Berre, N.; Durin, L.; Rousseau, H.; Frimat, L.; Thilly, N.; Pulcini, C. Microbiological epidemiology of preservation fluids in transplanted kidney: A nationwide retrospective observational study. *Clin. Microbiol. Infect.* **2020**, *26*, 475–484. [CrossRef] [PubMed]
38. Oriol, I.; Sabe, N.; Càmara, J.; Berbel, D.; Ballesteros, M.A.; Escudero, R.; Lopez-Medrano, F.; Linares, L.; Len, O.; Silva, J.T.; et al. The impact of culturing the organ preservation fluid on solid organ transplantation: A prospective multicenter cohort study. *Open Forum Infect. Dis.* **2019**, *6*, 1–7. [CrossRef]
39. Yu, X.; Wang, R.; Peng, W.; Huang, H.; Liu, G.; Yang, Q.; Zhou, J.; Zhang, X.; Lv, J.H.; Lei, W.; et al. Incidence, distribution and clinical relevance of microbial contamination of preservation solution in deceased kidney transplant recipients: A retrospective cohort study from China. *Clin. Microbiol. Infect.* **2019**, *25*, 595–600. [CrossRef]
40. Stern, S.; Bezinover, D.; Rath, P.M.; Paul, A.; Saner, F.H. Candida contamination in kidney and liver organ preservation solution: Does it matter? *J. Clin. Med.* **2021**, *10*, 2022. [CrossRef]
41. Sjekavica, I.; Novosel, L.; Rupčić, M.; Smiljanić, R.; Muršić, M.; Duspara, V.; Lušić, M.; Perkov, D.; Hrabak-Paar, M.; Zidanić, M.; et al. Radiological imaging in renal transplantation. *Acta Clin. Croat.* **2018**, *57*, 694–712. [CrossRef]

42. Sarier, M.; Callioglu, M.; Yuksel, Y.; Duman, E.; Emek, M.; Usta, S.S. Evaluation of the Renal Arteries of 2144 Living Kidney Donors Using Computed Tomography Angiography and Comparison with Intraoperative Findings. *Urol. Int.* **2020**, *104*, 637–640. [CrossRef]
43. Al-Adra, D.P.; Lambadaris, M.; Barbas, A.; Li, Y.; Selzner, M.; Singh, S.K.; Famure, O.; Kim, S.J.; Ghanekar, A. Donor kidney volume measured by computed tomography is a strong predictor of recipient eGFR in living donor kidney transplantation. *World J. Urol.* **2019**, *37*, 1965–1972. [CrossRef]
44. Fernandez, N.; Lorenzo, A.; Chua, M.; Koyle, M.A.; Farhat, W.; Matava, C. Real-time kidney graft perfusion monitoring using infrared imaging during pediatric kidney transplantation. *J. Pediatr. Urol.* **2019**, *15*, 222.e1–222.e7. [CrossRef]
45. Sucher, R.; Wagner, T.; Köhler, H.; Sucher, E.; Guice, H.; Recknagel, S.; Lederer, A.; Hau, H.M.; Rademacher, S.; Schneeberger, S.; et al. Hyperspectral Imaging (HSI) of Human Kidney Allografts. *Ann. Surg.* **2020**. [CrossRef]
46. Gerken, A.L.H.; Nowak, K.; Meyer, A.; Weiss, C.; Krüger, B.; Nawroth, N.; Karampinis, I.; Heller, K.; Apel, H.; Reissfelder, C.; et al. Quantitative Assessment of Intraoperative Laser Fluorescence Angiography with Indocyanine Green Predicts Early Graft Function after Kidney Transplantation. *Ann. Surg.* **2020**. [CrossRef] [PubMed]
47. Yu, Y.M.; Ni, Q.Q.; Wang, Z.J.; Chen, M.L.; Zhang, L.J. Multiparametric functional magnetic resonance imaging for evaluating renal allograft injury. *Korean J. Radiol.* **2019**, *20*, 894–908. [CrossRef] [PubMed]
48. Schutter, R.; Lantinga, V.A.; Borra, R.J.H.; Moers, C. MRI for diagnosis of post-renal transplant complications: Current state-of-the-art and future perspectives. *Magn. Reson. Mater. Physics Biol. Med.* **2020**, *33*, 49–61. [CrossRef] [PubMed]
49. Jehn, U.; Schuette-Nuetgen, K.; Kentrup, D.; Hoerr, V.; Reuter, S. Renal allograft rejection: Noninvasive ultrasound- and mri-based diagnostics. *Contrast Media Mol. Imaging* **2019**, *2019*, 3568067. [CrossRef] [PubMed]
50. Pajenda, S.; Rasul, S.; Hacker, M.; Wagner, L.; Geist, B.K. Dynamic 2-deoxy-2[18F] fluoro-D-glucose PET/MRI in human renal allotransplant patients undergoing acute kidney injury. *Sci. Rep.* **2020**, *10*, 8270. [CrossRef]
51. Jadoul, A.; Lovinfosse, P.; Bouquegneau, A.; Weekers, L.; Pottel, H.; Hustinx, R.; Jouret, F. Observer variability in the assessment of renal 18F-FDG uptake in kidney transplant recipients. *Sci. Rep.* **2020**, *10*, 4617. [CrossRef]
52. Cai, Y.; Li, Z.; Zuo, P.; Pfeuffer, J.; Li, Y.; Liu, F.; Liu, R. Diagnostic value of renal perfusion in patients with chronic kidney disease using 3D arterial spin labeling. *J. Magn. Reson. Imaging* **2017**, *46*, 589–594. [CrossRef]
53. Wang, W.; Yu, Y.; Li, X.; Chen, J.; Zhang, Y.; Zhang, L.; Wen, J. Early detection of subclinical pathology in patients with stable kidney graft function by arterial spin labeling. *Eur. Radiol.* **2021**, *31*, 2687–2695. [CrossRef]
54. Bontha, S.V.; Maluf, D.G.; Mueller, T.F.; Mas, V.R. Systems Biology in Kidney Transplantation: The Application of Multi-Omics to a Complex Model. *Am. J. Transplant.* **2017**, *17*, 11–21. [CrossRef] [PubMed]
55. Giraud, S.; Steichen, C.; Allain, G.; Couturier, P.; Labourdette, D.; Lamarre, S.; Ameteau, V.; Tillet, S.; Hannaert, P.; Thuillier, R.; et al. Dynamic transcriptomic analysis of Ischemic Injury in a Porcine Pre-Clinical Model mimicking Donors Deceased after Circulatory Death. *Sci. Rep.* **2018**, *8*, 5986. [CrossRef] [PubMed]
56. Boissier, R.; François, P.; Tellier, B.G.; Meunier, M.; Lyonnet, L.; Simoncini, S.; Magalon, J.; Legris, T.; Arnaud, L.; Giraudo, L.; et al. Perirenal Adipose Tissue Displays an Age-Dependent Inflammatory Signature Associated With Early Graft Dysfunction of Marginal Kidney Transplants. *Front. Immunol.* **2020**, *11*, 445. [CrossRef]
57. Hruba, P.; Krejcik, Z.; Dostalova Merkerova, M.; Klema, J.; Stranecky, V.; Slatinska, J.; Maluskova, J.; Honsova, E.; Viklicky, O. Molecular Fingerprints of Borderline Changes in Kidney Allografts Are Influenced by Donor Category. *Front. Immunol.* **2020**, *11*, 423. [CrossRef] [PubMed]
58. Han, F.; Wan, S.; Sun, Q.; Chen, N.; Li, H.; Zheng, L.; Zhang, N.; Huang, Z.; Hong, L.; Sun, Q. Donor Plasma Mitochondrial DNA Is Correlated with Posttransplant Renal Allograft Function. *Transplantation* **2019**, *103*, 2347–2358. [CrossRef]
59. Chen, H.-H.; Lan, Y.-F.; Li, H.-F.; Cheng, C.-F.; Lai, P.-F.; Li, W.-H.; Lin, H. Urinary miR-16 transactivated by C/EBPβ reduces kidney function after ischemia/reperfusion-induced injury. *Sci. Rep.* **2016**, *6*, 27945. [CrossRef]
60. Zhang, W.; Shu, L. Upregulation of miR-21 by Ghrelin Ameliorates Ischemia/Reperfusion-Induced Acute Kidney Injury by Inhibiting Inflammation and Cell Apoptosis. *DNA Cell Biol.* **2016**, *35*, 417–425. [CrossRef]
61. Song, T.; Chen, M.; Rao, Z.; Qiu, Y.; Liu, J.; Jiang, Y.; Huang, Z.; Wang, X.; Lin, T. miR-17-92 ameliorates renal ischemia reperfusion injury. *Kaohsiung J. Med. Sci.* **2018**, *34*, 263–273. [CrossRef]
62. Wang, Y.; Wang, D.; Jin, Z. miR-27a suppresses TLR4-induced renal ischemia-reperfusion injury. *Mol. Med. Rep.* **2019**, *20*, 967–976. [CrossRef]
63. Zhu, K.; Zheng, T.; Chen, X.; Wang, H. Bioinformatic analyses of renal ischaemia-reperfusion injury models: Identification of key genes involved in the development of kidney disease. *Kidney Blood Press. Res.* **2018**, *43*, 1898–1907. [CrossRef] [PubMed]
64. Su, M.; Hu, X.; Lin, J.; Zhang, L.; Sun, W.; Zhang, J.; Tian, Y.; Qiu, W. Identification of Candidate Genes Involved in Renal Ischemia/Reperfusion Injury. *DNA Cell Biol.* **2019**, *38*, 256–262. [CrossRef] [PubMed]
65. Liu, L.; Mao, L.; Wu, X.; Wu, T.; Liu, W.; Yang, Y.; Zhang, T.; Xu, Y. BRG1 regulates endothelial-derived IL-33 to promote ischemia-reperfusion induced renal injury and fibrosis in mice. *Biochim. Biophys. Acta Mol. Basis Dis.* **2019**, *1865*, 2551–2561. [CrossRef]
66. Cippà, P.E.; Sun, B.; Liu, J.; Chen, L.; Naesens, M.; McMahon, A.P. Transcriptional trajectories of human kidney injury progression. *JCI insight* **2018**, *3*, e123151. [CrossRef]
67. Hu, X.; Su, M.; Lin, J.; Zhang, L.; Sun, W.; Zhang, J.; Tian, Y.; Qiu, W. Corin is downregulated in renal ischemia/reperfusion injury and is associated with delayed graft function after kidney transplantation. *Dis. Markers* **2019**, *2019*, 9429323. [CrossRef]

68. Khalid, U.; Newbury, L.J.; Simpson, K.; Jenkins, R.H.; Bowen, T.; Bates, L.; Sheerin, N.S.; Chavez, R.; Fraser, D.J. A urinary microRNA panel that is an early predictive biomarker of delayed graft function following kidney transplantation. *Sci. Rep.* **2019**, *9*, 3584. [CrossRef]
69. Wang, J.; Li, X.; Wu, X.; Wang, Z.; Zhang, C.; Cao, G.; Yan, T. Expression Profiling of Exosomal miRNAs Derived from the Peripheral Blood of Kidney Recipients with DGF Using High-Throughput Sequencing. *Biomed. Res. Int.* **2019**, *2019*, 1759697. [CrossRef]
70. Mirzakhani, M.; Mohammadnia-Afrouzi, M.; Shahbazi, M.; Mirhosseini, S.A.; Hosseini, H.M.; Amani, J. The exosome as a novel predictive/diagnostic biomarker of rejection in the field of transplantation. *Clin. Immunol.* **2019**, *203*, 134–141. [CrossRef] [PubMed]
71. Milhoransa, P.; Montanari, C.C.; Montenegro, R.; Manfro, R.C. Micro RNA 146a-5p expression in Kidney transplant recipients with delayed graft function. *J. Bras. Nefrol.* **2019**, *41*, 242–251. [CrossRef] [PubMed]
72. Zmonarski, S.; Madziarska, K.; Banasik, M.; Mazanowska, O.; Magott-Procelewska, M.; Hap, K.; Krajewska, M. Expression of PBMC TLR4 in Renal Graft Recipients Who Experienced Delayed Graft Function Reflects Dynamic Balance Between Blood and Tissue Compartments and Helps Select a Problematic Patient. *Transplant. Proc.* **2018**, *50*, 1744–1749. [CrossRef]
73. Bi, H.; Zhang, M.; Wang, J.; Long, G. The mRNA landscape profiling reveals potential biomarkers associated with acute kidney injury AKI after kidney transplantation. *PeerJ* **2020**, *8*, e10441. [CrossRef]
74. Koo, T.Y.; Jeong, J.C.; Lee, Y.; Ko, K.-P.; Lee, K.-B.; Lee, S.; Park, S.J.; Park, J.B.; Han, M.; Lim, H.J.; et al. Pre-transplant evaluation of donor urinary biomarkers can predict reduced graft function after deceased donor kidney transplantation. *Medicine* **2016**, *95*, e3076. [CrossRef]
75. Reese, P.P.; Hall, I.E.; Weng, F.L.; Schröppel, B.; Doshi, M.D.; Hasz, R.D.; Thiessen-Philbrook, H.; Ficek, J.; Rao, V.; Murray, P.; et al. Associations between deceased-donor urine injury biomarkers and kidney transplant outcomes. *J. Am. Soc. Nephrol.* **2016**, *27*, 1534–1543. [CrossRef]
76. Schröppel, B.; Heeger, P.; Thiessen-Philbrook, H.; Hall, I.E.; Doshi, M.D.; Weng, F.L.; Reese, P.P.; Parikh, C.R. Donor Urinary C5a Levels Independently Correlate with Posttransplant Delayed Graft Function. *Transplantation* **2019**, *103*, e29–e35. [CrossRef] [PubMed]
77. Mansour, S.G.; Puthumana, J.; Reese, P.P.; Hall, I.E.; Doshi, M.D.; Weng, F.L.; Schröppel, B.; Thiessen-Philbrook, H.; Bimali, M.; Parikh, C.R. Associations Between Deceased-Donor Urine MCP-1 and Kidney Transplant Outcomes. *Kidney Int. Rep.* **2017**, *2*, 749–758. [CrossRef] [PubMed]
78. Mezzolla, V.; Pontrelli, P.; Fiorentino, M.; Stasi, A.; Franzin, R.; Rascio, F.; Grandaliano, G.; Stallone, G.; Infante, B.; Gesualdo, L.; et al. Emerging biomarkers of delayed graft function in kidney transplantation. *Transplant. Rev.* **2021**, *35*, 100629. [CrossRef] [PubMed]
79. Kostidis, S.; Bank, J.R.; Soonawala, D.; Nevedomskaya, E.; van Kooten, C.; Mayboroda, O.A.; de Fijter, J.W. Urinary metabolites predict prolonged duration of delayed graft function in DCD kidney transplant recipients. *Am. J. Transplant.* **2019**, *19*, 110–122. [CrossRef]
80. Braun, F.; Rinschen, M.; Buchner, D.; Bohl, K.; Plagmann, I.; Bachurski, D.; Späth, M.R.; Antczak, P.; Göbel, H.; Klein, C.; et al. The proteomic landscape of small urinary extracellular vesicles during kidney transplantation. *J. Extracell. Vesicles* **2020**, *10*, e12026. [CrossRef]
81. Li, L.; Li, N.; He, C.; Huang, W.; Fan, X.; Zhong, Z.; Wang, Y.; Ye, Q. Proteomic analysis of differentially expressed proteins in kidneys of brain dead rabbits. *Mol. Med. Rep.* **2017**, *16*, 215–223. [CrossRef]
82. Van Erp, A.C.; Rebolledo, R.A.; Hoeksma, D.; Jespersen, N.R.; Ottens, P.J.; Nørregaard, R.; Pedersen, M.; Laustsen, C.; Burgerhof, J.G.M.; Wolters, J.C.; et al. Organ-specific responses during brain death: Increased aerobic metabolism in the liver and anaerobic metabolism with decreased perfusion in the kidneys. *Sci. Rep.* **2018**, *8*, 4405. [CrossRef]
83. Huang, H.; Van Dullemen, L.F.A.; Akhtar, M.Z.; Faro, M.-L.L.; Yu, Z.; Valli, A.; Dona, A.; Thézénas, M.-L.; Charles, P.D.; Fischer, R.; et al. Proteo-metabolomics reveals compensation between ischemic and non-injured contralateral kidneys after reperfusion. *Sci. Rep.* **2018**, *8*, 8539. [CrossRef] [PubMed]
84. Malagrino, P.A.; Venturini, G.; Yogi, P.S.; Dariolli, R.; Padilha, K.; Kiers, B.; Gois, T.C.; Cardozo, K.H.M.; Carvalho, V.M.; Salgueiro, J.S.; et al. Proteome analysis of acute kidney injury—Discovery of new predominantly renal candidates for biomarker of kidney disease. *J. Proteomics* **2017**, *151*, 66–73. [CrossRef] [PubMed]
85. Moser, M.A.J.; Sawicka, K.; Sawicka, J.; Franczak, A.; Cohen, A.; Bil-Lula, I.; Sawicki, G. Protection of the transplant kidney during cold perfusion with doxycycline: Proteomic analysis in a rat model. *Proteome Sci.* **2020**, *18*, 3. [CrossRef] [PubMed]
86. Weissenbacher, A.; Huang, H.; Surik, T.; Faro, M.L.L.; Ploeg, R.J.; Coussios, C.C.; Friend, P.J.; Kessler, B.M. Urine recirculation prolongs normothermic kidney perfusion via more optimal metabolic homeostasis—a proteomics study. *Am. J. Transplant.* **2020**, *21*, 1740–1753. [CrossRef] [PubMed]
87. Williams, K.R.; Colangelo, C.M.; Hou, L.; Chung, L.; Belcher, J.M.; Abbott, T.; Hall, I.E.; Zhao, H.; Cantley, L.G.; Parikh, C.R. Use of a Targeted Urine Proteome Assay (TUPA) to identify protein biomarkers of delayed recovery after kidney transplant. *Proteomics Clin. Appl.* **2017**, *11*, 1600132. [CrossRef]
88. Lacquaniti, A.; Caccamo, C.; Salis, P.; Chirico, V.; Buemi, M.; Cernaro, V.; Noto, A.; Pettinato, G.; Santoro, D.; Bertani, T.; et al. Delayed graft function and chronic allograft nephropathy: Diagnostic and prognostic role of neutrophil gelatinase-associated lipocalin. *Biomarkers* **2016**, *21*, 371–378. [CrossRef]

89. Bank, J.R.; Ruhaak, R.; Soonawala, D.; Mayboroda, O.; Romijn, F.P.; Van Kooten, C.; Cobbaert, C.M.; De Fijter, J.W. Urinary TIMP-2 Predicts the Presence and Duration of Delayed Graft Function in Donation after Circulatory Death Kidney Transplant Recipients. *Transplantation* **2019**, *103*, 1014–1023. [CrossRef]
90. Van Erp, A.C.; Qi, H.; Jespersen, N.R.; Hjortbak, M.V.; Ottens, P.J.; Wiersema-Buist, J.; Nørregaard, R.; Pedersen, M.; Laustsen, C.; Leuvenink, H.G.D.; et al. Organ-specific metabolic profiles of the liver and kidney during brain death and afterwards during normothermic machine perfusion of the kidney. *Am. J. Transplant.* **2020**, *20*, 2425–2436. [CrossRef]
91. Nielsen, P.M.; Qi, H.; Bertelsen, L.B.; Laustsen, C. Metabolic reprogramming associated with progression of renal ischemia reperfusion injury assessed with hyperpolarized [1-^{13}C]pyruvate. *Sci. Rep.* **2020**, *10*, 8915. [CrossRef]
92. Chihanga, T.; Ma, Q.; Nicholson, J.D.; Ruby, H.N.; Edelmann, R.E.; Devarajan, P.; Kennedy, M.A. NMR spectroscopy and electron microscopy identification of metabolic and ultrastructural changes to the kidney following ischemia-reperfusion injury. *Am. J. Physiol. Ren. Physiol.* **2018**, *314*, F154–F166. [CrossRef] [PubMed]
93. Stryjak, I.; Warmuzińska, N.; Bogusiewicz, J.; Łuczykowski, K.; Bojko, B. Monitoring of the influence of long-term oxidative stress and ischemia on the condition of kidneys using solid-phase microextraction chemical biopsy coupled with liquid chromatography–high-resolution mass spectrometry. *J. Sep. Sci.* **2020**, *43*, 1867–1878. [CrossRef]
94. Stryjak, I.; Warmuzińska, N.; Łuczykowski, K.; Hamar, M.; Urbanellis, P.; Wojtal, E.; Masztalerz, M.; Selzner, M.; Włodarczyk, Z.; Bojko, B. Using a chemical biopsy for graft quality assessment. *J. Vis. Exp.* **2020**, e60946. [CrossRef]
95. Zheng, X.; Zhang, A.; Binnie, M.; McGuire, K.; Webster, S.P.; Hughes, J.; Howie, S.E.M.; Mole, D.J. Kynurenine 3-monooxygenase is a critical regulator of renal ischemia–reperfusion injury. *Exp. Mol. Med.* **2019**, *51*, 1–14. [CrossRef]
96. Beier, U.H.; Hartung, E.A.; Concors, S.; Hernandez, P.T.; Wang, Z.; Perry, C.; Baur, J.A.; Denburg, M.R.; Hancock, W.W.; Gade, T.P.; et al. Tissue metabolic profiling shows that saccharopine accumulates during renal ischemic-reperfusion injury, while kynurenine and itaconate accumulate in renal allograft rejection. *Metabolomics* **2021**, *16*, 65. [CrossRef]
97. Rao, S.; Walters, K.B.; Wilson, L.; Chen, B.; Bolisetty, S.; Graves, D.; Barnes, S.; Agarwal, A.; Kabarowski, J.H. Early lipid changes in acute kidney injury using SWATH lipidomics coupled with MALDI tissue imaging. *Am. J. Physiol. Ren. Physiol.* **2016**, *310*, F1136–F1147. [CrossRef]
98. Solati, Z.; Edel, A.L.; Shang, Y.; Karmin, O.; Ravandi, A. Oxidized phosphatidylcholines are produced in renal ischemia reperfusion injury. *PLoS ONE* **2018**, *13*, e0195172. [CrossRef]
99. van Smaalen, T.C.; Ellis, S.R.; Mascini, N.E.; Siegel, T.P.; Cillero-Pastor, B.; Hillen, L.M.; van Heurn, L.W.E.; Peutz-Kootstra, C.J.; Heeren, R.M.A. Rapid Identification of Ischemic Injury in Renal Tissue by Mass-Spectrometry Imaging. *Anal. Chem.* **2019**, *91*, 3575–3581. [CrossRef] [PubMed]
100. Wijermars, L.G.M.; Bakker, J.A.; de Vries, D.K.; van Noorden, C.J.F.; Bierau, J.; Kostidis, S.; Mayboroda, O.A.; Tsikas, D.; Schaapherder, A.F.; Lindeman, J.H.N. The hypoxanthine-xanthine oxidase axis is not involved in the initial phase of clinical transplantation-related ischemia-reperfusion injury. *Am. J. Physiol. Ren. Physiol.* **2017**, *312*, F457–F464. [CrossRef]
101. Lindeman, J.H.; Wijermars, L.G.; Kostidis, S.; Mayboroda, O.A.; Harms, A.C.; Hankemeier, T.; Bierau, J.; Gupta, K.B.S.S.; Giera, M.; Reinders, M.E.; et al. Results of an explorative clinical evaluation suggest immediate and persistent post-reperfusion metabolic paralysis drives kidney ischemia reperfusion injury. *Kidney Int.* **2020**, *98*, 1476–1488. [CrossRef]
102. Jochmans, I.; Brat, A.; Davies, L.; Hofker, H.S.; van de Leemkolk, F.E.M.; Leuvenink, H.G.D.; Knight, S.R.; Pirenne, J.; Ploeg, R.J. Oxygenated versus standard cold perfusion preservation in kidney transplantation (COMPARE): A randomised, double-blind, paired, phase 3 trial. *Lancet* **2020**, *396*, 1653–1662. [CrossRef]
103. Hosgood, S.A.; Hoff, M.; Nicholson, M.L. Treatment of transplant kidneys during machine perfusion. *Transpl. Int.* **2021**, *34*, 224–232. [CrossRef]
104. Resch, T.; Cardini, B.; Oberhuber, R.; Weissenbacher, A.; Dumfarth, J.; Krapf, C.; Boesmueller, C.; Oefner, D.; Grimm, M.; Schneeberger, S. Transplanting Marginal Organs in the Era of Modern Machine Perfusion and Advanced Organ Monitoring. *Front. Immunol.* **2020**, *11*, 631. [CrossRef]
105. Hamar, M.; Selzner, M. Ex-vivo machine perfusion for kidney preservation. *Curr. Opin. Organ. Transplant.* **2018**, *23*, 369–374. [CrossRef]
106. Coskun, A.; Baykal, A.T.; Kazan, D.; Akgoz, M.; Senal, M.O.; Berber, I.; Titiz, I.; Bilsel, G.; Kilercik, H.; Karaosmanoglu, K.; et al. Proteomic analysis of kidney preservation solutions prior to renal transplantation. *PLoS ONE* **2016**, *11*, e0168755. [CrossRef] [PubMed]
107. van Balkom, B.W.M.; Gremmels, H.; Ooms, L.S.S.; Toorop, R.J.; Dor, F.J.M.F.; de Jong, O.G.; Michielsen, L.A.; de Borst, G.J.; De Jager, W.; Abrahams, A.C.; et al. Proteins in preservation fluid as predictors of delayed graft function in kidneys from donors after circulatory death. *Clin. J. Am. Soc. Nephrol.* **2017**, *12*, 817–824. [CrossRef]
108. Wang, Z.; Yang, H.; Zhao, C.; Wei, J.; Wang, J.; Han, Z.; Tao, J.; Xu, Z.; Ju, X.; Tan, R.; et al. Proton nuclear magnetic resonance (1H-NMR)-based metabolomic evaluation of human renal allografts from donations after circulatory death. *Med. Sci. Monit.* **2017**, *23*, 5472–5479. [CrossRef]
109. Nath, J.; Smith, T.B.; Patel, K.; Ebbs, S.R.; Hollis, A.; Tennant, D.A.; Ludwig, C.; Ready, A.R. Metabolic differences between cold stored and machine perfused porcine kidneys: A 1H NMR based study. *Cryobiology* **2017**, *74*, 115–120. [CrossRef]
110. Adani, G.L.; Pravisani, R.; Crestale, S.; Baccarani, U.; Scott, C.A.; D'Alì, L.; Demaglio, G.; Tulissi, P.; Vallone, C.; Isola, M.; et al. Effects of delayed hypothermic machine perfusion on kidney grafts with a preliminary period of static cold storage and a total cold ischemia time of over 24 hours. *Ann. Transplant.* **2020**, *25*, e918997. [CrossRef]

111. Foucher, Y.; Fournier, M.-C.; Legendre, C.; Morelon, E.; Buron, F.; Girerd, S.; Ladrière, M.; Mourad, G.; Garrigue, V.; Glotz, D.; et al. Comparison of machine perfusion versus cold storage in kidney transplant recipients from expanded criteria donors: A cohort-based study. *Nephrol. Dial. Transplant.* **2020**, *35*, 1051–1059. [CrossRef] [PubMed]
112. Tejchman, K.; Sierocka, A.; Kotowski, M.; Zair, L.; Pilichowska, E.; Ostrowski, M.; Sieńko, J. Acid-Base Balance Disorders During Kidney Preservation in Cold Ischemia. *Transplant. Proc.* **2020**, *52*, 2036–2042. [CrossRef]
113. He, N.; Li, J.-H.; Jia, J.-J.; Xu, K.-D.; Zhou, Y.-F.; Jiang, L.; Lu, H.-H.; Yin, S.-Y.; Xie, H.-Y.; Zhou, L.; et al. Hypothermic Machine Perfusion's Protection on Porcine Kidney Graft Uncovers Greater Akt-Erk Phosphorylation. *Transplant. Proc.* **2017**, *49*, 1923–1929. [CrossRef] [PubMed]
114. Patel, K.; Smith, T.B.; Neil, D.A.H.; Thakker, A.; Tsuchiya, Y.; Higgs, E.B.; Hodges, N.J.; Ready, A.R.; Nath, J.; Ludwig, C. The Effects of Oxygenation on Ex Vivo Kidneys Undergoing Hypothermic Machine Perfusion. *Transplantation* **2019**, *103*, 314–322. [CrossRef]
115. Moser, M.A.J.; Sawicka, K.; Arcand, S.; O'Brien, P.; Luke, P.; Beck, G.; Sawicka, J.; Cohen, A.; Sawicki, G. Proteomic analysis of perfusate from machine cold perfusion of transplant kidneys: Insights into protection from injury. *Ann. Transplant.* **2017**, *22*, 730–739. [CrossRef] [PubMed]
116. Gómez-Dos-Santos, V.; Ramos-Muñoz, E.; García-Bermejo, M.L.; Ruiz-Hernández, M.; Rodríguez-Serrano, E.M.; Saiz-González, A.; Martínez-Perez, A.; Burgos-Revilla, F.J. MicroRNAs in Kidney Machine Perfusion Fluid as Novel Biomarkers for Graft Function. Normalization Methods for miRNAs Profile Analysis. *Transplant. Proc.* **2019**, *51*, 307–310. [CrossRef]
117. Tejchman, K.; Sierocka, A.; Kotfis, K.; Kotowski, M.; Dolegowska, B.; Ostrowski, M.; Sienko, J. Assessment of oxidative stress markers in hypothermic preservation of transplanted kidneys. *Antioxidants* **2021**, *10*, 1263. [CrossRef]
118. Longchamp, A.; Klauser, A.; Songeon, J.; Agius, T.; Nastasi, A.; Ruttiman, R.; Moll, S.; Meier, R.P.H.; Buhler, L.; Corpataux, J.-M.; et al. Ex Vivo Analysis of Kidney Graft Viability Using 31P Magnetic Resonance Imaging Spectroscopy. *Transplantation* **2020**, *104*, 1825–1831. [CrossRef]
119. Van Smaalen, T.C.; Beurskens, D.M.H.; Hoogland, E.R.P.; Winkens, B.; Christiaans, M.H.L.; Reutelingsperger, C.P.; van Heurn, L.W.E.; Nicolaes, G.A.F. Presence of Cytotoxic Extracellular Histones in Machine Perfusate of Donation after Circulatory Death Kidneys. *Transplantation* **2017**, *101*, e93–e101. [CrossRef]
120. Kaths, J.M.; Echeverri, J.; Chun, Y.M.; Cen, J.Y.; Goldaracena, N.; Linares, I.; Dingwell, L.S.; Yip, P.M.; John, R.; Bagli, D.; et al. Continuous Normothermic Ex Vivo Kidney Perfusion Improves Graft Function in Donation after Circulatory Death Pig Kidney Transplantation. *Transplantation* **2017**, *101*, 754–763. [CrossRef]
121. Tetschke, F.; Markgraf, W.; Gransow, M.; Koch, S.; Thiele, C.; Kulcke, A.; Malberg, H. Hyperspectral imaging for monitoring oxygen saturation levels during normothermic kidney perfusion. *J. Sensors Sens. Syst.* **2016**, *5*, 313–318. [CrossRef]
122. Markgraf, W.; Feistel, P.; Thiele, C.; Malberg, H. Algorithms for mapping kidney tissue oxygenation during normothermic machine perfusion using hyperspectral imaging. *Biomed. Tech.* **2018**, *63*, 557–566. [CrossRef] [PubMed]
123. Mariager, C.Ø.; Hansen, E.S.S.; Bech, S.K.; Munk, A.; Kjærgaard, U.; Lyhne, M.D.; Søberg, K.; Nielsen, P.F.; Ringgaard, S.; Laustsen, C. Graft assessment of the ex vivo perfused porcine kidney using hyperpolarized [1-^{13}C]pyruvate. *Magn. Reson. Med.* **2020**, *84*, 2645–2655. [CrossRef] [PubMed]
124. Hosgood, S.A.; Nicholson, M.L. An assessment of urinary biomarkers in a series of declined human kidneys measured during ex vivo normothermic kidney perfusion. *Transplantation* **2017**, *101*, 2120–2125. [CrossRef] [PubMed]

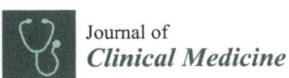

Review

The Impact of Recipient Demographics on Outcomes from Living Donor Kidneys: Systematic Review and Meta-Analysis †

Maria Irene Bellini [1,2,*], **Mikhail Nozdrin** [3], **Liset Pengel** [4], **Simon Knight** [4] **and Vassilios Papalois** [5]

1. Department of Emergency Medicine and Surgery, Azienda Ospedaliera San Camillo Forlanini, 00152 Rome, Italy
2. Department of Surgical Sciences, Sapienza University of Rome, 00161 Rome, Italy
3. Imperial College School of Medicine, London SW7 2AZ, UK; mikhail.nozdrin16@imperial.ac.uk
4. Centre for Evidence in Transplantation, Nuffield Department of Surgical Sciences, University of Oxford, Oxford OX3 7HE, UK; liset.pengel@nds.ox.ac.uk (L.P.); simon.knight@nds.ox.ac.uk (S.K.)
5. Department of Surgery and Cancer, Imperial College, London SW7 2AZ, UK; vassilios.papalois@nhs.net
* Correspondence: m.irene.bellini@gmail.com
† Meeting Presentation: European Society of Organ Transplantation Congress, 29 August–1 September 2021, Milan, Italy.

Abstract: *Background and Aims:* Recipient demographics affect outcomes after kidney transplantation. The aim of this study was to assess, for kidneys retrieved from living donors, the effect of recipient sex, ethnicity, and body mass index (BMI) on delayed graft function (DGF) and one-year graft function, incidence of acute rejection (AR), and recipient and graft survivals. *Methods:* A systematic review and meta-analysis was performed. EMBASE and MEDLINE databases were searched using algorithms through Ovid. Web of Science collection, BIOSIS, CABI, Korean Journal database, Russian Science Citation Index, and SciELO were searched through Web of Science. Cochrane database was also searched. Risk of bias was assessed using the NHBLI tools. Data analysis was performed using Revman 5.4. Mean difference (MD) and risk ratio (RR) were used in analysis. *Results:* A total of 5129 studies were identified; 24 studies met the inclusion criteria and were analysed. Female recipients were found to have a significantly lower serum creatinine 1-year-post renal transplantation (MD: −0.24 mg/dL 95%CI: −0.18 to −0.29 $p < 0.01$) compared to male recipients. No significant difference in survival between male and female recipients nor between Caucasians and Africans was observed ($p = 0.08$). However, Caucasian recipients had a higher 1-year graft survival compared to African recipients (95% CI 0.52−0.98) with also a lower incidence of DGF (RR = 0.63 $p < 0.01$) and AR (RR = 0.55 $p < 0.01$). Recipient obesity (BMI > 30) was found to have no effect on 1-year recipient ($p = 0.28$) and graft survival ($p = 0.93$) compared to non-obese recipients although non-obese recipients had a lower rate of DGF (RR = 0.65 $p < 0.01$) and AR (RR = 0.81 $p < 0.01$) compared to obese recipients. *Conclusions:* Gender mismatch between male recipients and female donors has negative impact on graft survival. African ethnicity and obesity do not to influence recipient and graft survival but negatively affect DGF and AR rates.

Keywords: BMI; ethnicity; living donation; kidney transplant; recipient's demographics

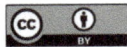

1. Introduction

In kidney transplantation, the relative contribution of donor versus other factors on clinical outcomes is considered a main criterion to allocate an organ [1].

Living kidney donation (LKD) represents the optimal treatment for kidney failure [2,3]. Previous reports on deceased donation indicate that the donor constitution has small or moderate effect on post-transplant clinical outcomes [4], while it is widely accepted that a living donor (LD) kidney tends to function immediately, reducing the risk of hospitalisation and renal replacement therapy after transplantation to less than 4% [5] and thus setting up the recipient for the best possible result.

In the context of living donation, recipient demographics are considered equally important and are constantly evaluated as potential contraindications for an LD to come forward. For instance, there is still an ongoing debate whether or not to use a body mass index (BMI) cut-off [6], especially if that specific recipient has already one or more LDs under evaluation, in consideration of the risks related to LKD and the hypothesized inferior outcomes related to obesity [7,8].

Additionally, growing attention is being attributed to donor-recipient gender match [9] and ethnicity, in consideration of the fact that African and Asian candidates face prolonged waiting times due to difficulties in the matching process, mostly because of the scarcity of donors from these minority groups [10].

The aim of this study was to assess, for kidneys retrieved from LDs, the effect of recipient sex, ethnicity, and BMI on short- and long-term graft outcomes.

2. Methods

The study was registered with PROSPERO (CRD42020221109) before commencement of the literature search. The review was conducted and reported according to PRISMA guidelines [5].

2.1. Search Strategy

Literature searches were performed in Ovid (EMBASE, MEDLINE), Web of Science, and Cochrane databases, using combinations of free text and keyword terms for living kidney donation and donor demographics of interest. A full search strategy is shown in Appendix A (Tables A1–A3). Searches were conducted on 14/11/20 and according to the PRISMA flowchart (Figure 1)

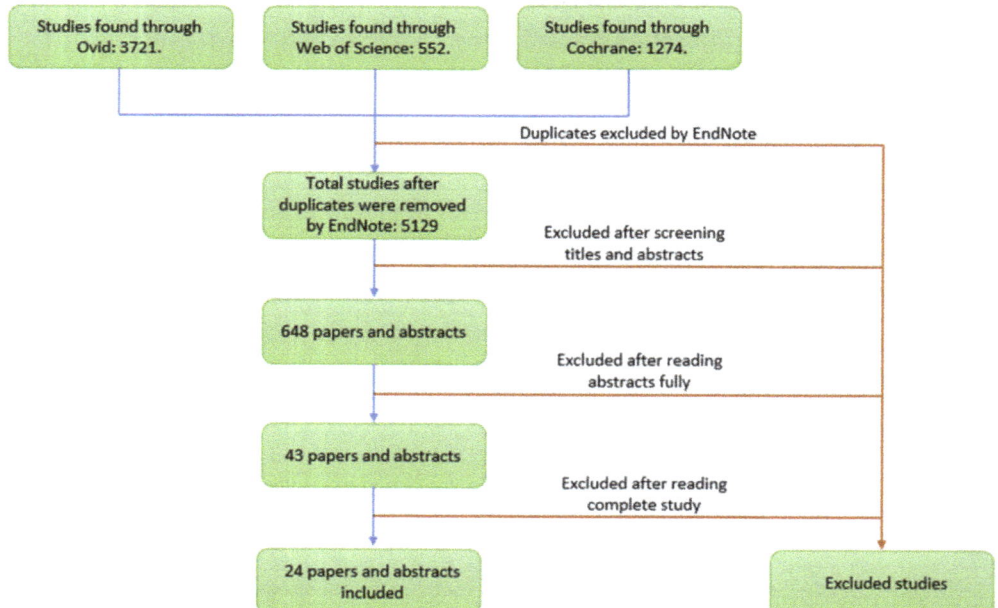

Figure 1. PRISMA Flowchart.

2.2. Inclusion/Exclusion Criteria

Any study relating to recipient's demographic characteristics on graft outcomes after LKD were eligible for inclusion, including full articles and meeting abstracts. Only studies in English were included for the analysis.

2.3. Outcomes of Interest

The primary objective was to assess the effect of recipient demographics of ethnicity, BMI, and sex on kidney function evaluated using estimated glomerular filtration rate (eGFR) adjusted for body surface area, serum creatinine, and proteinuria incidence, where reported.

The secondary objectives included assessing effect of the above-mentioned recipient demographics on patient and graft survival, incidence of delayed graft function (DGF), and acute rejection (AR).

2.4. Screening and Data Extraction

Study identification and data extraction were performed in three stages: the first stage included downloading the studies identified by the search strategy from Cochrane, Ovid, and Web of Science databases into EndNote reference management software. The reference management software was then used to remove duplicate studies. The second stage included two independent researchers (M.I.B. and M.N.) screening the titles and abstracts of long-listed studies. The researchers then each produced a list of studies eligible for the review. The two lists were compared to produce a single short-list of studies selected for full text review. The third stage of data extraction included the researchers fully read of the short-listed studies to identify the studies meeting the inclusion criteria. Data extraction was performed by two independent reviewers (M.I.B. and M.N.), and disagreements were solved by discussion or consulting a third reviewer. Data were extracted into a Microsoft Excel sheet.

2.5. Risk of Bias Assessment

Risk of bias assessment was performed using National Institute of Health National Heart, Lung and Blood Institute (NIH NHBLI) quality assessment tool [6], as shown in Appendix B. Two independent reviewers, M.I.B. and M.N., judged the quality of the articles and compared their results.

2.6. Meta-Analysis

All data analyses were performed in Revman 5.4.1 and IBM SPSS Statistics 26. Meta-analysis of mean difference was used for continuous data. Random effect models were used for all meta-analyses due to the heterogeneous and small study samples. Mean differences with a 95% confidence interval were calculated for the summary effect. The Z test was performed to calculate p-values. Where p-values were <0.05, and 95% CI did not include 0, a statistically significant difference between the two groups was recorded. Forest plots were created in Revman 5.4.1. Heterogeneity of the data was assessed using the I2 test, where the I2 value greater than 0.5 heterogeneity of the data was assumed to be high and where the I2 value lower than 0.5 heterogeneity of the data was assumed to be low.

3. Results

A total of 5129 studies were identified; 24 studies met the inclusion criteria and were analysed.

3.1. Recipient Sex

Jacobs et al. [11] compared graft survival between male and female transplant recipients at one- and three-years post-transplantation. Wafa et al. [12] compared graft survival between male and female recipients at five- and 10- years post-transplantation. Both studies found no significant difference in short- and long-term graft survivals between male and female transplant recipients, also showing no significant difference between graft survival in transplant recipients who were the same gender as the donor and transplant recipients who were of a opposite gender as their donor. More in detail, Wafa et al. [12] found no difference between graft survival in male recipients who had received their kidney from a male or female donor, both five years and 10 years after receiving a renal transplant. The same findings were confirmed by Jacobs et al. [11], who reported no difference between graft survival in male recipients who had received their kidney from a male or female donor at one year post-transplantation; however, at three years of follow up, male recipients who had received a transplant from a male donor were 65% less likely to lose a graft compared to male recipients who received graft from a female donor (RR = 0.35; chi-square $p = 0.006$). In both studies, there was no significant difference in graft survival between females who received grafts from male and female donors.

Four studies [9,11,13,14] investigated the effect of recipient gender on the post-transplantation serum creatinine. Naderi et al. [9], Jacobs et al. [11], and Villeda-Sandoval et al. [13] compared one-year post-transplantation serum creatinine between male and female recipients of LD kidney grafts. Figure 2a shows how female recipients on average had a serum creatinine 0.24 mg/dL (0.18 to 0.29) lower than male recipients ($p < 0.00001$).

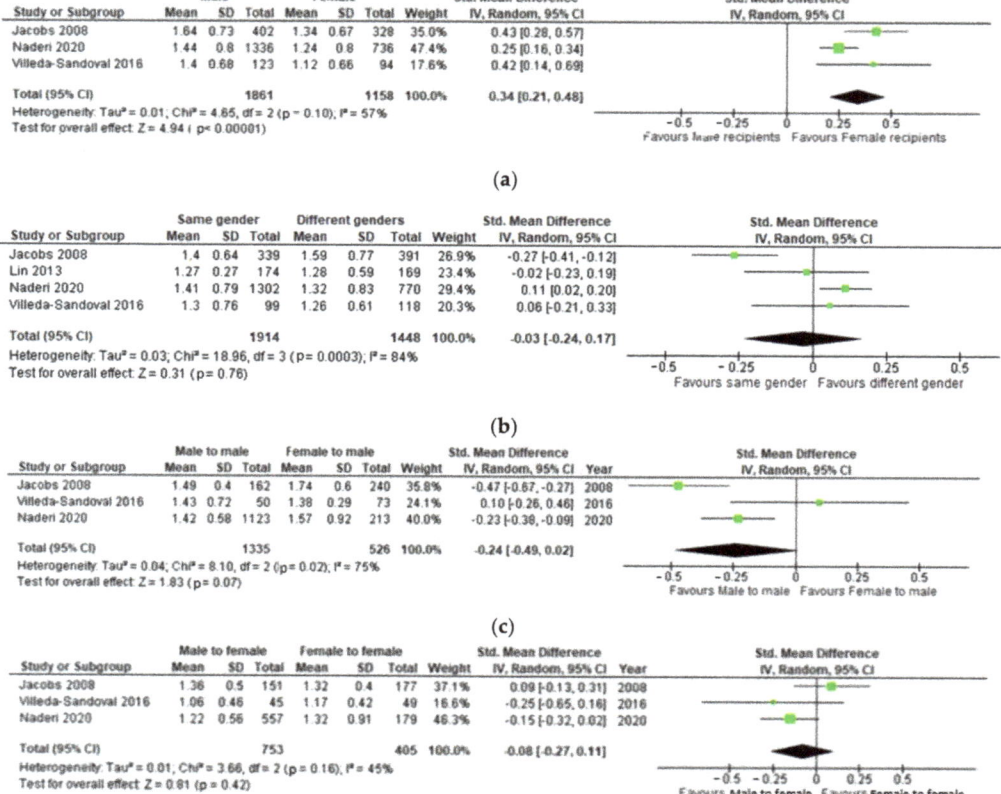

Figure 2. Cont.

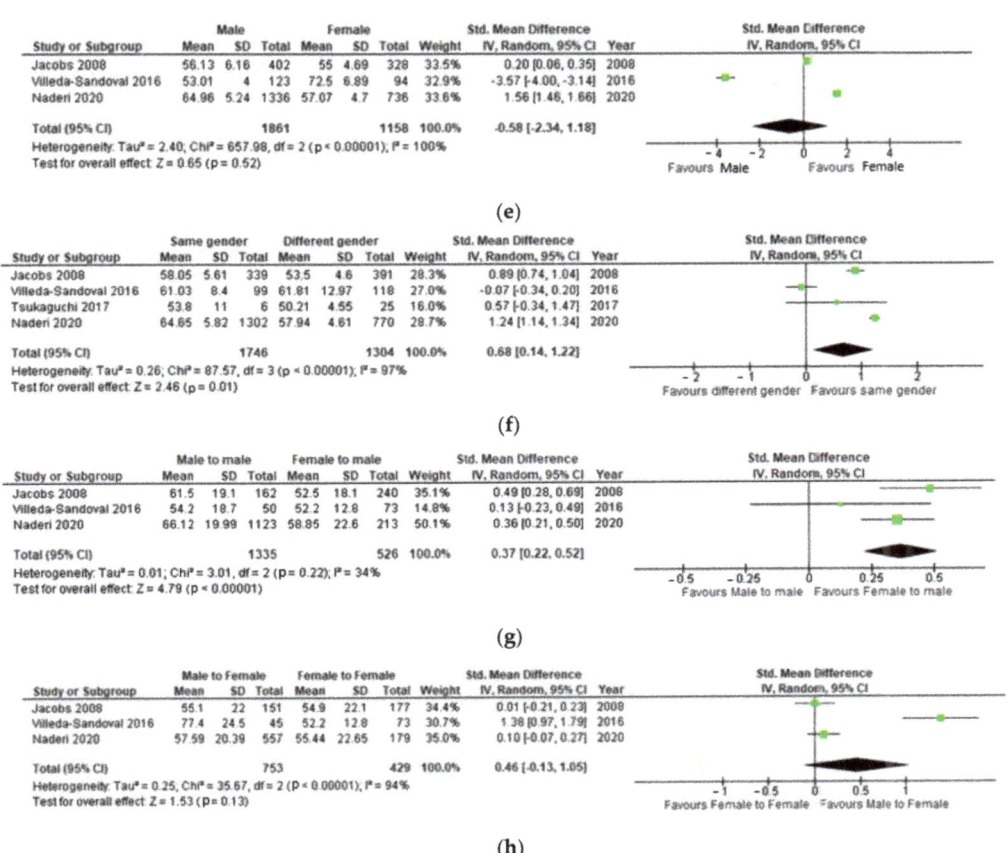

Figure 2. (a) Effect of recipient gender on serum creatinine 1-year post-transplantation. (b) Effect of matching genders between recipient and donor on 1-year post-transplantation serum creatinine. (c) One-year post-transplantation serum creatinine in male renal transplant recipients based on the gender of their donor. (d) One-year post-transplantation serum creatinine in female renal transplant recipients based on the gender of their donor. (e) One-year post-transplantation eGFR in male renal transplant recipients compared to female recipients. (f) Effect of matching genders of renal donor and recipient on 1-year post-transplantation eGFR. (g) One-year post-transplantation eGFR in male renal transplant recipients based on the gender of their donor. (h) One-year post-transplantation eGFR in female renal transplant recipients based on the gender of their donor.

All four studies [9,11,13,14] compared one-year post-transplantation serum creatinine in recipients of kidney grafts from the same gender donors and opposite gender donors. No significant difference between recipients of renal transplants from the same gender donors and opposite gender donors ($p = 0.78$), (Figure 2b).

Three studies [8,10,12] compared one-year post-transplantation serum creatinine in male recipients receiving a transplant from male and female donors. No significant was found in one-year post-transplantation serum creatinine male recipients recovering a graft from female donors and male donors $p = 0.06$ (Figure 2c).

No significant difference in one-year post-transplantation serum creatinine was found between female recipients who had received their transplant from a male donor and female recipients who had received their transplant from a female donor ($p = 0.22$), as represented in Figure 2d.

Three studies [8,10,12] compared eGFR between male and female recipients of renal transplantation following a donation from either same gender or opposite gender donor. No significant difference in eGFR ($p = 0.52$) was found one-year post-transplantation between male and female renal transplant recipients (Figure 2e).

In Figure 2f, an important finding is that patients who received a graft from same sex donor had a significantly higher eGFR compared to recipients who received a graft from a donor of opposite sex ($p < 0.00001$). The effect size of the difference between 2 means was medium (95%CI: 0.14 to 1.22).

More in detail, male recipients who received a transplant from a male donor had a significantly higher eGFR compared to male recipients who received a transplant from a female donor ($p < 0.00001$), as represented in Figure 2g, while on the contrary, there was no significant difference in eGFR one-year post-transplantation between female recipients who received their graft from a male donor compared to those who received a graft from a female donor ($p = 0.13$) (Figure 2h).

Two studies [15,16] investigated the effect of recipient gender on the development of diabetes mellitus on grafts retrieved from LKDs. Xu et al. [15] compared the incidence of diabetes at three months of follow up, whereas Xie et al. [16] followed patients up 53.5 ± 10.4. Both studies found no significant difference between the incidence of diabetes in male and female renal transplant recipients.

Two studies [17,18] compared proteinuria between four groups: male recipients who received a transplant from a male, male recipients who received a transplant from a female, female recipients who received a transplant from male, and female recipients who received a transplant from a female. Oh et al. [18] found no significant difference in proteinuria 24 h after surgery between the four groups. On the other hand, Yanishi et al. [17] found proteinuria to be significantly lower in female recipients who had received a graft from a male donor compared to recipients who had received a transplant from the donor of the same gender as them and to male recipients who had received a renal graft from a female donor (Table 1).

Table 1. Effect of donor-recipient sex match on the graft proteinuria.

Proteinuria	Male to Male	Male to Female	Female to Female	Female to Male	Outcomes Reported in the Paper
Oh et al. Protein excretion (mg/d), 24 h urine post-op.	MM ($n = 65$): $23.4 +/- 61.6$	MF ($n = 34$): $81.9 +/- 354.4$	FF (=29): $9.7 +/- 51.6$	FM ($n = 67$): $36.1 +/- 123.8$	Independent sample t-test: MM-FM ($p = 0.461$), MF-FF ($p = 0.282$); MM-MF ($p = 0.198$), FM-FF: ($p = 0.273$).
Yanishi et al. (mg/day). Recipient proteinuria at 1-year post-surgery.	Group 1(same gender) $n = 6$: 135.2 ± 98.1	Group 2: (male donor to female recipient) ($n = 8$). 63.7 ± 28.7	Group 1(same gender) $n= 6$: 135.2 ± 98.1	Group 3: female donor to male recipient ($n = 17$): 205.5 ± 35.2	ANOVA between the 3 groups found the lowest proteinuria to be in the Male to Female group ($p < 0.01$).

3.2. Recipient Ethnicity

Four studies [19–22] compared recipient survival one-year post-transplantation in Caucasian and African renal transplant recipients. There was no significant statistical difference between the recipient survival in Caucasian and African recipients ($p = 0.88$) (Figure 3a).

Williams et al. [22] and Isaacs et al. [23] compared the incidence of acute rejection in Caucasian and African recipients (Figure 3b), the latter finding a significantly lower incidence of acute rejection in Caucasian transplant recipients compared to African recipients. On the contrary, Williams et al. [11] found a higher rate of acute rejection in Caucasian recipients compared to African recipients; however, this finding was non-significant. Overall, the incidence of acute rejection post-transplantation was found to be 45% lower in Caucasian group compared to the African group; this difference was significant ($p < 0.00001$) [24].

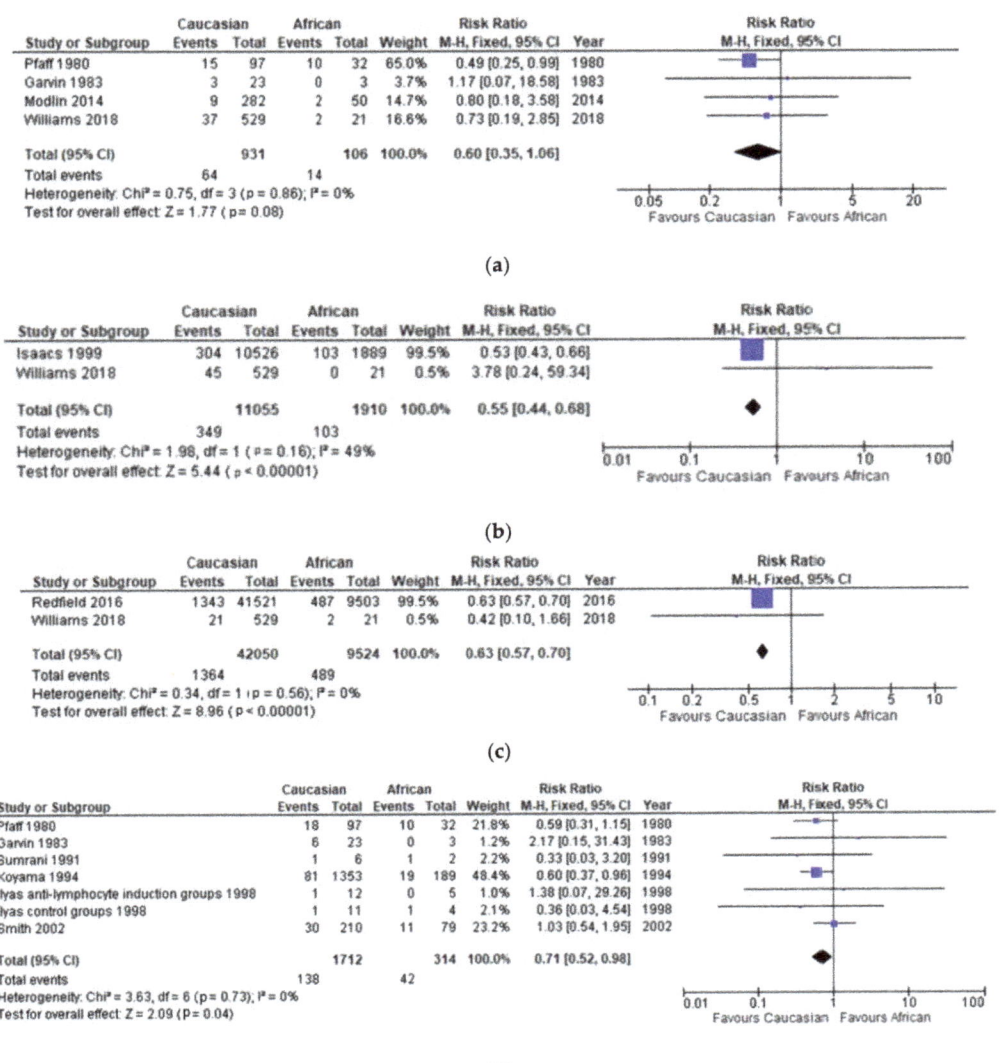

Figure 3. (a) Effect of recipient ethnicity on 1-year post-transplantation recipient survival. (b) Effect of recipient ethnicity on the incidence of acute rejection. (c) Effect of recipient ethnicity on the incidence of delayed graft function. (d) Effect of recipient ethnicity on 1-year graft survival.

Two studies by Williams [22] and Redfield [5] compared the incidence of DGF between Caucasian ethnicity and African ethnicity transplant recipients. Caucasian recipients were found to have a 47% lower rate of DGF following renal transplantation compared to African recipients ($p \leq 0.00001$), as shown in Figure 3c.

Six studies compared rates of graft survival one year following renal transplantation between Caucasian and African recipients [19,20,24–27]. Ilyas et al. further split the cohorts of Caucasian and African ethnicity donors into sub-groups by whether they received anti-lymphocyte induction treatment or not. Overall, Caucasian recipients had a 29% reduced risk of losing the graft within the first year after transplantation compared to African recipients, and this difference was significant $p = 0.04$ (Figure 3d).

3.3. Recipient Body Mass Index

Four studies investigated effect of recipient BMI on the post-transplantation one-year recipient and graft survival [28–31], finding no significant difference in obese and non-obese recipients ($p = 0.28$) (Figure 4a).

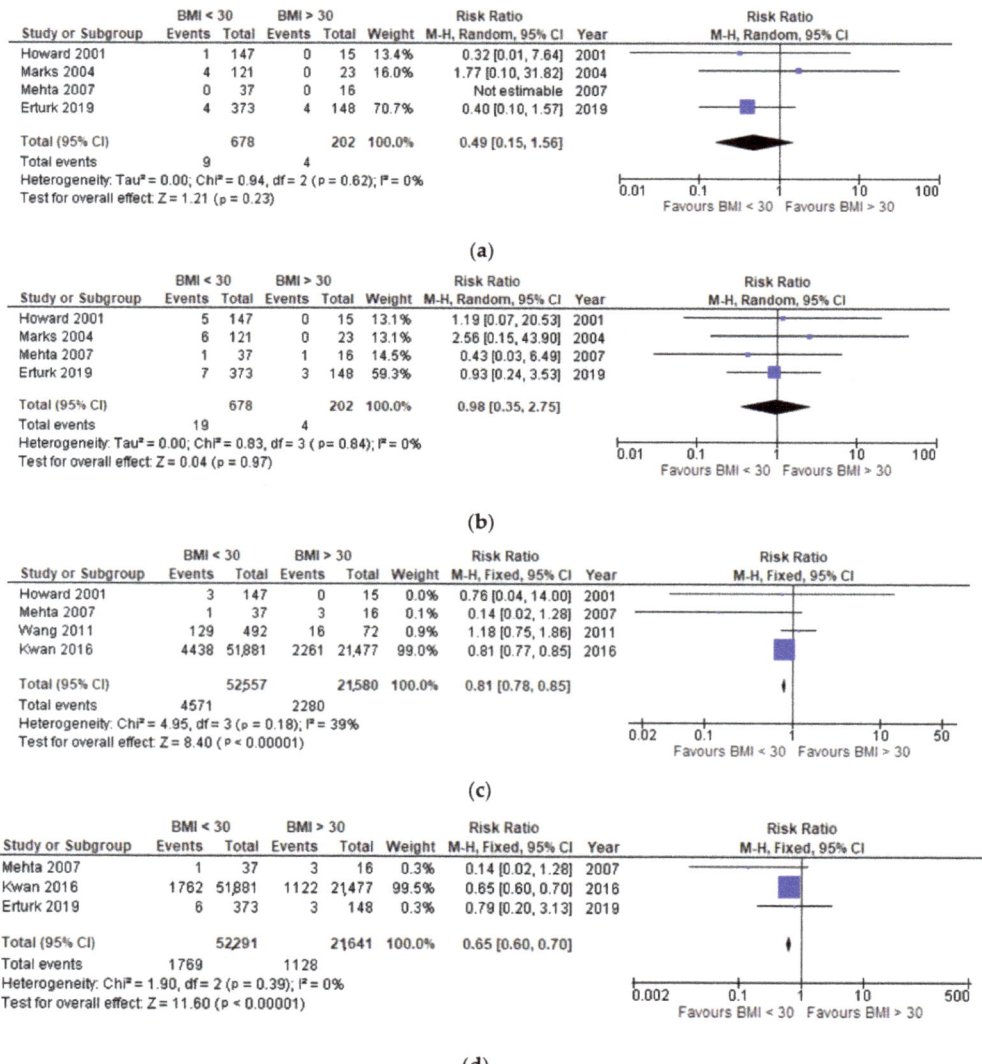

Figure 4. (a) Effect of recipient BMI on 1-year post-transplantation recipient survival. (b) Effect of recipient BMI on 1-year post-transplantation graft survival. (c) Effect of recipient BMI on the development of acute rejection. (d) Effect of recipient BMI on the development of delayed graft function.

There was no significant difference between one-year graft survival in the obese and non-obese groups ($p = 0.93$), as observed in Figure 4b.

In Figure 4c, four studies [28,30,32,33] were compared to look at the difference in the acute rejection incidence between non-obese and obese recipients.

It was found that non-obese donors were 19% less likely to develop acute transplant rejection compared to obese recipients ($p < 0.00001$) (Figure 4c). Non-obese donors were also 35% less likely to develop DGF compared to obese donors ($p < 0.00001$) (Figure 4d).

4. Discussion

The survival advantages of transplantation over long-term dialysis are known if a given patient with end-stage kidney disease is suitable for a transplant. A major challenge is to optimize modifiable variables that could improve long-term survival [34], and with the present study, we aimed to assess the impact of recipient demographic characteristics of sex, ethnicity, and BMI on kidney grafts retrieved from LDs.

With regards to sex, an interesting finding of our meta-analysis was that at three years follow up, male recipients who had received a transplant from a male donor were 65% less likely to lose a graft compared to male recipients who have received grafts from female donors. This result might lead to think there is a nephron mass effect playing an increasing role in the medium and long-term graft function, as a female kidney could be in general of lower weight and therefore with less functional nephrons, demonstrated also by a lower eGFR in women in the general population [35].

In addition to this, the graft survival advantage for male recipients of male donor kidneys was previously also reported by Kayler et al. [36], who analysed the Scientific Registry of Transplant Recipients database between 1990 and 1999 and who pointed out the gender disparities in LD transplantation, with a higher proportion of wife-to-husband donations and disproportionate female-to-male donations among biological relatives and unrelated pairs.

In the present meta-analyses, we found no significant difference in graft survival among female recipients according to the sex of their donors. To this regard, as a risk factor for inferior outcomes in women, it is worth to mention the theory related to the sex-determined minor histocompatibility antigen (H-Y antigen), firstly described in 1976 on a female recipient who rejected the bone marrow transplant from her HLA-identical brother [37]. More recently, the highest number of H-Y antibodies detected in the blood of female recipients transplanted with kidneys from male donors in comparison to other sex combinations was reported to significantly correlate with the higher occurrence of acute rejection [38]. This consideration implies a careful evaluation of every possible intervention and consequent risk of sensitization in transplant patients [39]. In literature, this is supported for both deceased and living donation, as sustained by Tan et al. [40], who recommend a major focus on clinical detection of markers for minor histocompatibility loci.

Although almost significant ($p = 0.06$), the above finding was confirmed in one-year post transplant serum creatinine, with male recipients recovering better from a graft from male donors. In this view, the use of sex as a biological variable in medical research is increasingly recognized as an important modulator to better understand the complex pathophysiology of several diseases [41] and better address the future health needs. Furthermore, our study adds to the evidence that in transplantation, relevant sex-specific issues are underrecognized factors influencing patient and transplant outcomes: it is already known that women are less likely to access kidney transplantation in general, as well as transplantation from LD; therefore, whenever possible, a better gender matching is advisable for better outcomes.

This approach with a close eye to diversity and inclusion extends also to individuals from minority backgrounds: interventions to ameliorate the effects of demographic discrepancies, different ethnicity, and cultural backgrounds may improve access to transplantation [42,43] as well as transplant outcomes. From our analysis, Caucasian recipients were found to have a 47% lower rate of DGF following renal transplantation compared to African recipients ($p = <0.00001$) as well as lower AR incidence. Reasons unpinning this discrepancy are several, from different socio-economic status to prevalence of metabolic diseases [44], although a better and more inclusive allocation policy as well sensibilization of Black and Asian minorities to donate could represent an important key to improve ethnicity-related outcomes [42]; in fact, from our meta-analysis, Caucasian recipients had a 29% recused risk of losing the graft within the first year after transplantation.

Finally, the same discourse regarding discrimination could be raised with regards to high BMI recipients who are denied access to the waiting list because of their body weight only. From the present meta-analysis, the four studies investigating the effect of recipient BMI on the post-transplantation one-year recipient and graft survival [28–31] found no significant difference in obese and non-obese recipients ($p = 0.28$); therefore, even if it is true that bridge interventions, such as bariatric surgery [45], are increasingly being adopted to overcome this barrier, we think that obese patients should have the same chance as their non-obese counterparts, at least for LD renal transplantation. We also believe that obesity, as a metabolic and systemic disease, leads to higher AR and DGF rates, as per our findings; therefore, an additional effort trying to maximize all the adding risk factors to graft and patient loss is advisable, with a tailored immunosuppression [7].

5. Limitations

The retrospective nature of the studies analysed has limited the level of evidence we could achieve, based on observational registry data, small number of studies, and great deal of heterogeneity. Longer-term follow up reports should be also warranted to better analyse any potential relationship between the other contributing factors and the recipients' demographics.

6. Conclusions

In conclusion, gender mismatch between male recipients and female donors has a negative impact on graft survival, with male recipients who received a transplant from a male donor 65% less likely to lose a graft compared to male recipients who have received grafts from female donors. African ethnicity increases DGF and AR rates compared to the Caucasian, and no significant difference between one-year graft survival in the obese and non-obese groups has been observed; therefore, BMI-only cut-offs to waitlist are not considered appropriate.

Author Contributions: Conceptualization, M.I.B. and V.P.; methodology, M.I.B., M.N., L.P., S.K.; software and formal analysis M.N.; investigation and data curation M.I.B. and M.N.; writing—original draft preparation, M.I.B.; writing—review and editing, L.P., S.K. and V.P. All authors have read and agreed to the published version of the manuscript.

Funding: Not applicable.

Institutional Review Board Statement: The study, performed in accordance to the Declaration of Helsinki principles, is a retrospective analysis. The data used were anonymised; the study did not require patient or public involvement nor affected patient care. The study fell under the category of research through the use of anonymised data of existing databases which, based on the Health Research Authority criteria, does not require proportional or full ethics review and approval.

Informed Consent Statement: As a meta-analysis of published data, no informed consent was required.

Data Availability Statement: The data used to support the findings of this study are included within the article.

Conflicts of Interest: The authors declare no conflict of interest.

Abbreviations

Abbreviations

AR, acute rejection; BMI, body mass index; DGF, delayed graft function; eGFR, estimated glomerular filtration rate; LD, living donor; LKD, living kidney donation.

Appendix A Search Strategy

EMBASE and MEDLINE databases were searched through Ovid on 14/11/2020, the search algorithm used is shown in Table A1. English language filter was applied to the search.

Table A1. Search algorithm used to search EMBASE and MEDLINE databases through Ovid.

Step	Input
1	gender/ or "gender and sex"/
2	sex/ or sex difference/
3	sex
4	age/
5	ethnicit*
6	ethnic minorit*
7	BAME
8	exp "ethnic or racial aspects"/
9	BMI/
10	BMI or weight
11	genetic relationship/
12	1 or 2 or 3 or 4
13	5 or 6 or 7 or 8 or 9 or 10 or 11
14	12 and 13
15	exp kidney donor/
16	kidney transplantation/
17	living donor/
18	exp graft recipient/
19	15 or 16 or 17 or 18
20	14 and 19

Web of Science core collection, BIOSIS (1950-2008), CABI, Korean Journal database, Russian Science Citation Index and SciELO were searched through Web of Science search engine on 14/11/2020. The search algorithm used is shown in Table A2.

Table A2. Search algorithm used to search Web of Science core collection, BIOSIS (1950-2008), CABI, Korean Journal database, Russian Science Citation Index and SciELO through Web of Science.

Step	Input
1	TS=(sex or gender)
2	TS=(sex and difference)
3	TS=age
4	TS=(ethnicit* or ethnic minorit*)
5	TS=BAME
6	TS=(ethnic* or race)
7	TS=(BMI or weight)
8	TS=genetic relationship
9	#1 or #2 or #3
10	#4 or #5 or #6 or #7 or #8
11	#9 and #10
12	TS=kidney
13	TS=transplantation
14	TS=(living or live or non-deceased)
15	TS=(donor)
16	TS=graft
17	TS=recipient
18	#12 and #13 and #14 and #15 and #16 and #17
19	#11 and #18

Cochrane library database was searched on 14/11/2020. The search algorithm used is shown in Table A3.

Table A3. Search algorithm used to search the Cochrane library database.

Step	Input
1	MeSH descriptor: [Gender Identity] this term only
2	MeSH descriptor: [Sex] this term only
3	MeSH descriptor: [Sex Characteristics] this term only
4	(sex):ti,ab,kw
5	MeSH descriptor: [Age Factors] this term only
6	ethnicit*
7	ethnic minorit*
8	BAME
9	BMI
10	weight
11	MeSH descriptor: [Family] explode all trees
12	genetic relationship
13	MeSH descriptor: [Ethnic Groups] explode all trees
14	MeSH descriptor: [Continental Population Groups] explode all trees
15	#1 or #2 or #3 or #4 or #5
16	#6 or #7 or #8 or #9 or #10 or #11 or #12 or #13 or #14
17	#15 or #16
18	MeSH descriptor: [Kidney] explode all trees
19	MeSH descriptor: [Tissue Donors] explode all trees
20	MeSH descriptor: [Transplantation] explode all trees
21	MeSH descriptor: [Transplant Recipients] explode all trees
22	#18 and #19
23	#18 and #20
24	#18 and #21
25	#22 or #23 or #24
26	Kidney 51158
27	donor or transplantation or recipient or transplant
28	#26 and #27
29	#17 AND #25
30	#17 AND #28
31	#29 or #30

Appendix B. Risk of Bias Assessment

Reference number	Country of study	Authors	1. Was the research question clearly stated?	2. Was the study population clearly specified and defined?	3. Was the participation of eligible persons at least 50%?	4. Were inclusion and exclusion criteria for being in the study prespecified and applied uniformly to all participants?	5. Was a sample size justification, power description, or variance and effect estimates provided?	6. For the analyses in this paper, were the exposure(s) of interest measured prior to the outcome(s) being measured?	7. Was the timeframe sufficient so that one could reasonably expect to see an association between exposure and outcome if it existed?	8. For exposures that can vary in amount or level, did the study examine different levels of the exposure as related to the outcome (e.g., categories of exposure, or exposure measured as continuous variable)?	9. Were the exposure measures (independent variables) clearly defined, valid, reliable, and implemented consistently across all study participants?	10. Was the exposure(s) assessed more than once over time?	11. Were the outcome measures (dependent variables) clearly defined, valid, reliable, and implemented consistently across all study participants?	12. Were the outcome assessors blinded to the exposure status of participants?	13. Was loss to follow-up after baseline 20% or less?	14. Were key potential confounding variables measured and adjusted statistically for their impact on the relationship between exposure(s) and outcome(s)?	Quality Rating (Good, Fair or Poor)
[5]	USA	Redfield, R.R., et al.	Yes	Yes	Yes	Yes	Yes	Yes	Yes	No	Yes	Not applicable	Yes	No	Yes	Yes	Good
[9]	Iran	Naderi, G., et al.	Yes	Yes	Yes	Yes	No	Yes	Yes	Not applicable	Yes	Not applicable	Yes	No	Yes	No	Fair
[11]	USA	Jacobs, S.C., et al.	Yes	Yes	Yes	Yes	No	Yes	Yes	Not applicable	Yes	Not applicable	Yes	No	Yes	Yes	Good
[12]	Egypt	Wafa, E.W., et al.	Yes	Yes	Yes	Yes	No	Yes	Yes	Not applicable	Yes	Not applicable	Yes	No	Yes	No	Fair

Reference number	Country of study	Authors	1. Was the research question clearly stated?	2. Was the study population clearly specified and defined?	3. Was the participation of eligible persons at least 50%?	4. Were inclusion and exclusion criteria for being in the study prespecified and applied uniformly to all participants?	5. Was a sample size justification, power description, or variance and effect estimates provided?	6. For the analyses in this paper, were the exposure(s) of interest measured prior to the outcome(s) being measured?	7. Was the timeframe sufficient so that one could reasonably expect to see an association between exposure and outcome if it existed?	8. For exposures that can vary in amount or level, did the study examine different levels of the exposure as related to the outcome (e.g., categories of exposure, or exposure measured as continuous variable)?	9. Were the exposure measures (independent variables) clearly defined, valid, reliable, and implemented consistently across all study participants?	10. Was the exposure(s) assessed more than once over time?	11. Were the outcome measures (dependent variables) clearly defined, valid, reliable, and implemented consistently across all study participants?	12. Were the outcome assessors blinded to the exposure status of participants?	13. Was loss to follow-up after baseline 20% or less?	14. Were key potential confounding variables measured and adjusted statistically for their impact on the relationship between exposure(s) and outcome(s)?	Quality Rating (Good, Fair or Poor)
[13]	Mexico	Villeda-Sandoval, C.I., et al.	Yes	Yes	Yes	Yes	No	Yes	Yes	Not applicable	Yes	Not applicable	Yes	No	Yes	No	Fair
[14]	China	Lin, J., et al.	Yes	Yes	Yes	Yes	No	Yes	Yes	Not applicable	Yes	Not applicable	Yes	No	Yes	No	Fair
[15]	China	Xu, J., et al.	Yes	Yes	Yes	Yes	No	Yes	Yes	Not applicable	Yes	Not applicable	Yes	No	Yes	No	Fair
[16]	China	Xie, L., et al.	Yes	Yes	Yes	Yes	No	Yes	Yes	Not applicable	Yes	Not applicable	Yes	No	Yes	No	Fair
[17]	Japan	Yanishi, M., et al.	Yes	Yes	Yes	Yes	No	Yes	Yes	Not applicable	Yes	Not applicable	Yes	No	Yes	No	Fair

Reference number	Country of study	Authors	1. Was the research question clearly stated?	2. Was the study population clearly specified and defined?	3. Was the participation of eligible persons at least 50%?	4. Were inclusion and exclusion criteria for being in the study prespecified and applied uniformly to all participants?	5. Was a sample size justification, power description, or variance and effect estimates provided?	6. For the analyses in this paper, were the exposure(s) of interest measured prior to the outcome(s) being measured?	7. Was the timeframe sufficient so that one could reasonably expect to see an association between exposure and outcome if it existed?	8. For exposures that can vary in amount or level, did the study examine different levels of the exposure as related to the outcome (e.g., categories of exposure, or exposure measured as continuous variable)?	9. Were the exposure measures (independent variables) clearly defined, valid, reliable, and implemented consistently across all study participants?	10. Was the exposure(s) assessed more than once over time?	11. Were the outcome measures (dependent variables) clearly defined, valid, reliable, and implemented consistently across all study participants?	12. Were the outcome assessors blinded to the exposure status of participants?	13. Was loss to follow-up after baseline 20% or less?	14. Were key potential confounding variables measured and adjusted statistically for their impact on the relationship between exposure(s) and outcome(s)?	Quality Rating (Good, Fair or Poor)
[18]	South Korea	Oh, C.-K., et al.	Yes	Yes	Yes	Yes	No	Yes	Yes	Not applicable	Yes	Not applicable	Yes	No	Yes	No	Fair
[19]	USA	Pfaff, W.W., et al.	No	Yes	Yes	Yes	No	Yes	Yes	No	Yes	Not applicable	Yes	No	Yes	No	Fair
[20]	USA	Garvin, P.J., et al.	Yes	Yes	Yes	Yes	No	Yes	Yes	No	Yes	Not applicable	Yes	No	Yes	No	Fair
[21]	USA	Modlin, C.S., et al.	YEs	Yes	Yes	Yes	No	Yes	Yes	No	Yes	Not applicable	Yes	No	Yes	Yes	Good
[22]	UK	Williams, A., et al.	Yes	Yes	Yes	Yes	Yes	Yes	Yes	No	Yes	Not applicable	Yes	No	Yes	Yes	Good

Reference number	Country of study	Authors	1. Was the research question clearly stated?	2. Was the study population clearly specified and defined?	3. Was the participation of eligible persons at least 50%?	4. Were inclusion and exclusion criteria for being in the study prespecified and applied uniformly to all participants?	5. Was a sample size justification, power description, or variance and effect estimates provided?	6. For the analyses in this paper, were the exposure(s) of interest measured prior to the outcome(s) being measured?	7. Was the timeframe sufficient so that one could reasonably expect to see an association between exposure and outcome if it existed?	8. For exposures that can vary in amount or level, did the study examine different levels of the exposure as related to the outcome (e.g., categories of exposure, or exposure measured as continuous variable)?	9. Were the exposure measures (independent variables) clearly defined, valid, reliable, and implemented consistently across all study participants?	10. Was the exposure(s) assessed more than once over time?	11. Were the outcome measures (dependent variables) clearly defined, valid, reliable, and implemented consistently across all study participants?	12. Were the outcome assessors blinded to the exposure status of participants?	13. Was loss to follow-up after baseline 20% or less?	14. Were key potential confounding variables measured and adjusted statistically for their impact on the relationship between exposure(s) and outcome(s)?	Quality Rating (Good, Fair or Poor)
[23]	USA	Isaacs, R.B., et al.	Yes	Yes	Yes	Yes	Yes	Yes	Yes	No	Yes	Not applicable	Yes	No	Yes	yes	Good
[24]	USA	Ilyas, M., et al.	Yes	Yes	Yes	Yes	No	Yes	Yes	No	Yes	Not applicable	Yes	No	Yes	No	Fair
[26]	USA	Koyama, H. et al.	Yes	Yes	Yes	Yes	Yes	Yes	Yes	No	Yes	Not applicable	Yes	No	Yes	Yes	Good
[27]	USA	Smith, S.R. et al.	Yes	Yes	Yes	Yes	No	Yes	Yes	No	Yes	Not applicable	Yes	No	Yes	Yes	Good
[28]	USA	Howard, R.J., et al.	YEs	Yes	No	Yes	No	Yes	Yes	No	Yes	Not applicable	Yes	No	Not stated	No	Fair

Reference number	Country of study	Authors	1. Was the research question clearly stated?	2. Was the study population clearly specified and defined?	3. Was the participation of eligible persons at least 50%?	4. Were inclusion and exclusion criteria for being in the study prespecified and applied uniformly to all participants?	5. Was a sample size justification, power description, or variance and effect estimates provided?	6. For the analyses in this paper, were the exposure(s) of interest measured prior to the outcome(s) being measured?	7. Was the timeframe sufficient so that one could reasonably expect to see an association between exposure and outcome if it existed?	8. For exposures that can vary in amount or level, did the study examine different levels of the exposure as related to the outcome (e.g., categories of exposure, or exposure measured as continuous variable)?	9. Were the exposure measures (independent variables) clearly defined, valid, reliable, and implemented consistently across all study participants?	10. Was the exposure(s) assessed more than once over time?	11. Were the outcome measures (dependent variables) clearly defined, valid, reliable, and implemented consistently across all study participants?	12. Were the outcome assessors blinded to the exposure status of participants?	13. Was loss to follow-up after baseline 20% or less?	14. Were key potential confounding variables measured and adjusted statistically for their impact on the relationship between exposure(s) and outcome(s)?	Quality Rating (Good, Fair or Poor)
[29]	USA	Marks, W.H., et al.	Yes	Yes	Yes	Yes	No	Yes	Yes	No	Yes	Not applicable	Yes	No	Yes	No	Fair
[30]	USA	Mehta, R., et al.	Yes	Yes	Yes	Yes	No	Yes	Yes	No	Yes	Not applicable	Yes	No	Yes	No	Fair
[31]	Turkey	Erturk, T. et al.	Yes	Yes	Yes	Yes	No	Yes	Yes	No	Yes	Not applicable	Yes	No	Not stated	No	Fair
[32]	China	Wang, K. et al.	No	Yes	Yes	Yes	No	Yes	Yes	No	Yes	Not applicable	Yes	No	Yes		
[33]	USA	Kwan, J.M., et al.	Yes	Yes	Yes	Yes	Yes	Yes	Yes	No	Yes	Not applicable	Yes	No	Yes	Yes	Good

References

1. Policies and Guidance ODT. Available online: https://www.odt.nhs.uk/transplantation/tools-policies-and-guidance/policies-and-guidance/ (accessed on 18 November 2021).
2. LaPointe, R.D.; Hays, R.; Baliga, P.; Cohen, D.J.; Cooper, M.; Danovitch, G.M.; Dew, M.A.; Gordon, E.J.; Mandelbrot, D.A.; McGuire, S.; et al. Consensus conference on best practices in live kidney donation: Recommendations to optimize education, access, and care. American journal of transplantation. *Am. J. Transplant.* **2015**, *15*, 914–922. [CrossRef] [PubMed]
3. Bellini, M.I.; Courtney, A.E.; McCaughan, J.A. Living Donor Kidney Transplantation Improves Graft and Recipient Survival in Patients with Multiple Kidney Transplants. *J. Clin. Med.* **2020**, *9*, 2118. [CrossRef]
4. Kerr, K.F.; Morenz, E.R.; Thiessen-Philbrook, H.; Coca, S.G.; Wilson, F.P.; Reese, P.P.; Parikh, C.R. Quantifying Donor Effects on Transplant Outcomes Using Kidney Pairs from Deceased Donors. *Clin. J. Am. Soc. Nephrol.* **2019**, *14*, 1781–1787. [CrossRef]
5. Redfield, R.R.; Scalea, J.R.; Zens, T.J.; Muth, B.; Kaufman, D.B.; Djamali, A.; Astor, B.C.; Mohamed, M. Predictors and outcomes of delayed graft function after living-donor kidney transplantation. *Transpl. Int.* **2016**, *29*, 81–87. [CrossRef]
6. Bellini, M.I.; Paoletti, F.; Herbert, P.E. Obesity and bariatric intervention in patients with chronic renal disease. *J. Int. Med. Res.* **2019**, *47*, 2326–2341. [CrossRef] [PubMed]
7. Bellini, M.I.; Koutroutsos, K.; Galliford, J.; Herbert, P.E. One-Year Outcomes of a Cohort of Renal Transplant Patients Related to BMI in a Steroid-Sparing Regimen. *Transpl. Direct* **2017**, *3*, e330. [CrossRef]
8. Bellini, M.I.; Koutroutsos, K.; Nananpragasam, H.; Deurloo, E.; Galliford, J.; Herbert, P.E. Obesity affects graft function but not graft loss in kidney transplant recipients. *J. Int. Med. Res.* **2020**, *48*, 300060519895139. [CrossRef]
9. Naderi, G.; Azadfar, A.; Yahyazadeh, S.R.; Khatami, F.; Aghamir, S.M.K. Impact of the donor-recipient gender matching on the graft survival from live donors. *BMC Nephrol.* **2020**, *21*, 5. [CrossRef] [PubMed]
10. Purnell, T.S.; Luo, X.; Cooper, L.A.; Massie, A.B.; Kucirka, L.M.; Henderson, M.L.; Gordon, E.J.; Crews, D.C.; Boulware, E.; Segev, D.L. Association of Race and Ethnicity With Live Donor Kidney Transplantation in the United States From 1995 to 2014. *Jama* **2018**, *319*, 49–61. [CrossRef]
11. Jacobs, S.C.; Nogueira, J.M.; Phelan, M.W.; Bartlett, S.T.; Cooper, M. Transplant recipient renal function is donor renal mass- and recipient gender-dependent. *Transpl. Int.* **2008**, *21*, 340–345. [CrossRef] [PubMed]
12. Wafa, E.W.; Shokeir, A.; Akl, A.; Hassan, M.; Fouda, M.A.; El Dahshan, K.; Ghoneim, M.A. Effect of donor and recipient variables on the long-term live-donor renal allograft survival in children. *Arab. J. Urol.* **2011**, *9*, 85–91. [CrossRef]
13. Villeda-Sandoval, C.I.; Rodríguez-Covarrubias, F.; Martinez, A.G.-C.Y.; Lara-Nuñez, D.; Guinto-Nishimura, G.Y.; González-Sánchez, B.; Magaña-Rodríguez, J.D.; Alberú-Gómez, J.; Vilatobá-Chapa, M.; Gabilondo-Pliego, B. The impact of donor-to-recipient gender match and mismatch on the renal function of living donor renal graft recipients. *Gac. Med. Mex.* **2016**, *152*, 645–650.
14. Lin, J.; Zheng, X.; Xie, Z.-L.; Sun, W.; Zhang, L.; Tian, Y.; Guo, Y.-W. Factors potentially affecting the function of kidney grafts. *Chin. Med. J.* **2013**, *126*, 1738–1742. [PubMed]
15. Xu, J.; Xu, L.; Wei, X.; Li, X.; Cai, M. Incidence and Risk Factors of Posttransplantation Diabetes Mellitus in Living Donor Kidney Transplantation: A Single-Center Retrospective Study in China. *Transplant. Proc.* **2018**, *50*, 3381–3385. [CrossRef] [PubMed]
16. Xie, L.; Tang, W.; Wang, X.; Wang, L.; Lu, Y.; Lin, T. Pretransplantation Risk Factors Associated With New-onset Diabetes After Living-donor Kidney Transplantation. *Transplant. Proc.* **2016**, *48*, 3299–3302. [CrossRef] [PubMed]
17. Yanishi, M.; Tsukaguchi, H.; Huan, N.T.; Koito, Y.; Taniguchi, H.; Yoshida, K.; Mishima, T.; Sugi, M.; Kinoshita, H.; Matsuda, T. Correlation of whole kidney hypertrophy with glomerular over-filtration in live, gender-mismatched renal transplant allografts. *Nephrology* **2017**, *22*, 1002–1007. [CrossRef] [PubMed]
18. Oh, C.-K.; Lee, B.M.; Jeon, K.O.; Kim, H.J.; Pelletier, S.J.; Kim, S.I.; Kim, Y.S. Gender-related differences of renal mass supply and metabolic demand after living donor kidney transplantation. *Clin. Transplant.* **2006**, *20*, 163–170. [CrossRef] [PubMed]
19. Pfaff, W.W.; Morehead, R.A.; Fennell, R.S.; Mars, D.R.; Thomas, J.M.; Brient, B.W. The role of various risk factors in living related donor renal transplant success. *Ann. Surg.* **1980**, *191*, 617–625. [CrossRef]
20. Garvin, P.J.; Castaneda, M.; Codd, J.E.; Mauller, K. Recipient race as a risk factor in renal transplantation. *Arch. Surg.* **1983**, *118*, 1441–1444. [CrossRef]
21. Modlin, C.S.; Alster, J.M.; Saad, I.R.; Tiong, H.Y.; Mastroianni, B.; Savas, K.M.; Zaramo, C.E.; Kerr, H.L.; Goldfarb, D.; Flechner, S.M. Renal Transplantations in African Americans: A Single-center Experience of Outcomes and Innovations to Improve Access and Results. *Urology* **2014**, *84*, 68–77. [CrossRef] [PubMed]
22. Williams, A.; Richardson, C.; McCready, J.; Anderson, B.; Khalil, K.; Tahir, S.; Nath, J.; Sharif, A. Black Ethnicity is Not a Risk Factor for Mortality or Graft Loss After Kidney Transplant in the United Kingdom. *Exp. Clin. Transpl.* **2018**, *16*, 682–689.
23. Isaacs, R.B.; Nock, S.L.; Spencer, C.E.; Connors, A.F.; Wang, X.-Q.; Sawyer, R.; Lobo, P.I. Racial disparities in renal transplant outcomes. *Am. J. Kidney Dis.* **1999**, *34*, 706–712. [CrossRef]
24. Ilyas, M.; Ammons, J.D.; Gaber, A.O.; Iii., S.R.; Batisky, D.L.; Chesney, R.W.; Jones, D.P.; Wyatt, R. Comparable renal graft survival in African-American and Caucasian recipients. *Pediatric Nephrol.* **1998**, *12*, 534–539. [CrossRef] [PubMed]

25. Sumrani, N.; Delaney, V.; Hong, J.H.; Daskalakis, P.; Markell, M.; Friedman, E.A.; Sommer, B.G. Racial differences in renal transplant outcome of insulin-dependent diabetic recipients in the cyclosporine era. *ASAIO Trans.* **1991**, *37*, M304–M305. [PubMed]
26. Koyama, H.; Cecka, J.M.; Terasaki, P.I. Kidney transplants in black recipients. HLA matching and other factors affecting long-term graft survival. *Transplantation* **1994**, *57*, 1064–1068. [CrossRef]
27. Smith, S.R.; Butterly, D.W. Declining influence of race on the outcome of living-donor renal transplantation. *Am. J. Transpl.* **2002**, *2*, 282–286. [CrossRef]
28. Howard, R.J.; Thai, V.B.; Patton, P.R.; Hemming, A.W.; Reed, A.; Van Der Werf, W.J.; Fujita, S.; Karlix, J.L.; Scornik, J.C. Obesity does not portend a bad outcome for kidney transplant recipients. *Transplantation* **2002**, *73*, 53–55. [CrossRef] [PubMed]
29. Marks, W.H.; Florence, L.S.; Chapman, P.H.; Precht, A.F.; Perkinson, D.T. Morbid obesity is not a contraindication to kidney transplantation. *Am. J. Surg.* **2004**, *187*, 635–638. [CrossRef] [PubMed]
30. Mehta, R.; Shah, G.; Leggat, J.; Hubbell, C.; Roman, A.; Kittur, D.; Narsipur, S. Impact of recipient obesity on living donor kidney transplant outcomes: A single-center experience. *Transpl. Proc.* **2007**, *39*, 1421–1423. [CrossRef]
31. Erturk, T.; Berber, I.; Cakir, U. Effect of Obesity on Clinical Outcomes of Kidney Transplant Patients. *Transpl. Proc.* **2019**, *51*, 1093–1095. [CrossRef] [PubMed]
32. Wang, K.; Liu, Q.Z. Effect Analysis of 1-Year Posttransplant Body Mass Index on Chronic Allograft Nephropathy in Renal Recipients. *Transplant. Proc.* **2011**, *43*, 2592–2595. [CrossRef]
33. Kwan, J.M.; Hajjiri, Z.; Metwally, A.; Finn, P.W.; Perkins, D.L. Effect of the Obesity Epidemic on Kidney Transplantation: Obesity Is Independent of Diabetes as a Risk Factor for Adverse Renal Transplant Outcomes. *PLoS ONE* **2016**, *11*, e0165712. [CrossRef]
34. Hariharan, S.; Israni, A.K.; Danovitch, G. Long-Term Survival after Kidney Transplantation. *N. Engl. J. Med.* **2021**, *385*, 729–743. [CrossRef] [PubMed]
35. Piccoli, G.B.; Alrukhaimi, M.; Liu, Z.-H.; Zakharova, E.; Levin, A. What We Do and Do Not Know about Women and Kidney Diseases; Questions Unanswered and Answers Unquestioned: Reflection on World Kidney Day and International Women's Day. *Nephron* **2018**, *138*, 249–260. [CrossRef] [PubMed]
36. Kayler, L.K.; Rasmussen, C.S.; Dykstra, D.M.; Ojo, A.O.; Port, F.K.; Wolfe, R.A.; Merion, R.M. Gender imbalance and outcomes in living donor renal transplantation in the United States. *Am. J. Transpl.* **2003**, *3*, 452–458. [CrossRef]
37. Tan, J.C.; Wadia, P.P.; Coram, M.; Grumet, F.C.; Kambham, N.; Miller, K.; Pereira, S.; Vayntrub, T.; Miklos, D.B. H-Y antibody development associates with acute rejection in female patients with male kidney transplants. *Transplantation* **2008**, *86*, 75–81. [CrossRef] [PubMed]
38. Graňák, K.; Kováčiková, L.; Skálová, P.; Vnučák, M.; Miklušica, J.; Laca, .; Mokáň, M.; Dedinská, I. Kidney Transplantation and "Sex Mismatch": A 10-Year Single-Center Analysis. *Ann. Transpl.* **2020**, *25*, e921117. [CrossRef]
39. Bellini, M.I.; Charalmpidis, S.; Brookes, P.; Hill, P.; Dor, F.J.M.F.; Papalois, V. Bilateral Nephrectomy for Adult Polycystic Kidney Disease Does Not Affect the Graft Function of Transplant Patients and Does Not Result in Sensitisation. *Biomed Res. Int.* **2019**, *2019*, 7423158. [CrossRef]
40. Tan, J.C.; Kim, J.P.; Chertow, G.M.; Grumet, F.C. Donor–Recipient Sex Mismatch in Kidney Transplantation. *Gend. Med.* **2012**, *9*, 335–347. [CrossRef]
41. Bairey Merz, C.N.; Dember, L.M.; Ingelfinger, J.R.; Vinson, A.; Neugarten, J.; Sandberg, K.L.; Sullivan, J.C.; Maric-Bilkan, C.; Rankin, T.L.; et al.; on behalf of the participants of the National Institute of Diabetes and Digestive and Kidney Diseases Workshop on "Sex and the Kidneys". Sex and the kidneys: Current understanding and research opportunities. *Nat. Rev. Nephrol.* **2019**, *15*, 776–783. [CrossRef]
42. Taylor, D.M.; Bradley, J.A.; Bradley, C.; Draper, H.; Dudley, C.; Fogarty, D.; Fraser, S.D.; Johnson, R.; Leydon, G.M.; Metcalfe, W.; et al. Limited health literacy is associated with reduced access to kidney transplantation. *Kidney Int.* **2019**, *95*, 1244–1252. [CrossRef] [PubMed]
43. Bellini, M.I.; Charalampidis, S.; Stratigos, I.; Dor, F.; Papalois, V. The Effect of Donors' Demographic Characteristics in Renal Function Post-Living Kidney Donation. Analysis of a UK Single Centre Cohort. *J. Clin. Med.* **2019**, *8*, 883. [CrossRef] [PubMed]
44. Pruthi, R.; Robb, M.L.; Oniscu, G.C.; Tomson, C.; Bradley, A.; Forsythe, J.L.; Metcalfe, W.; Bradley, C.; Dudley, C.; Johnson, R.J.; et al. Inequity in Access to Transplantation in the United Kingdom. *Clin. J. Am. Soc. Nephrol.* **2020**, *15*, 830–842. [CrossRef]
45. Ku, E.; McCulloch, C.E.; Roll, G.R.; Posselt, A.; Grimes, B.A.; Johansen, K.L. Bariatric surgery prior to transplantation and risk of early hospital re-admission, graft failure, or death following kidney transplantation. *Am. J. Transpl.* **2021**, *21*, 3750–3757. [CrossRef] [PubMed]

MDPI
St. Alban-Anlage 66
4052 Basel
Switzerland
Tel. +41 61 683 77 34
Fax +41 61 302 89 18
www.mdpi.com

Journal of Clinical Medicine Editorial Office
E-mail: jcm@mdpi.com
www.mdpi.com/journal/jcm

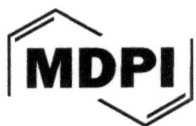

www.ingramcontent.com/pod-product-compliance
Lightning Source LLC
LaVergne TN
LVHW070646100526
838202LV00013B/894